Fluids & Electrolytes

A 2-in-1 Reference for Nurses

Fluids & Electrolytes

A 2-in-1 Reference for Nurses

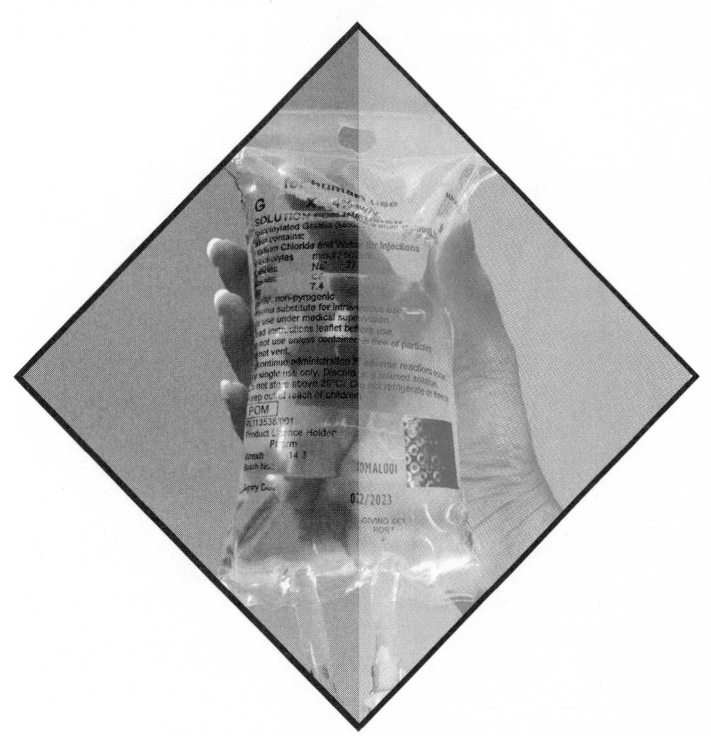

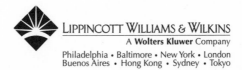

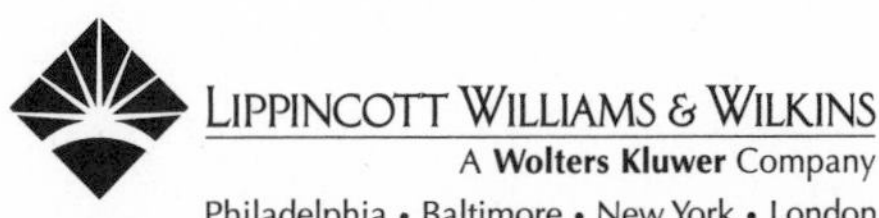

Philadelphia • Baltimore • New York • London
Buenos Aires • Hong Kong • Sydney • Tokyo

STAFF

Executive Publisher
Judith A. Schilling McCann, RN, MSN

Editorial Director
H. Nancy Holmes

Clinical Director
Joan M. Robinson, RN, MSN

Senior Art Director
Arlene Putterman

Editorial Project Manager
William Welsh

Clinical Project Manager
Beverly Ann Tscheschlog, RN, BS

Editor
Julie Munden

Clinical Editor
Jana Sciarra, RN, MSN CRNP

Copy Editors
Kimberly Bilotta (supervisor), Carolyn Petersen, Kelly Taylor, Pamela Wingrod

Designers
Linda Jovinelly Franklin (project manager), Gail Wagner

Digital Composition Services
Diane Paluba (manager), Joyce Rossi Biletz, Donna S. Morris

Manufacturing
Patricia K. Dorshaw (director), Beth J. Welsh

Editorial Assistants
Megan L. Aldinger, Karen J. Kirk, Linda K. Ruhf

Indexer
Barbara Hodgson

F&E2IN1 — D N O S A J J M A M
07 06 05 10 9 8 7 6 5 4 3 2 1

Library of Congress Cataloging-in Publication Data

Fluids & electrolytes : a 2-in-1 reference for nurses.
p. ; cm.
Includes bibliographical references and index.
1. Water-electrolyte imbalances—Nursing. 2. Water-electrolyte balance (Physiology) I. Lippincott Williams & Wilkins. II. Title: Fluids and electrolytes.
[DNLM: 1. Water-Electrolyte Imbalance—nursing. 2. Water-Electrolyte Imbalance—prevention & control. 3. Water-Electrolyte Balance. WY 100 F646 2006]
RC630.F588 2006
616.3'9920231—dc22
ISBN 1-58255-425-0 (alk. paper) 2004028215

Contents

Contributors and consultants

Cheryl L. Brady, RN, MSN
Adjunct Faculty
Kent State University
East Liverpool, Ohio

Shari Regina Cammon, RN, MSN, CCRN
Clinical Risk Management & Safety Surveillance Associate
Merck & Co., Inc.
West Point, Pa.

Helen Fu, RN, MSN, FNP
Family Nurse Practitioner
Soteria Family Health Center
Plymouth, Minn.

Margaret M. Gingrich, RN, MSN
Associate Professor
Harrisburg (Pa.) Area Community College

David J. Hartman, RN, MSN, CCRN
Nurse Practitioner
University of Pennsylvania Health System
Philadelphia

Dawna Martich, RN, MSN
Clinical Trainer
American Healthways
Pittsburgh

Valerie Mignatti, RN, BSN
Cardiovascular Clinical Nurse
University of Pennsylvania Medical Center
Philadelphia

Sharon D. O'Kelley, RN, ADN, OCN
Clinical Nurse III
Duke University Hospital
Durham, N.C.

Sherry A. Parmenter, RD, LD
Clinical Dietitian
Fairfield Medical Center
Lancaster, Ohio

Abby Plambeck, RN, BSN
Freelance Writer
Milwaukee

Theresa Pulvano, RN, BSN
Practical Nursing Instructor
Ocean County Vocational Technical School
Lakehurst, N.J.

Monica Narvaez Ramirez, RN, MSN
Instructor
University of the Incarnate Word School of Nursing & Health Professions
San Antonio, Tex.

Patricia Weiskittel, RN, MSN, APRN, BC, CNN
Primary Care Nurse Practitioner
Veterans Administration Hospital
Cincinnati

Foreword

The human body continually strives for homeostasis — the state of equilibrium that can only be achieved through the complex balancing of the body's fluids and electrolytes. In healthy people, it's a naturally occurring, self-regulating process. However, in people with such disorders as heart failure, cancer, and hyperthyroidism, achieving homeostasis is a daunting challenge that requires the utmost in quality patient care.

In this era of rising health care costs and dwindling health care dollars, nurses play an incredibly vital role in helping patients maintain this all-important equilibrium. With the demand from hospital administrators to delay admissions and to promote early discharge, nurses must possess superior patient assessment skills. In some instances, the early detection of subtle changes in a patient's fluid and electrolyte balance may prevent a costly acute care admission, a protracted hospital stay, and prolonged patient suffering. However, without proper guidance, nurses find it difficult to dispel their confusion about this troublesome subject.

Fluids & Electrolytes: A 2-in-1 Reference for Nurses greatly assists today's nurses to fight through their uncertainty. This text is an exceptional resource for nursing students as well as established nurses because of its unique two-column format. The book's inner column contains narrative text that provides clear, in-depth descriptions of the basic physiology of fluid, electrolyte, and acid-base homeostasis as well as comprehensive discussions of the pathophysiology underlying imbalances. In addition, signs and symptoms associated with these imbalances are detailed in a clear, concise manner. The book's outer column presents succinct summaries and bulleted points related to the text located on the adjoining page to facilitate rapid review.

You won't find such an accommodating read-and-review format anywhere.

This expertly designed book also effectively organizes this cumbersome topic into well-constructed parts and chapters. Part one, Balancing basics, presents the basics of fluid, electrolyte, and acid-base balance. Part two, Imbalances, devotes specific chapters to the understanding of all the different fluid and electrolyte imbalances that a body can experience. Part three, Disorders causing imbalances, addresses heat syndromes, heart failure, respiratory failure, excessive GI fluid losses, renal failure, and burns. Part four, Treatment, focuses on I.V. fluid replacement therapy, total parenteral nutrition, and blood component therapy.

Fluids & Electrolytes: A 2-in-1 Reference for Nurses is also distinguished by helpful tables and illustrations that help bring clarity to concepts and by eye-catching icons that highlight important information. *Danger* highlights potentially life-threatening conditions or critical situations. *Closer look* describes the underlying pathophysiologic mechanism for a specific imbalance or condition. *Charting checklist* calls attention to vital documentation practices and procedures that you may otherwise overlook. *Age alert* identifies life span changes that may influence fluid and electrolyte balance. In addition, appendices dedicated to common fluid and electrolyte imbalances in pediatric and elderly patients not only expand the scope of this book, but also clearly accentuate the critical differences in the fluid, electrolyte, and acid-base status and assessment of patients of varying ages.

In the performance of high quality, holistic patient care, nurses must be especially proficient, vigilant, and knowledgeable. Acutely ill patients and fragile patients in all health care settings require careful assessment and monitoring of their fluids, electrolytes, and acid-base balance. *Fluids & Electrolytes: A 2-in-1 Reference for Nurses* is an invaluable resource for all nurses providing this care. It's a part of my reference library, and I hope that it becomes part of yours.

Pamela R. Cangelosi, RN, PhD
Assistant Professor
George Mason University
College of Nursing and Health Science
Fairfax, Va.

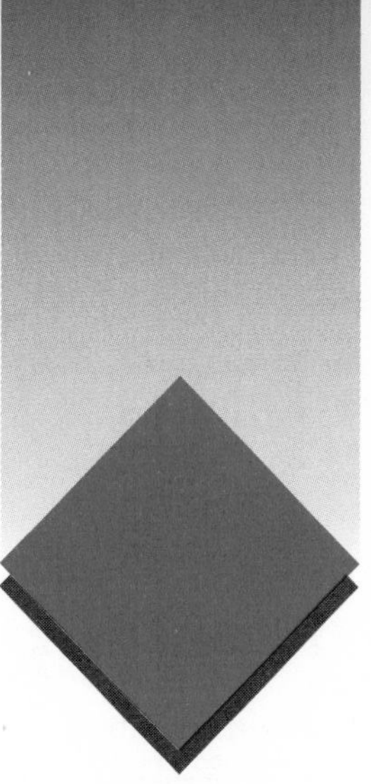

Part one

Balancing basics

Fluid balance

Fluids
- Maintain temperature and cell shape
- Transport nutrients, gases, and wastes

A LOOK AT FLUIDS

Fluids are vital to all forms of life. In the human body, they help maintain temperature and cell shape and also help transport nutrients, gases, and wastes. This chapter tells you what you need to know about fluids and the way the body balances them.

The skin, the lungs, and the kidneys — just about all major organs — work together to maintain the proper balance of fluid, or homeostasis. To maintain that balance, the amount of fluid gained throughout the day must equal the amount lost. Maintaining this equilibrium would be easy if all losses could be measured, but they can't.

Fluid losses
- Measurable (sensible) — from urination, defecation, and wounds
- Immeasurable (insensible) — from skin and lungs

FLUID LOSSES

Fluid losses are either measurable, referred to as *sensible losses,* or immeasurable, referred to as *insensible losses.* Sensible losses include losses from urination, defecation, and wounds. Insensible losses include losses from the skin and the lungs. (See *Sites involved in fluid loss.*)

A typical adult loses 100 to 200 ml/day through defecation. However, in a patient with severe diarrhea, losses may exceed 5,000 ml/day. Insensible losses from the skin, though fairly constant, can vary depending on changes in humidity levels and a person's body surface area (BSA).

Sites involved in fluid loss

Each day, the body gains and loses fluid through several different processes. This illustration shows the primary sites of fluid losses and gains as well as their average amounts. Gastric, intestinal, pancreatic, and biliary secretions are almost completely reabsorbed and aren't usually counted in daily fluid losses and gains.

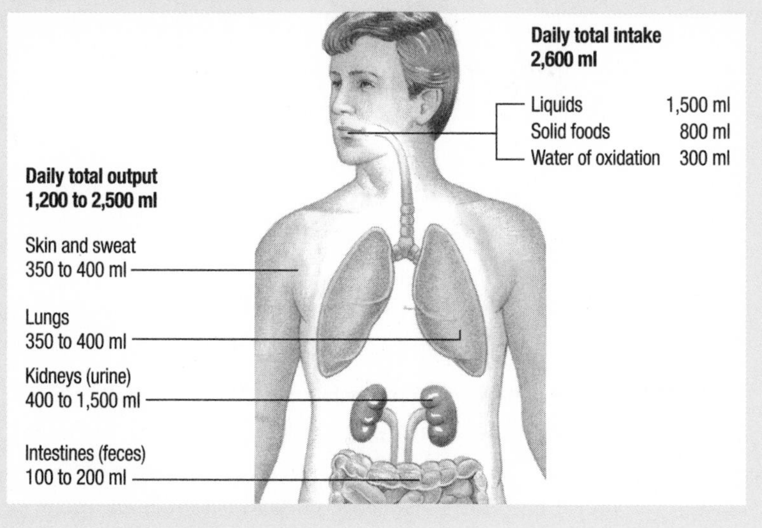

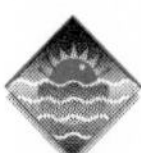

AGE ALERT *The BSA of an infant is greater than that of an adult relative to their respective weights. As a result, infants typically lose more water from the skin than adults do.*

Respiratory rate and depth can affect the amount of fluid lost through the lungs. Tachypnea, for example, causes more water to be lost; bradypnea, less. Fever increases insensible losses of fluid from both the skin and lungs.

Fluid distribution

The body holds fluid in two basic areas, or compartments — inside the cells and outside the cells. Fluid found inside the cells is called *intracellular fluid;* fluid found outside the cells, *extracellular fluid.* Capillary walls and cell membranes separate the intracellular and extracellular compartments. (See *Understanding fluid compartments,* page 4.)

To maintain proper fluid balance, the distribution of fluid between the two compartments must remain relatively constant. In an adult, the total amount of intracellular fluid averages 40% of the person's body weight,

Fluid distribution

- Fluid held in two different compartments: inside cells (intracellular fluid) and outside cells (extracellular fluid)

Understanding fluid compartments

This illustration shows the primary fluid compartments in the body: intracellular and extracellular. Extracellular compartments are further divided into interstitial and intravascular compartments. Capillary walls and cell membranes separate intracellular fluids from extracellular fluids.

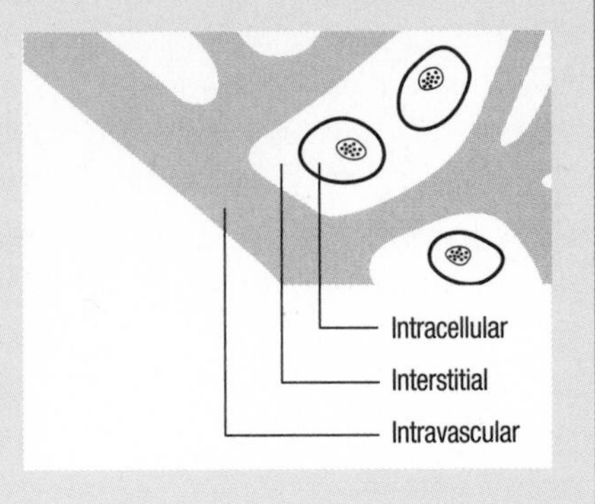

Fluid distribution *(continued)*

Extracellular fluid

- Comprised of interstitial fluid (surrounds cells) and intravascular fluid or plasma (liquid portion of blood)

Age alert

- Greater percentage of body water in infants than in adults
- Full-term neonates: Water equals 80% of body weight
- Premature neonates: Water equals 90% of body weight
- Lean adult male: Water equals 60% of body weight

or about 28 L. The total amount of extracellular fluid averages 20% of the person's body weight, or about 14 L.

Extracellular fluid can be broken down further into interstitial fluid, which surrounds the cells, and intravascular fluid, or plasma, which is the liquid portion of blood. In an adult, interstitial fluid accounts for about 75% of the extracellular fluid. Plasma accounts for the remaining 25%.

Skeletal muscle cells hold much of the body's water content; fat cells contain little of it. Women, who normally have a higher ratio of fat to skeletal muscle than men, typically have a lower relative water content than men. Likewise, a person who's obese may have a relative water content level as low as 45%. Accumulated body fat in these individuals increases weight without boosting the body's water content.

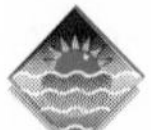

AGE ALERT *Fluid distribution within the body varies with age. Compared with adults, infants have a greater percentage of body water stored in interstitial spaces. About 80% of a full-term neonate's body weight is water. About 90% of a premature neonate's body weight is water. The amount of water as a percentage of body weight decreases with age until puberty. In a typical 154-lb (69.8-kg), lean adult male, about 60% (93 lb [42.2 kg]) of body weight is water. (See* Fluid changes with aging.*)*

The body contains other fluids, called *transcellular fluids,* in the cerebrospinal column, pleural cavity, lymphatic system, joints, and eyes. These fluids generally aren't subject to significant gains and losses throughout the day.

AGE ALERT

Fluid changes with aging

The risk of suffering a fluid imbalance increases with age. Skeletal muscle mass declines, and the proportion of fat within the body increases. After age 60, water content drops to about 45%.

Likewise, the distribution of fluid within the body changes with age. For instance, about 15% of a typical young adult's total body weight is made up of interstitial fluid. That percentage progressively decreases with age.

About 5% of the body's total fluid volume is made up of plasma, yet plasma volume remains stable throughout life.

Fluid changes with aging

- Skeletal muscle mass declines
- Proportion of fat increases
- Water content drops to 45% at age 60
- Distribution changes

FLUID TYPES

Fluids in the body generally aren't found in pure forms. They're usually found in three types of solutions: isotonic, hypotonic, and hypertonic.

Fluid types

- Three types: isotonic, hypotonic, hypertonic

Isotonic solutions

An isotonic solution has the same solute concentration as another solution. For instance, if two fluids in adjacent compartments are equally concentrated, they're already in balance, so the fluid inside each compartment stays put. No imbalance means no net fluid shift.

Normal saline solution is considered isotonic because the concentration of sodium in the solution nearly equals the concentration of sodium in the blood. (See *Understanding isotonic solutions.*)

Isotonic solutions

- Have equal solute concentrations
- In adjacent compartments, result in no net fluid shift
- Example: normal saline solution

Understanding isotonic solutions

No net fluid shifts occur between isotonic solutions because the solutions are equally concentrated.

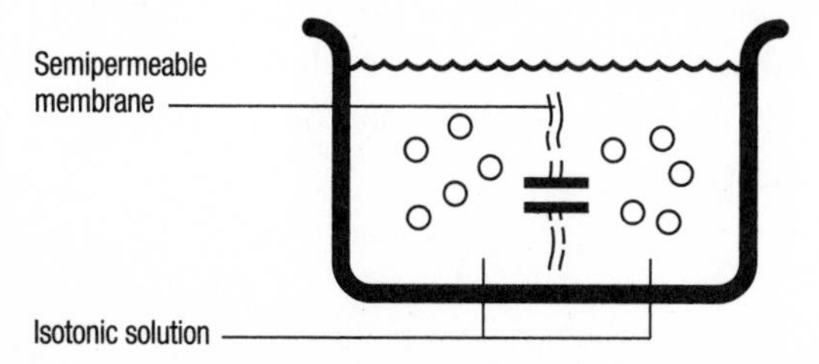

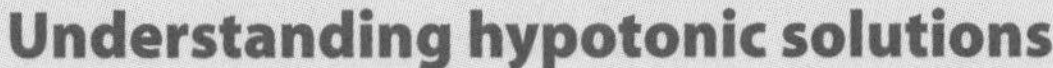

Understanding hypotonic solutions

When a less concentrated, or hypotonic, solution is placed next to a more concentrated solution, fluid shifts from the hypotonic solution into the more concentrated compartment to equalize concentrations.

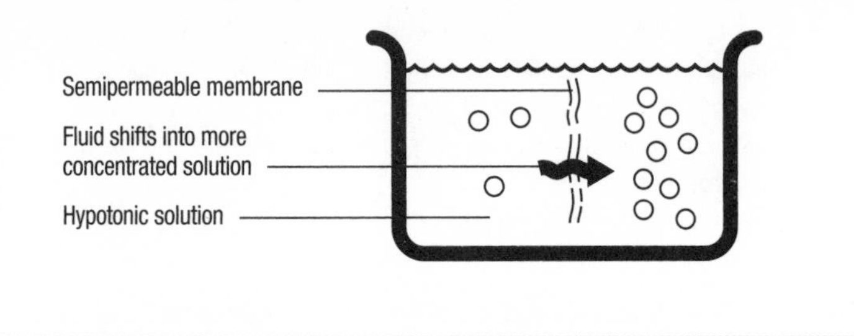

Hypotonic solutions
- Have lower solute concentrations than other solutions
- In adjacent compartments, result in fluid shifting from the compartment with the lower concentration to the compartment with the higher concentration
- Example: half-normal saline solution

Hypotonic solutions

A hypotonic solution has a lower solute concentration than another solution. For instance, if one solution contains only a little sodium and another solution contains more, the first solution is hypotonic compared with the second solution. As a result, fluid from the hypotonic solution would shift into the second solution until the two solutions had equal concentrations.

Half-normal saline solution is considered hypotonic because the concentration of sodium in the solution is lower than the concentration of sodium in the patient's blood. (See *Understanding hypotonic solutions.*)

Hypertonic solutions
- Have higher solute concentrations than other solutions
- In adjacent compartments, result in fluid shifting from the compartment with the lower concentration to the compartment with the higher concentration

Hypertonic solutions

A hypertonic solution has a higher solute concentration than another solution. For instance, one solution contains a large amount of sodium and a second solution contains hardly any. The first solution is hypertonic compared with the second solution. As a result, fluid from the second solution would shift into the hypertonic solution until the two solutions had equal concentrations.

Understanding hypertonic solutions

If one solution has more solutes than an adjacent solution, it has less fluid relative to the adjacent solution. Fluid will move out of the less concentrated solution into the more concentrated, or hypertonic, solution until both solutions have the same amount of solutes and fluid.

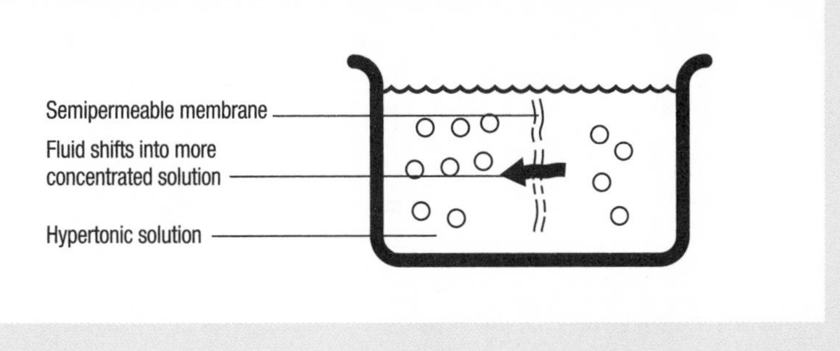

A solution of dextrose 5% in normal saline solution is considered hypertonic because the concentration of solutes in the solution is greater than the concentration of solutes in the patient's blood. (See *Understanding hypertonic solutions.*)

Hypertonic solutions ***(continued)***

- Example: dextrose 5% in normal saline solution

FLUID MOVEMENT

Just as the heart constantly beats, fluids and solutes constantly move within the body. This movement allows the body to maintain homeostasis, the constant state of balance the body seeks. (See *Shifting fluids,* page 8.)

Fluid movement

- Fluids and solutes constantly move
- Helps maintain homeostasis across intracellular, interstitial, and intravascular compartments

AT THE CELLULAR LEVEL

Solutes within the intracellular, interstitial, and intravascular compartments of the body move through cell membranes, separating those compartments in different ways. Cell membranes are semipermeable, meaning that they allow some solutes to pass through but not others. The different ways that fluids and solutes move through membranes at the cellular level are called *diffusion, active transport,* and *osmosis.*

At the cellular level

- Cell membranes allow select solutes through (semipermeable)
- Different ways fluids and solutes move through membranes at cellular level called *diffusion, active transport,* and *osmosis*

Shifting fluids

Fluids, along with nutrients and waste products, constantly shift within the body's compartments — from the cells to the interstitial spaces, to the blood vessels, and back again. A change in one compartment can affect all of the others.

KEEPING TRACK OF FLUID SHIFTS

That continuous shifting of fluids can have important implications in the care of patients. For example, if a hypotonic fluid is given to a patient, it may cause too much fluid to move from the veins into the cells, causing the cells to swell. On the other hand, if a hypertonic solution is given to a patient, it may cause too much fluid to be pulled from cells into the bloodstream, causing the cells to shrink.

At the cellular level *(continued)*

Diffusion

- Occurs when solutes move from area of higher concentration to area of lower concentration
- Results in equal distribution of solutes
- Form of passive transport

Diffusion

In diffusion, solutes move from an area of higher concentration to an area of lower concentration, eventually resulting in an equal distribution of solutes within the two areas. Diffusion is a form of passive transport because no energy is required to make it happen; it just happens. Like swimming with a river's current, solutes simply go with the flow. (See *Understanding diffusion.*)

Understanding diffusion

In diffusion, solutes move from areas of higher concentration to areas of lower concentration until the concentration in both areas equalizes.

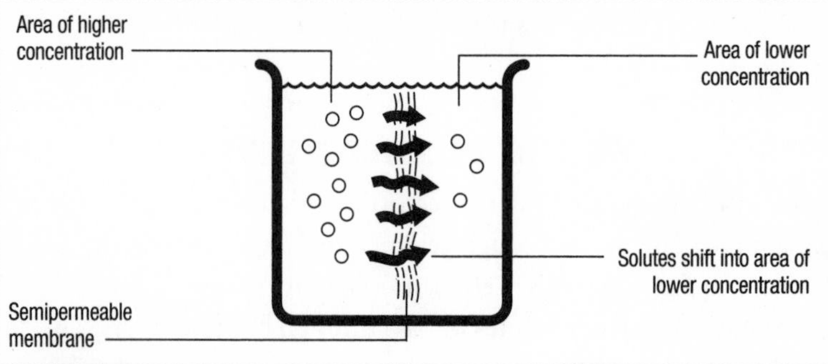

Area of higher concentration
Area of lower concentration
Solutes shift into area of lower concentration
Semipermeable membrane

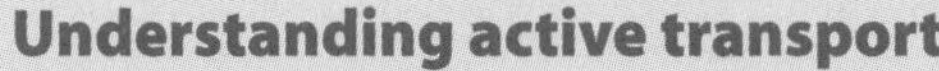

Understanding active transport

During active transport, energy from the molecule adenosine triphosphate (ATP) moves solutes from an area of lower concentration to an area of higher concentration.

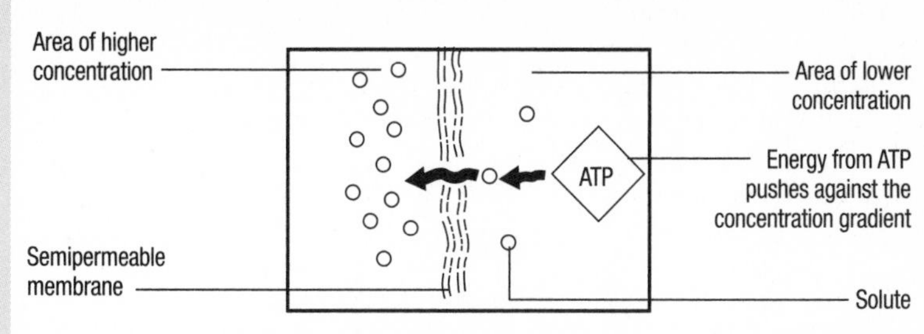

Active transport

In active transport, solutes move from an area of lower concentration to an area of higher concentration. Like swimming against the current, active transport requires energy to make it happen. Adenosine triphosphate (ATP), which is stored in all cells, supplies this energy. (See *Understanding active transport.*)

Some solutes, such as sodium and potassium, use ATP to move in and out of cells in a form of active transport called the *sodium-potassium pump.* Other solutes that require active transport to cross cell membranes include calcium ions, hydrogen ions, amino acids, and certain sugars.

Osmosis

Osmosis refers to the passive movement of fluid across a membrane from an area of lower solute concentration and comparatively more fluid into an area of higher solute concentration and comparatively less fluid. Osmosis stops when enough fluid has moved through the membrane to equalize the solute concentration on both sides of the membrane. (See *Understanding osmosis,* page 10.)

Within the vascular system

Within the vascular system, only capillaries have walls thin enough to let solutes pass through. This movement of fluids and solutes through capillary walls — called *capillary filtration* — plays a critical role in the body's fluid balance.

At the cellular level *(continued)*

Active transport

- Occurs when solutes move from area of lower concentration to area of higher concentration
- Requires energy supplied by adenosine triphosphate

Osmosis

- Occurs when fluid moves from area of lower solute concentration and comparatively more fluid into area of higher solute concentration and comparatively less fluid
- Stops when solute concentration equalizes

Within the vascular system

- Only capillaries have walls thin enough to let solutes through
- Capillary filtration — the movement of fluids and solutes through capillary walls

Understanding osmosis

In osmosis, fluid moves passively from areas with more fluid (and fewer solutes) to areas with less fluid (and more solutes). Remember: In osmosis, fluid moves; in diffusion, solutes move.

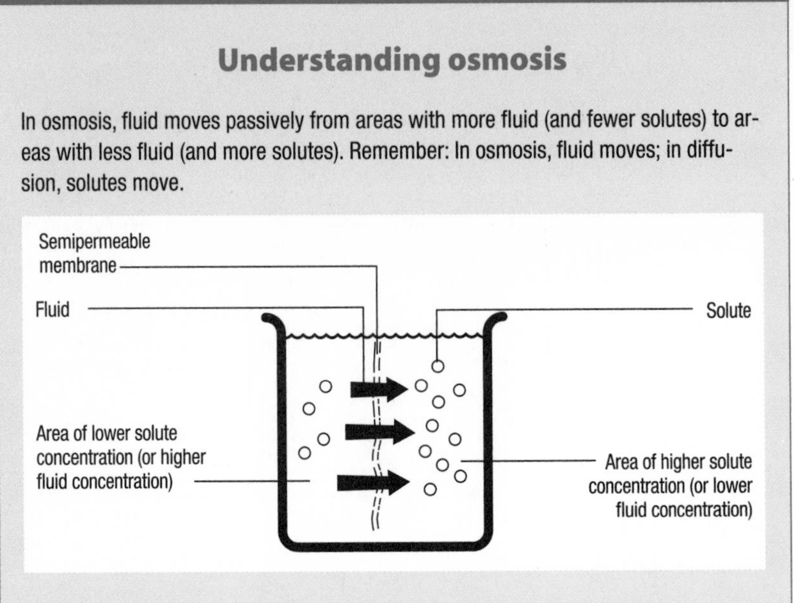

Capillary filtration

- Results from hydrostatic (fluid-pushing) pressure
- Reabsorption — prevents too much fluid from leaving capillaries
- Plasma colloid osmotic pressure — osmotic (pulling) force of albumin in intravascular space
- If hydrostatic pressure exceeds plasma colloid osmotic pressure, water and solutes leave capillaries and enter interstitial fluid
- If plasma colloid osmotic pressure exceeds hydrostatic pressure, water and solutes return to capillaries

Capillary filtration

Capillary filtration results from blood pushing against the walls of the capillary. That pressure, called *hydrostatic* (or fluid-pushing) *pressure,* forces fluids and solutes through the capillary wall. When the hydrostatic pressure inside a capillary is greater than the pressure in the surrounding interstitial space, fluids and solutes inside the capillary are forced out into the interstitial space. When the pressure inside the capillary is less than the pressure outside of it, fluids and solutes move back into the capillary. (See *Fluid movement through capillaries.*)

A process called *reabsorption* prevents too much fluid from leaving the capillaries no matter how much hydrostatic pressure exists within the capillaries. When fluid filters through a capillary, the protein albumin — a large molecule that normally can't pass through the capillary membranes — remains behind in the diminishing volume of water. As the concentration of albumin inside a capillary increases, fluid begins to move back into the capillaries through osmosis. The osmotic, or pulling, force of albumin in the intravascular space is called the *plasma colloid osmotic pressure.* In the arteries, it averages about 25 mm Hg.

As long as capillary blood pressure (the hydrostatic pressure) exceeds plasma colloid osmotic pressure, water and solutes can leave the capillaries and enter the interstitial fluid. When capillary blood pressure falls be-

Fluid movement through capillaries

When hydrostatic pressure builds inside a capillary, it forces fluids and solutes out through capillary walls and into the interstitial fluid, as shown below.

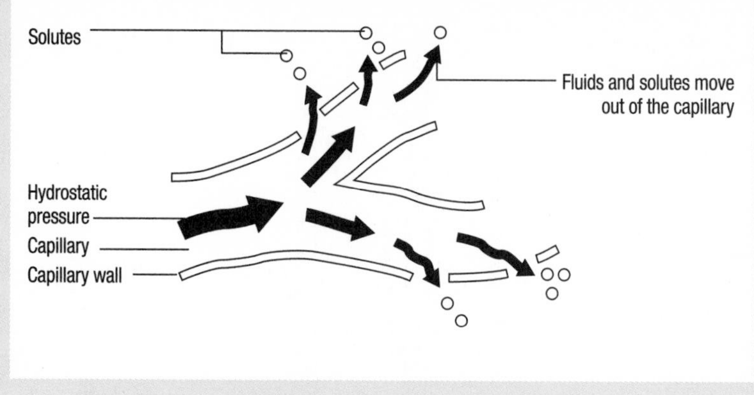

low plasma colloid osmotic pressure, water and diffusible solutes return to the capillaries.

Normally, blood pressure in a capillary exceeds plasma colloid osmotic pressure in the arteriole end and falls below it in the venule end. As a result, capillary filtration occurs along the first half of the vessel; reabsorption, along the second. As long as capillary blood pressure and plasma albumin levels remain normal, the amount of water that moves into the vessel equals the amount that moves out.

Occasionally, extra fluid filters out of the capillary. When that happens, the excess fluid shifts into the lymphatic vessels located just outside the capillaries and eventually returns to the heart for recirculation.

MAINTAINING FLUID BALANCE

Many organs in the body work together to maintain fluid balance. Because one problem can affect the entire fluid-maintenance system, it's important to keep all body systems in check. The kidneys, various hormones, and thirst are what make maintaining and balancing fluids in the body possible.

Maintaining fluid balance

- Responsibility of kidneys, various hormones, and thirst

Looking at a nephron

A nephron filters blood, produces urine, and excretes excess solutes, electrolytes, fluids, and metabolic waste products while keeping blood composition and volume constant.

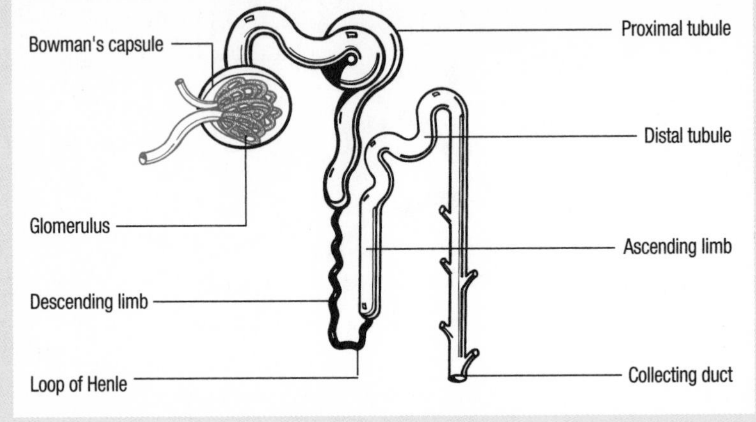

The kidneys

Nephrons

- ✦ Filter blood, produce urine, excrete excess waste, and constantly work to maintain fluid balance
- ✦ Consist of glomerulus (cluster of capillaries that filters blood) and tubule (ends in collecting duct)
- ✦ Bowman's capsule — surrounds glomerulus

Physiology

- ✦ Capillary blood pressure forces fluid through capillary walls and into Bowman's capsule
- ✦ Depending on body's needs, water and electrolytes either excreted or retained along tubule
- ✦ Resulting filtrate eventually flows into the bladder as urine

Key facts

- ✦ Glomerular filtration rate — the rate at which nephrons filter blood (normally, about 125 ml of blood every minute, or about 180 L/day)
- ✦ Produce 1 to 2 L of urine per day
- ✦ Must excrete at least 20 ml of urine per hour to eliminate body wastes

The kidneys

The kidneys play a vital role in fluid balance: If they don't work properly, the body has a difficult time controlling fluid balance. The nephrons, the workhorse of the kidneys, filter blood, produce urine, and excrete excess waste, as well as constantly work to maintain fluid balance.

A nephron consists of a glomerulus and a tubule. The tubule, sometimes convoluted, ends in a collecting duct. The glomerulus is a cluster of capillaries that filters blood. Like a vascular cradle, Bowman's capsule surrounds the glomerulus. (See *Looking at a nephron.*)

Capillary blood pressure forces fluid through the capillary walls and into Bowman's capsule at the proximal end of the tubule. Along the length of the tubule, water and electrolytes are either excreted or retained depending on the body's needs. If the body needs more fluid, for instance, it retains more. If it needs less, it reabsorbs less and excretes more. Electrolytes, such as sodium and potassium, are either filtered or reabsorbed throughout the same area. The resulting filtrate, which eventually becomes urine, flows through the tubule into the collecting ducts and eventually into the bladder.

The nephrons filter about 125 ml of blood every minute, or about 180 L/day. That rate, called the *glomerular filtration rate,* leads to the production of 1 to 2 L of urine per day. The nephrons reabsorb the remaining 178 L (or more) of fluid.

If the body loses even 1% to 2% of its fluid, the kidneys take steps to conserve water. Perhaps the most important step involves reabsorbing more water from the filtrate, which produces a more concentrated urine.

The kidneys must continue to excrete at least 20 ml of urine every hour (about 500 ml/day) to eliminate body wastes. A urine excretion rate that's less than 20 ml/hour usually indicates renal disease. The minimum urine excretion rate varies with age.

AGE ALERT *Urine excretion in infants and young children occurs at a higher rate than adults due to their higher metabolic rates, which produce more waste. Also, infants can't concentrate urine until about age 3 months, and their kidneys remain less efficient than an adult's kidneys until about age 2 years.*

The kidneys respond to fluid excesses by excreting a more dilute urine, which rids the body of fluid and conserves electrolytes.

Antidiuretic hormone

Several hormones affect fluid balance, among them a water retainer called *antidiuretic hormone* (ADH), which is sometimes referred to as *vasopressin.* The hypothalamus produces ADH, but the posterior pituitary gland stores and releases it. ADH restores blood volume by reducing diuresis and increasing water retention. (See *How antidiuretic hormone works.*)

How antidiuretic hormone works

Antidiuretic hormone (ADH) regulates fluid balance through a series of steps, which are outlined here.

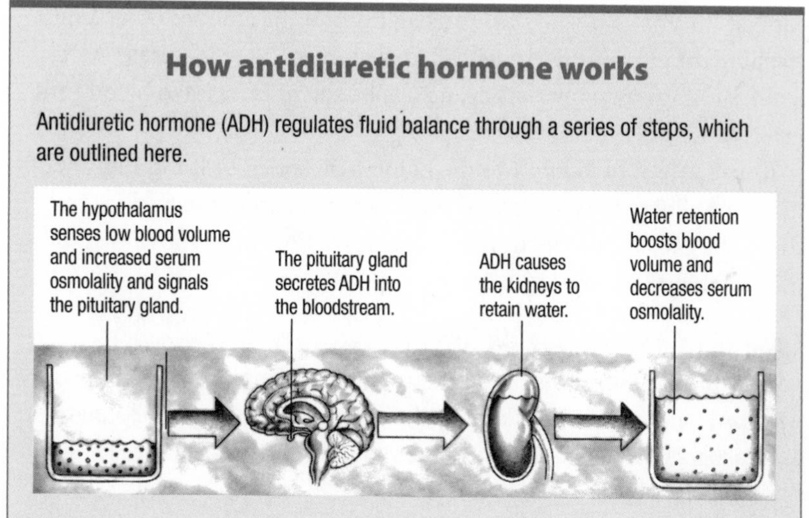

The hypothalamus senses low blood volume and increased serum osmolality and signals the pituitary gland.
The pituitary gland secretes ADH into the bloodstream.
ADH causes the kidneys to retain water.
Water retention boosts blood volume and decreases serum osmolality.

Antidiuretic hormone

- Sometimes referred to as *vasopressin*
- Produced by hypothalamus
- Stored and released by posterior pituitary gland
- Restores blood volume and increases urine concentration by reducing diuresis and increasing water retention
- Release can be stimulated by increased serum osmolality (decreased blood volume)
- Release can be inhibited by decreased serum osmolality (increased blood volume), resulting in less water reabsorption and less concentrated urine

Increased serum osmolality, or decreased blood volume, can stimulate the release of ADH, which in turn increases the kidneys' reabsorption of water and results in more concentrated urine.

Likewise, decreased serum osmolality, or increased blood volume, inhibits the release of ADH and causes less water to be reabsorbed, making the urine less concentrated. The amount of ADH released varies throughout the day, depending on the body's needs. The body holds water when fluid levels drop and releases it when fluid levels rise. It's a constant cycle that keeps fluid levels in balance all day long.

Renin-angiotensin-aldosterone system

To help the body maintain a balance of sodium and water as well as a healthy blood volume and blood pressure, the juxtaglomerular cells near each glomerulus secrete an enzyme called *renin.* Through a complex series of steps, renin leads to the production of angiotensin II, a powerful vasoconstrictor that causes peripheral vasoconstriction and stimulates the production of aldosterone. Both actions raise blood pressure. (See *Understanding aldosterone production.*)

As soon as the blood pressure reaches a normal level, the body stops releasing renin, and this feedback cycle of renin to angiotensin to aldosterone stops.

Renin secretion

The amount of renin secreted depends on blood flow and the level of sodium in the bloodstream. If blood flow to the kidneys diminishes, as happens in a patient who's hemorrhaging, or if the amount of sodium reaching the glomerulus drops, the juxtaglomerular cells secrete more renin, causing vasoconstriction and a subsequent increase in blood pressure.

Conversely, if blood flow to the kidneys increases, or if the amount of sodium reaching the glomerulus increases, juxtaglomerular cells secrete less renin, causing a reduction in vasoconstriction and a subsequent decrease in blood pressure.

Sodium and water regulation

The hormone aldosterone also plays a role in maintaining blood pressure and fluid balance. Secreted by the adrenal cortex, aldosterone regulates the reabsorption of sodium and water within the nephron. (See *How aldosterone works.*)

Renin-angiotensin-aldosterone system

Physiology

- Juxtaglomerular cells secrete renin to help maintain sodium and water balance, blood volume, blood pressure
- Renin secretion leads to production of angiotensin II, causing peripheral vasoconstriction and aldosterone production and raising blood pressure

Renin secretion

- Amount secreted depends on blood flow and blood level of sodium
- Increase (and increased blood pressure) caused by diminished blood flow to kidneys or decreased amounts of sodium reaching glomerulus
- Decrease (and decreased blood pressure) caused by increased blood flow to kidneys or increased amounts of sodium reaching glomerulus

Sodium and water regulation

- Aldosterone regulates reabsorption of sodium and water within nephron

Understanding aldosterone production

This illustration shows the steps involved in the production of aldosterone, which helps to regulate fluid balance through the renin-angiotensin-aldosterone system.

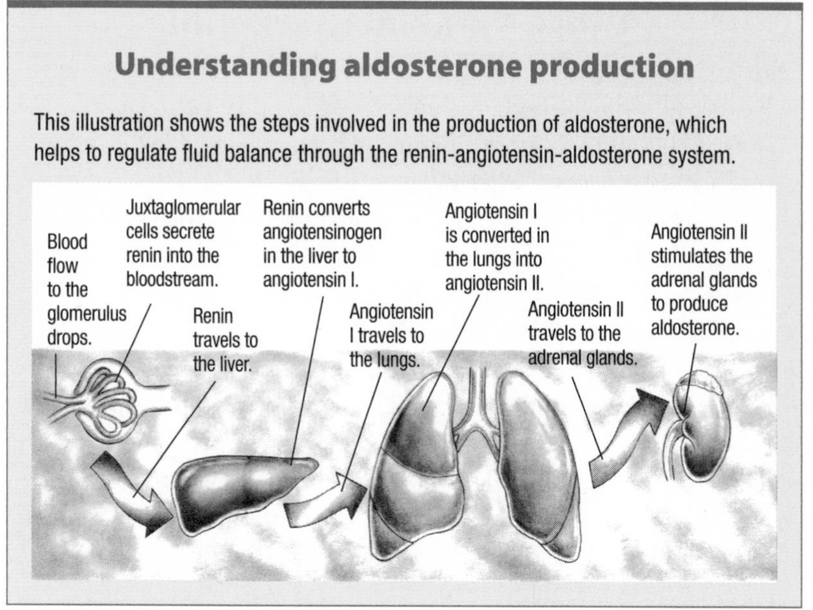

Renin travels to the liver.

Angiotensin I travels to the lungs.

Active transport initiation

When blood volume drops, aldosterone initiates the active transport of sodium from the distal tubules and the collecting ducts into the bloodstream. When sodium is forced into the bloodstream, more water is reabsorbed and blood volume expands.

How aldosterone works

Aldosterone, produced as a result of the renin-angiotensin-aldosterone system, regulates fluid volume as depicted here.

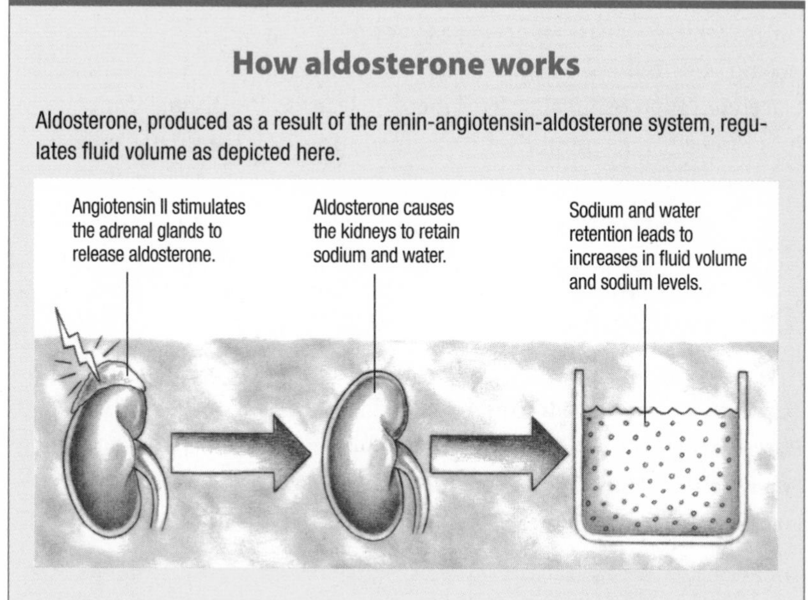

Angiotensin II stimulates the adrenal glands to release aldosterone.
Aldosterone causes the kidneys to retain sodium and water.
Sodium and water retention leads to increases in fluid volume and sodium levels.

Atrial natriuretic peptide

- ✦ Cardiac hormone stored in atrial cells
- ✦ Released when atrial pressure increases
- ✦ Suppresses serum renin levels
- ✦ Decreases aldosterone release
- ✦ Increases glomerular filtration
- ✦ Decreases ADH release
- ✦ Causes vasodilation

Atrial natriuretic peptide

The renin-angiotensin-aldosterone system isn't the only factor working to balance fluids in the body. A cardiac hormone called *atrial natriuretic peptide* (ANP) also helps to maintain that balance. Stored in the cells of the atria, ANP is released when atrial pressure increases. The hormone counteracts the effects of the renin-angiotensin-aldosterone system by decreasing blood pressure and reducing intravascular blood volume.

ANP is a powerful hormone that:

- ✦ suppresses serum renin levels
- ✦ decreases aldosterone release from the adrenal glands
- ✦ increases glomerular filtration, which increases urine excretion of sodium and water
- ✦ decreases ADH release from the posterior pituitary gland
- ✦ reduces vascular resistance by causing vasodilation.

The amount of ANP that the atria release rises in response to several conditions, including chronic renal failure and heart failure.

Causes of atrial stretching, such as orthostatic changes, atrial tachycardia, high sodium intake, sodium chloride infusions, and use of drugs that cause vasoconstriction, can also lead to increases in the amount of ANP released.

Thirst

- ✦ Simplest mechanism for maintaining fluid balance
- ✦ Stimulated by increases in extracellular fluid osmolality that lead to drying of mucus membranes in mouth
- ✦ Ingested fluid absorbed from intestine into bloodstream, leading to increase in body fluid and decrease in solute concentration

Thirst

Perhaps the simplest mechanism for maintaining fluid balance is the thirst mechanism. Thirst occurs as a result of even small losses of fluid. Losing body fluids or eating highly salty foods leads to an increase in extracellular fluid osmolality. This increase leads to the drying of mucus membranes in the mouth, which in turn stimulates the thirst center in the hypothalamus.

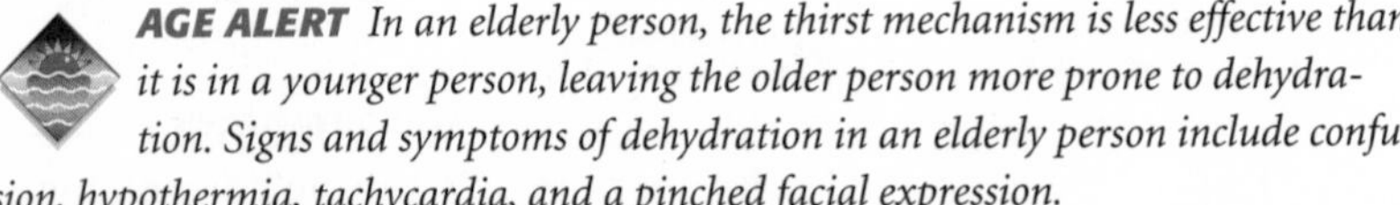

AGE ALERT *In an elderly person, the thirst mechanism is less effective than it is in a younger person, leaving the older person more prone to dehydration. Signs and symptoms of dehydration in an elderly person include confusion, hypothermia, tachycardia, and a pinched facial expression.*

The normal response when a person is thirsty is to drink fluid. The ingested fluid is absorbed from the intestine into the bloodstream, where it moves freely between fluid compartments. This movement leads to an increase in the amount of fluid in the body and a decrease in the concentration of solutes, thus balancing fluid levels throughout the body.

Electrolyte balance

A LOOK AT ELECTROLYTES

Electrolytes work with fluids to maintain health and well-being and are crucial for nearly every cellular reaction and function. They're found in various concentrations, depending on whether they're inside or outside the cells. Knowing their basics — what they are, how they function, and what upsets their balance — is essential to providing effective patient care.

Electrolytes
- ✦ Work with fluids to maintain health and well-being
- ✦ Crucial for nearly every cellular reaction and function
- ✦ Found in various concentrations

Ions

Electrolytes are substances that, when in a solution, separate (or dissociate) into electrically charged particles called ions. Some ions are positively charged; others, negatively charged. Several pairs of oppositely charged ions — such as sodium and chloride and calcium and phosphorus — are so closely linked that a problem with one ion causes a problem with the other.

Various disorders can disrupt the normal balance of electrolytes in the body. Understanding electrolytes and recognizing imbalances can make your patient assessment more accurate.

Ions
- ✦ Electrically charged particles created by electrolyte dissociation when in a solution
- ✦ Can be positively or negatively charged

Anions and cations

- Anions — electrolytes that generate positive charge
- Cations — electrolytes that generate negative charge

Error

ANIONS AND CATIONS

Anions are electrolytes that generate a negative charge; cations are electrolytes that produce a positive charge. These charges enable normal cell function. (See *Differentiating anions and cations.*)

Understanding how electrolytes work

- Operate in extracellular and intracellular fluid compartments

UNDERSTANDING HOW ELECTROLYTES WORK

Electrolytes operate outside the cell in extracellular fluid compartments and inside the cell in intracellular fluid compartments. Individual electrolytes differ in concentration, but anions and cations balance to achieve a neutral electrical charge called *electroneutrality.* Most electrolytes interact with hydrogen ions to maintain acid-base balance. The body's major electrolytes have specialized functions that contribute to metabolism and fluid and electrolyte balance.

Major electrolytes outside the cell

Sodium
- Affects serum osmolality and extracellular fluid
- Helps nerve and muscle cells interact

Chloride
- Maintains osmotic pressure
- Needed by gastric mucosal cells to produce hydrochloric acid

Calcium
- Major cation involved in structure and function of bones and teeth
- Stabilizes cell membrane and reduces its permeability to sodium
- Transmits nerve impulses
- Contracts muscles

Bicarbonate
- Base produced by kidneys
- Central buffering agent in blood

MAJOR ELECTROLYTES OUTSIDE THE CELL

Sodium and chloride, the major electrolytes in extracellular fluid, exert most of their influence outside the cell. Sodium concentration affects serum osmolality (solute concentration in 1 L of water) and extracellular fluid volume. Sodium also helps nerve and muscle cells interact. Chloride helps maintain osmotic pressure (water-pulling pressure), and gastric mucosal cells need chloride to produce hydrochloric acid, which breaks down food into absorbable components.

Calcium and bicarbonate are two other major electrolytes found in extracellular fluid. Calcium is the major cation involved in the structure and function of bones and teeth. It's needed to:
- stabilize the cell membrane and reduce its permeability to sodium
- transmit nerve impulses
- contract muscles
- coagulate blood
- form bone and teeth.

Bicarbonate plays a vital role in acid-base balance. It's a base produced by the kidneys that acts as a central buffering agent in the blood.

& pancreas

Differentiating anions and cations

Electrolytes can be either anions or cations. Anions generate a negative charge; cations produce a positive charge.

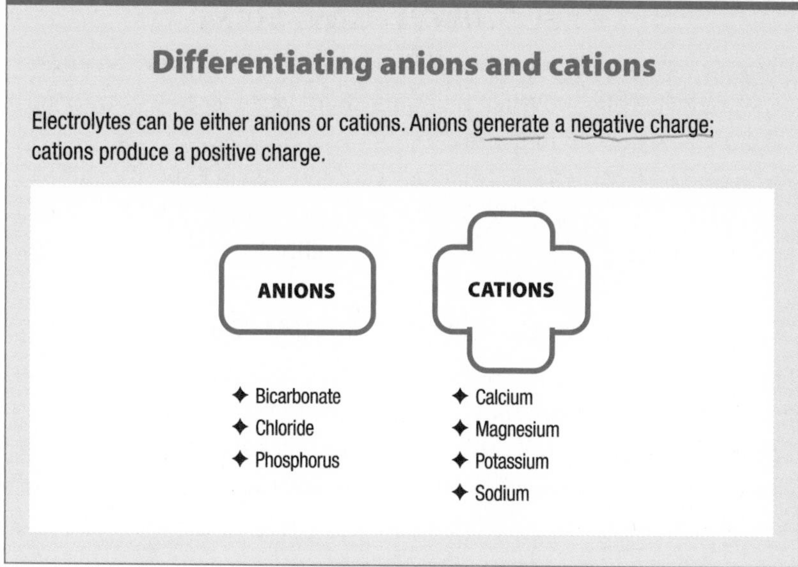

Major electrolytes inside the cell

Potassium, phosphorus, and magnesium are among the most abundant electrolytes inside the cell.

Potassium

Potassium plays an important role in:
- ✦ cell excitability regulation
- ✦ nerve impulse conduction
- ✦ resting membrane potential
- ✦ muscle contraction and myocardial membrane responsiveness
- ✦ intracellular osmolality control.

Phosphorus

The body contains phosphorus in the form of phosphate salts. Phosphate, used interchangeably with phosphorus, is essential for energy metabolism. Combined with calcium, phosphate plays a key role in bone and tooth mineralization. It also helps maintain acid-base balance.

Magnesium

Magnesium acts as a catalyst for enzyme reactions. It regulates neuromuscular contraction, promotes normal functioning of the nervous and cardiovascular systems, and aids in protein synthesis and sodium and potassium ion transportation.

Major electrolytes inside the cell

Potassium
- ✦ Important for cell excitability regulation, nerve impulse conduction, resting membrane potential, muscle contraction, myocardial membrane responsiveness, and intracellular osmolality control

Phosphorus
- ✦ Essential for energy metabolism
- ✦ Key role in bone and tooth mineralization
- ✦ Maintains acid-base balance

Magnesium
- ✦ Catalyst for enzyme reactions
- ✦ Regulates neuromuscular contraction
- ✦ Promotes normal functioning of nervous and cardiovascular systems
- ✦ Aids in protein synthesis and sodium and potassium ion transportation

Electrolyte movement

When cells die, their contents spill into the extracellular area and upset the electrolyte balance. When this happens, elevated levels of intracellular electrolytes are found in plasma.

Although electrolytes are generally concentrated in a specific compartment, they aren't confined to these areas. Like fluids, they move around trying to maintain balance and electroneutrality.

Electrolyte balance

- Affected by fluid intake and output, acid-base balance, hormone secretion, and normal cell function

Electrolyte balance

Fluid intake and output, acid-base balance, hormone secretion, and normal cell function influence electrolyte balance. (See *Understanding electrolytes.*) Because electrolytes function both collaboratively with other electrolytes and individually, imbalances in one electrolyte can affect balance in others.

Electrolyte levels

- Only levels outside cell in bloodstream are measured
- Frequency of measurements determined by patient's condition
- Before intervening for imbalance, important to assess patient history and symptoms

Electrolyte levels

Even though electrolytes exist inside and outside the cell, only the levels outside the cell in the bloodstream are measured. Although serum levels remain fairly stable throughout a person's life span, understanding which levels are normal and which are abnormal is critical to reacting quickly and appropriately to a patient's electrolyte imbalance.

The patient's condition determines how often electrolyte levels are checked. Results for many laboratory tests are reported in milliequivalents per liter (mEq/L), which is a measure of the ion's chemical activity, or its power. (See *Interpreting serum electrolyte test results,* page 22.)

When you see an abnormal laboratory test result, consider what you know about the patient. For example, a serum potassium level of 7 mEq/L for a patient with previously normal serum potassium levels and no apparent reason for the increase may be an inaccurate result. Perhaps the patient's blood sample was hemolyzed from trauma to the cells.

It's crucial to look at the whole picture before you act, including what you know about the patient, his symptoms, and his electrolyte levels. (See *Documenting electrolyte imbalances,* page 23.)

Understanding electrolytes

Electrolytes help regulate water distribution, manage acid-base balance, and transmit nerve impulses. They also contribute to energy generation and blood clotting. This table summarizes the functions of each of the body's major electrolytes. The illustration below shows how electrolytes are distributed in and around the cell.

Calcium (Ca)
- A major cation
- Found in teeth and bones and in fairly equal concentrations in intracellular fluid (ICF) and extracellular fluid (ECF)
- Also found in cell membranes, where it helps cells adhere to one another and maintain their shape
- Acts as an enzyme activator within cells (muscles must have Ca to contract)
- Aids coagulation
- Affects cell membrane permeability and firing level

Chloride (Cl)
- Main ECF anion
- Helps maintain normal ECF osmolality
- Affects body pH
- Plays a vital role in maintaining acid-base balance; combines with hydrogen ions to produce hydrochloric acid

Bicarbonate (HCO_3^-)
- Present in ECF
- Regulates acid-base balance

Magnesium (Mg)
- A leading ICF cation
- Contributes to many enzymatic and metabolic processes, particularly protein synthesis
- Modifies nerve impulse transmission and skeletal muscle response (unbalanced Mg concentrations dramatically affect neuromuscular processes)

Phosphorus (P)
- Main ICF anion
- Promotes energy storage and carbohydrate, protein, and fat metabolism
- Acts as a hydrogen buffer

Potassium (K)
- Main ICF cation
- Regulates cell excitability
- Permeates cell membranes, thereby affecting the cell's electrical status
- Helps to control ICF osmolality and, consequently, ICF osmotic pressure

Sodium (Na)
- Main ECF cation
- Helps govern normal ECF osmolality (a shift in Na concentrations triggers a fluid volume change to restore normal solute and water ratio)
- Helps maintain acid-base balance
- Activates nerve and muscle cells
- Influences water distribution (with chloride)

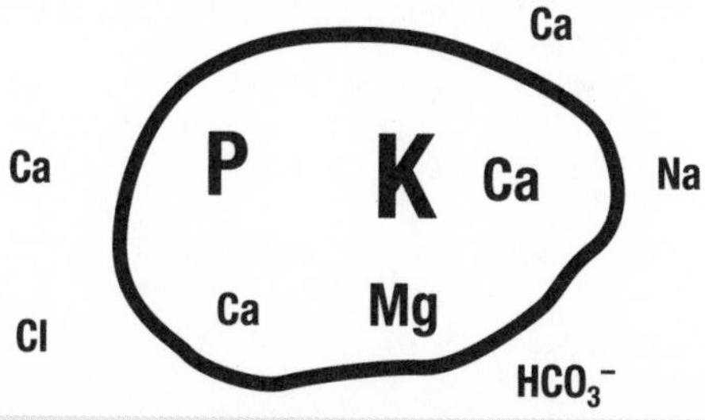

Interpreting serum electrolyte test results

Use the quick-reference chart to interpret serum electrolyte test results in adult patients. This chart also includes disorders that can cause imbalances.

Electrolyte	Results	Implications	Common causes
Calcium	8.9 to 10.1 mg/dl	Normal	
	< 8.9 mg/dl	Hypocalcemia	Acute pancreatitis
	> 10.1 mg/dl	Hypercalcemia	Hyperparathyroidism
Calcium, ionized	4.5 to 5.1 mg/dl	Normal	
	< 4.5 mg/dl	Hypocalcemia	Massive transfusion
	> 5.1 mg/dl	Hypercalcemia	Acidosis
Chloride	96 to 106 mEq/L	Normal	
	< 96 mEq/L	Hypochloremia	Prolonged vomiting
	> 106 mEq/L	Hyperchloremia	Hypernatremia
Magnesium	1.5 to 2.5 mEq/L	Normal	
	< 1.5 mEq/L	Hypomagnesemia	Malnutrition
	> 2.5 mEq/L	Hypermagnesemia	Renal failure
Phosphates	2.5 to 4.5 mg/dl or 1.8 to 2.6 mEq/L	Normal	
	< 2.5 mg/dl or 1.8 mEq/L	Hypophosphatemia	Diabetic ketoacidosis
	> 4.5 mg/dl or 2.6 mEq/L	Hyperphosphatemia	Renal insufficiency
Potassium	3.5 to 5 mEq/L	Normal	
	< 3.5 mEq/L	Hypokalemia	Diarrhea
	> 5 mEq/L	Hyperkalemia	Burns and renal failure
Sodium	135 to 145 mEq/L	Normal	
	< 135 mEq/L	Hyponatremia	Syndrome of inappropriate antidiuretic hormone
	> 145 mEq/L	Hypernatremia	Diabetes insipidus

CHARTING CHECKLIST

Documenting electrolyte imbalances

If your patient has an electrolyte imbalance, make sure you document:

- ❑ assessment findings
- ❑ laboratory results pertaining to the imbalance
- ❑ related nursing diagnoses
- ❑ notification of the physician
- ❑ interventions and treatment, including safety measures
- ❑ patient's response to interventions
- ❑ patient teaching.

FLUID REGULATION

Many activities within the body and certain drugs, such as diuretics and I.V. fluids, regulate fluid and electrolyte balance. A quick review of some of the basics will help you better understand this regulation.

Fluid and solute movement

Active transport moves solutes across semipermeable membranes and requires pumps within the body to move the substances from areas of lower concentration to areas of higher concentration — against a concentration gradient. Adenosine triphosphate is the energy that moves solutes across semipermeable membranes.

The sodium-potassium pump, an example of an active transport mechanism, moves sodium ions from intracellular fluid (an area of lower concentration) to extracellular fluid (an area of higher concentration). With potassium, the reverse happens: A large amount of potassium in intracellular fluid causes an electrical potential at the cell membrane. As ions rapidly shift in and out of the cell, electrical impulses are conducted. These impulses are essential for maintaining life.

Fluid and solute movement

- ✦ Accomplished by active transport
- ✦ Requires pumps within body to move substances from areas of lower concentration to areas of higher concentration
- ✦ Adenosine triphosphate provides energy to move solutes across semipermeable membranes

Organ and gland involvement

Most major organs and glands in the body — the lungs, liver, adrenal glands, kidneys, heart, hypothalamus, pituitary gland, skin, GI tract, parathyroid glands, and thyroid gland — help to regulate fluid and electrolyte balance.

Organ and gland involvement

Lungs and liver

- ✦ Regulate sodium, water balance, and blood pressure

Organ and gland involvement *(continued)*

Adrenal glands

- Secrete aldosterone, influencing kidney sodium and potassium balance

Heart

- Secretes atrial natriuretic peptide, causing sodium excretion

Hypothalamus and posterior pituitary gland

- Produce and secrete antidiuretic hormone, causing water retention

Parathyroid glands

- Secrete parathyroid hormone, drawing calcium into blood from bones, intestines, and kidneys and helping move phosphorus from blood to kidneys

Thyroid gland

- Secretes calcitonin, which lowers elevated calcium levels by preventing calcium release from bone and decreasing intestinal absorption and kidney reabsorption of calcium

Kidney involvement

- Perform filtration — process of removing particles from solution by allowing liquid portion to pass through membrane

As part of the renin-angiotensin-aldosterone system, the lungs and liver help regulate sodium and water balance as well as blood pressure. The adrenal glands secrete aldosterone, which influences sodium and potassium balance in the kidneys. These levels are affected because the kidneys excrete potassium, or hydrogen ions, in exchange for retained sodium.

The heart counteracts the renin-angiotensin-aldosterone system when it secretes atrial natriuretic peptide, causing sodium excretion. The hypothalamus and posterior pituitary gland produce and secrete an antidiuretic hormone that causes the body to retain water, which affects solute concentration in the blood.

Sodium, potassium, chloride, and water are lost in sweat and from the GI tract; however, electrolytes are also absorbed from the GI tract, affecting their balance.

The parathyroid glands also play a role in electrolyte balance, specifically the balance of calcium and phosphorus. The parathyroid glands (usually two pairs) are located behind and to the side of the thyroid gland. They secrete parathyroid hormone, which draws calcium into the blood from the bones, intestines, and kidneys and helps move phosphorus from the blood to the kidneys, where it's excreted in urine.

The thyroid gland is also involved in electrolyte balance by secreting calcitonin. This hormone lowers an elevated calcium level by preventing calcium release from bone and decreasing intestinal absorption and kidney reabsorption of calcium.

Kidney involvement

The kidneys perform the vital function of filtration — the process of removing particles from a solution by allowing the liquid portion to pass through a membrane. Filtration occurs in the nephron (the anatomic and functional unit of the kidneys). As blood circulates through the glomerulus (a tuft of capillaries), fluids and electrolytes are filtered and collected in the nephron's tubule.

Some fluids and electrolytes are reabsorbed through capillaries at various points along the nephron; others are secreted. (See *How the nephron regulates fluids and electrolytes.*) Age can play an important role in the way kidneys function — or malfunction.

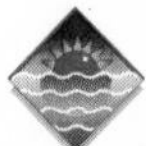

AGE ALERT *The immature kidneys of an infant can't concentrate urine or reabsorb electrolytes the way the kidneys of an adult can, so infants are at a higher risk for electrolyte imbalances. Older adults are also at risk for elec-*

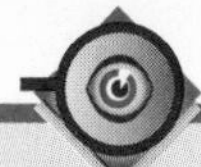

CLOSER LOOK

How the nephron regulates fluids and electrolytes

In this illustration, the nephron has been stretched to show where and how fluids and electrolytes are regulated.

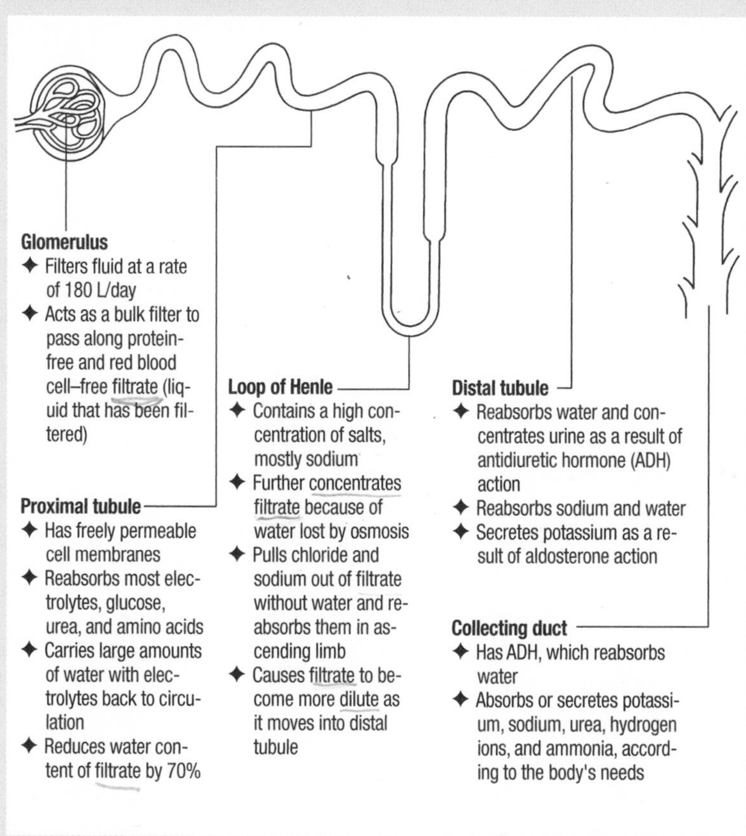
Glomerulus
✦ Filters fluid at a rate of 180 L/day
✦ Acts as a bulk filter to pass along protein-free and red blood cell–free filtrate (liquid that has been filtered)
Proximal tubule
✦ Has freely permeable cell membranes
✦ Reabsorbs most electrolytes, glucose, urea, and amino acids
✦ Carries large amounts of water with electrolytes back to circulation
✦ Reduces water content of filtrate by 70%
Loop of Henle
✦ Contains a high concentration of salts, mostly sodium
✦ Further concentrates filtrate because of water lost by osmosis
✦ Pulls chloride and sodium out of filtrate without water and reabsorbs them in ascending limb
✦ Causes filtrate to become more dilute as it moves into distal tubule
Distal tubule
✦ Reabsorbs water and concentrates urine as a result of antidiuretic hormone (ADH) action
✦ Reabsorbs sodium and water
✦ Secretes potassium as a result of aldosterone action
Collecting duct
✦ Has ADH, which reabsorbs water
✦ Absorbs or secretes potassium, sodium, urea, hydrogen ions, and ammonia, according to the body's needs

trolyte imbalances because their kidneys have fewer functional nephrons, a decreased glomerular filtration rate, and a diminished ability to concentrate.

A vital part of the kidneys' job is to regulate electrolyte levels in the body. Normally functioning kidneys maintain the correct fluid level in the body. Sodium and fluid balance are closely related. When too much sodium is released, the body's fluid level drops.

Parts of the nephron

- ✦ Glomerulus — filters fluid at rate of 180 L/day
- ✦ Proximal tubule — reabsorbs most electrolytes, glucose, urea, and amino acids
- ✦ Loop of Henle — causes filtrate to become more dilute as it moves into distal tubule
- ✦ Distal tubule — reabsorbs water and concentrates urine
- ✦ Collecting duct — reabsorbs water and absorbs or secretes potassium, sodium, hydrogen ions, and ammonia

Kidney involvement *(continued)*

- ✦ Regulate electrolyte levels
- ✦ Eliminate excess potassium

The kidneys also rid the body of excess potassium. When the kidneys fail, potassium builds up in the body—and high levels of potassium in the blood can be fatal.

Diuretic involvement
- ✦ Used to treat such disorders as hypertension, heart failure, electrolyte imbalances, and kidney disease

Diuretic involvement

Many patients—whether in a health care facility or at home—take a diuretic to increase urine production. Diuretics are used to treat many disorders, such as hypertension, heart failure, electrolyte imbalances, and kidney disease.

The health care team should monitor the effects of a diuretic, including its effect on electrolyte balance. A diuretic causes electrolyte loss, whereas an I.V. fluid causes electrolyte gain. Older adults, who are at risk for fluid and electrolyte imbalances, require careful monitoring because a diuretic can worsen an existing imbalance.

When you know how the nephron functions normally, you can predict a diuretic's effects on your patient by knowing where along the nephron the drug acts. This knowledge and understanding can help you provide optimal care for a patient taking a diuretic. (See *How drugs affect nephron activity*.)

I.V. fluid involvement
- ✦ Remember: When administering I.V. fluids, keep in mind patient's normal electrolyte requirements

Three questions to ask
- ✦ Is I.V. fluid providing correct amount of electrolytes?
- ✦ How long has patient been receiving I.V. fluids?
- ✦ Is patient receiving oral electrolyte supplementation?

I.V. fluid involvement

Like diuretics, I.V. fluids affect fluid and electrolyte balance in the body. (See *I.V. fluids components,* page 28.) When providing I.V. fluid, keep in mind the patient's normal electrolyte requirements. For example, the patient may require:

- ✦ 1 to 2 mEq/kg/day of sodium
- ✦ 0.5 to 1 mEq/kg/day of potassium
- ✦ 1 to 2 mEq/kg/day of chloride.

To evaluate I.V. fluid treatment, ask yourself these questions:

- ✦ Is the I.V. fluid providing the correct amount of electrolytes?
- ✦ How long has the patient been receiving I.V. fluids?
- ✦ Is the patient receiving oral supplementation of electrolytes?

How drugs affect nephron activity

Here's a look at how certain diuretics and other drugs affect the nephron's regulation of fluid and electrolyte balance.

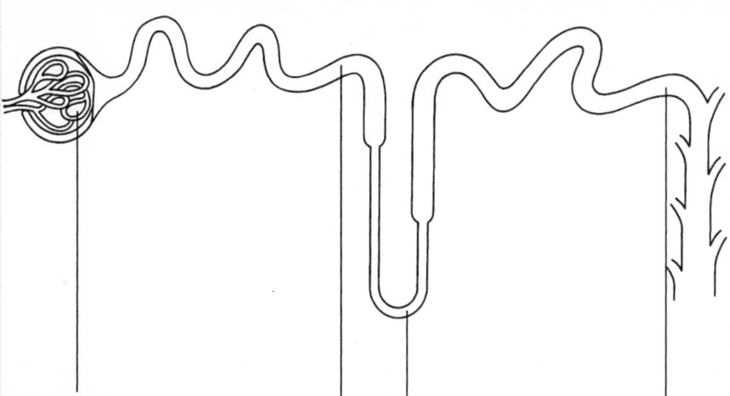

Glomerulus

✦ *Dopamine.* Dopamine may increase urine output. Dopaminergic receptor sites exist along the afferent arterioles (tiny vessels that bring blood to the glomerulus). In low doses (0.5 to 3 mcg/kg/minute), dopamine dilates these vessels in the glomerulus to increase blood flow to it. This, in turn, increases filtration in the nephron.

Proximal tubule

✦ *Carbonic anhydrase inhibitors* (acetazolamide [Diamox]). These drugs reduce hydrogen ion (acid) concentration in the tubule, which causes increased excretion of bicarbonate, water, sodium, and potassium.

✦ *Glucose.* High blood levels of osmotic diuretic cause excess glucose to spill over into the tubules. The osmotic effect of glucose also results in increased urine output.

✦ *Mannitol.* Osmotic diuretic mannitol isn't reabsorbed in the tubule; it remains in high concentrations throughout its journey, increasing filtrate osmolality and hindering water, sodium, and chloride reabsorption, thereby increasing their excretion.

Loop of Henle

✦ *Loop diuretics* (furosemide [Lasix], bumetanide [Bumex], and ethacrynic acid [Edecrin]). Loop diuretics act on the ascending loop of Henle to prevent water and sodium reabsorption. As a result, volume in the tubules is increased and blood volume is decreased. Potassium and chloride are also excreted here.

Distal tubule

✦ *Potassium-sparing diuretics* (spironolactone [Aldactone]). These diuretics interfere with sodium and chloride reabsorption in the tubule. Potassium is spared, and sodium, chloride, and water are excreted. Urine output increases, and the body retains potassium.

✦ *Thiazide diuretics* (hydrochlorothiazide [HydroDIURIL] and metolazone [Zaroxolyn]). Thiazide diuretics act high in the distal tubule to prevent sodium reabsorption, which increases the amount of tubular fluid and electrolytes farther down the nephron. Blood volume decreases, aldosterone increases sodium reabsorption and, in exchange, potassium is lost from the body.

Drugs affecting nephron activity

Dopamine

✦ May increase urine output

Loop diuretics

✦ Prevent water and sodium reabsorption in ascending loop of Henle, resulting in increased tubular volume and decreased blood volume

Osmotic diuretics

✦ Carbonic anhydrase inhibitors — cause increased excretion of bicarbonate, water, sodium, and potassium

✦ Glucose — increases urine output

✦ Mannitol — increases filtrate osmolality and hinders water, sodium, and chloride reabsorption, increasing their excretion

Potassium-sparing diuretics

✦ Increase sodium, chloride, and water absorption in the tubule

✦ Increase urine output

✦ Retain potassium

Thiazide diuretics

✦ Prevent sodium reabsorption high in distal tubule, increasing amount of tubular fluid and electrolytes farther down nephron

✦ Result in decrease in blood volume and body potassium and increase in sodium reabsorption

I.V. fluid components

This table lists the electrolyte content of some commonly used I.V. fluids.

I.V. SOLUTION	ELECTROLYTE	AMOUNT
Dextrose	None	—
Sodium chloride		
5%	Sodium chloride	855 mEq/L
3%	Sodium chloride	513 mEq/L
0.9%	Sodium chloride	154 mEq/L
0.45%	Sodium chloride	77 mEq/L
Dextrose and sodium chloride		
5% dextrose and 0.9% sodium chloride	Sodium chloride	154 mEq/L
5% dextrose and 0.45% sodium chloride	Sodium chloride	77 mEq/L
Ringer's solution (plain)		
	Chloride	156 mEq/L
	Sodium	147 mEq/L
	Calcium	4.5 mEq/L
	Potassium	4 mEq/L
Lactated Ringer's solution		
	Sodium	130 mEq/L
	Chloride	109 mEq/L
	Lactate	28 mEq/L
	Potassium	4 mEq/L
	Calcium	3 mEq/L

Acid-base balance

A LOOK AT ACIDS AND BASES

The chemical reactions that sustain life depend on a delicate balance—known as *homeostasis*—between acids and bases in the body. Even a slight imbalance can profoundly affect metabolism and essential body functions. Several conditions, such as infection or trauma, and medications can affect homeostasis, which is why it's important for every nurse to understand some basic chemistry.

UNDERSTANDING pH

Understanding acids and bases requires an understanding of pH, a calculation based on the percentage of hydrogen ions (H^+) in a solution as well as the amount of acids and bases. Acids consist of molecules that can give up, or donate, H^+ to other molecules. Carbonic acid is an acid that occurs naturally in the body. Bases consist of molecules that can accept H^+; bicarbonate (HCO_3^-) is an example.

To understand how pH is measured, know that a solution that contains more base than acid has fewer H^+ and a higher pH. A solution with a pH above 7 is a base, or alkaline. In contrast, a solution that contains more acid than base has more H^+ and a lower pH. A solution with a pH below 7 is an acid, or acidic.

You can assess a patient's acid-base balance if you know the pH of his blood. Because arterial blood is usually used to measure pH, this discus-

Understanding pH

Acids

- Consist of molecules that can yield H^+ to other molecules
- Have pH < 7 (acidic)
- Example: Carbonic acid

Bases

- Consist of molecules that can accept pH
- Have pH > 7 (alkaline)
- Example: bicarbonate

Measuring pH

- Solution containing more base than acid has fewer H^+ and higher pH
- Solution containing more acid than base has more H^+ and lower pH

Interpreting normal pH
- Normal pH (7.35 to 7.45) — amount of acid is balanced with amount of base
- pH < 7.35 abnormally acidic
- pH > 7.45 abnormally alkaline

Acidosis
- Decrease in pH below 7.35
- May be caused by increase in blood's H^+ concentration or decrease in blood's HCO_3^- level

Alkalosis
- Increase in pH above 7.45
- May be caused by increase in blood's HCO_3^- level or decrease in blood's H^+ concentration

Regulating acids and bases
- Proper regulation of pH necessary for maintaining health
- Deviation in pH can compromise electrolyte balance, activity of critical enzymes, muscle contraction, and basic cellular function

Interpreting normal pH

This illustration shows that blood pH normally stays slightly alkaline, between 7.35 to 7.45. At that point, the amount of acid (H) is balanced with the amount of base (represented here as bicarbonate). A pH below 7.35 is abnormally acidic; a pH above 7.45, abnormally alkaline.

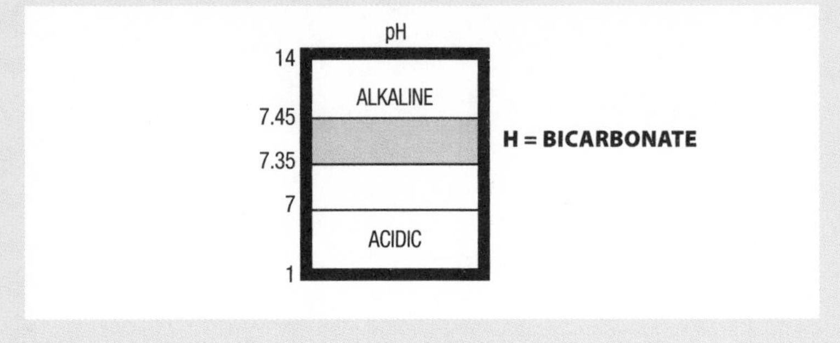

sion focuses on arterial samples. Arterial blood is normally slightly alkaline, with a pH ranging from 7.35 to 7.45. A pH level within that range represents a balance between the percentage of H^+ and HCO_3^-. Generally, pH is maintained in a ratio of 20 parts HCO_3^- to 1 part carbonic acid. A pH below 6.8 or above 7.8 is usually fatal. (See *Interpreting normal pH.*)

Acidosis

Under certain conditions, the pH of arterial blood may deviate significantly from its normal narrow range. If the blood's H^+ concentration increases or HCO_3^- level decreases, pH may decrease. In either case, a decrease in pH below 7.35 signals acidosis. (See *Recognizing acidosis.*)

Alkalosis

If the blood's HCO_3^- level increases or H^+ concentration of the blood decreases, pH may increase. In either case, an increase in pH above 7.45 signals alkalosis. (See *Recognizing alkalosis.*)

REGULATING ACIDS AND BASES

A person's well-being depends on his ability to maintain a normal pH. A deviation in pH can compromise essential body processes, including electrolyte balance, activity of critical enzymes, muscle contraction, and basic cellular function. The body normally maintains pH within a narrow

Recognizing acidosis

Acidosis, a condition in which pH is below 7.35, occurs when acids (H) accumulate or bases, such as bicarbonate, are lost.

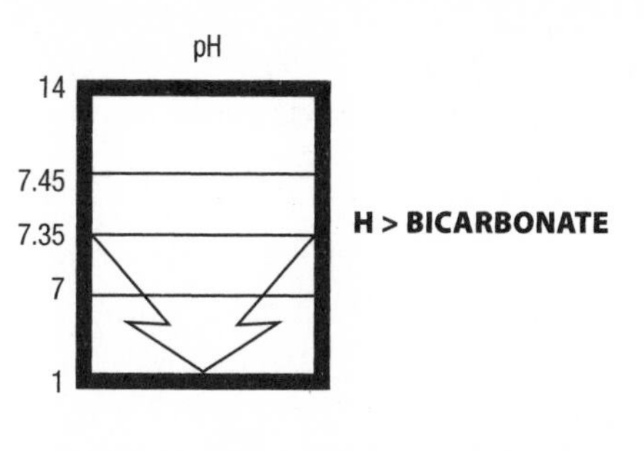

Recognizing alkalosis

Alkalosis, a condition in which pH is higher than 7.45, occurs when bases, such as bicarbonate, accumulate or acids (H) are lost.

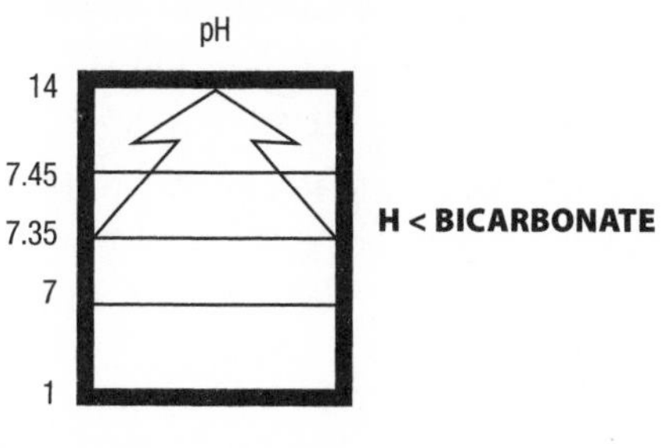

range by carefully balancing acidic and alkaline elements. When one aspect of that balance breaks down, the body can't maintain a healthy pH as easily, and problems develop.

The body regulates acids and bases to avoid potentially serious consequences. Therefore, when pH rises or falls, three regulatory systems come into play:

Regulating acids and bases *(continued)*

- Three systems regulate pH: Chemical buffers, respiratory system, and kidneys

- Chemical buffers act immediately to protect tissues and cells. These buffers instantly combine with the offending acid or base, neutralizing harmful effects until other regulators take over.
- The respiratory system uses hypoventilation or hyperventilation as needed to regulate excretion or retention of acids within minutes of a change in pH.
- The kidneys excrete or retain acids and bases as needed. Renal regulation can restore normal H^+ concentration within hours or days.

Chemical buffers

The body maintains a healthy pH in part through chemical buffers, substances that minimize changes in pH by combining with excess acids or bases. Chemical buffers in the blood, intracellular fluid, and interstitial fluid serve as the body's most efficient pH-balancing weapon. The main chemical buffers are HCO_3^-, phosphate, and protein.

Bicarbonate buffers

HCO_3^- buffers make up the body's primary buffer system. They are mainly responsible for buffering blood and interstitial fluid. These buffers rely on a series of chemical reactions in which pairs of weak acids and bases (such as carbonic acid and HCO_3^-) combine with stronger acids (such as hydrochloric acid) and bases to weaken them.

Decreasing the strength of potentially damaging acids and bases reduces the danger those chemicals pose to pH balance. The kidneys assist HCO_3^- buffers by regulating HCO_3^- production. The lungs assist by regulating the carbonic acid production, which results from combining carbon dioxide (CO_2) and water.

Phosphate buffers

Like HCO_3^- buffers, phosphate buffers depend on a series of chemical reactions to minimize pH changes. Phosphate buffers react with either acids or bases to form compounds that slightly alter pH, which can provide extremely effective buffering. Phosphate buffers prove especially effective in renal tubules, where phosphates exist in greater concentrations.

Protein buffers

Protein buffers, the most plentiful buffers in the body, work inside and outside cells. They're made up of hemoglobin as well as other proteins. Behaving chemically like HCO_3^- buffers, protein buffers bind with acids and bases to neutralize them. In red blood cells, for instance, hemoglobin combines with H^+ to act as a buffer.

Chemical buffers
- Substances that minimize changes in pH by combining with excess acids or bases
- Body's most efficient pH-balancing weapons
- Main buffers: HCO_3^-, phosphate, and protein

HCO_3^- buffers
- Body's primary buffer system
- Buffer blood and interstitial fluid
- Rely on pairs of weak acids and bases to combine with stronger acids and bases to weaken them

Phosphate buffers
- Provide extremely effective buffering
- React with acids or bases to form compounds that slightly alter pH
- Especially effective in renal tubules

Protein buffers
- Most plentiful buffers in body
- Work inside and outside cells
- Bind with acids and bases to neutralize them

Respiratory system

The respiratory system serves as the second line of defense against acid-base imbalances. The lungs regulate blood levels of CO_2, a gas that combines with water to form carbonic acid. Increased levels of carbonic acid lead to a decrease in pH.

Chemoreceptors in the medulla of the brain sense those pH changes and vary the rate and depth of breathing to compensate. Breathing faster or deeper eliminates more CO_2 from the lungs, and the CO_2 level in the blood drops. The more CO_2 that's lost, the less carbonic acid that's made and, as a result, pH rises. The body regulates such a pH change by breathing slower or less deeply, thereby reducing CO_2 excretion.

To assess the effectiveness of ventilation, look at the partial pressure of carbon dioxide in arterial blood ($Paco_2$). A normal $Paco_2$ level in the body is 35 to 45 mm Hg. $Paco_2$ values reflect CO_2 levels in the blood. As those levels increase, so does $Paco_2$.

As a buffer, the respiratory system can maintain acid-base balance twice as effectively as chemical buffers because it can handle twice the amount of acids and bases. Although the respiratory system responds to pH changes within minutes, it can restore normal pH only temporarily. The kidneys are responsible for long-term adjustments to pH.

Respiratory system

- Second line of defense against acid-base imbalances
- Regulates blood levels of CO_2 by varying rate and depth of breathing to compensate for pH changes
- Breathing faster or deeper eliminates CO_2, thereby increasing pH

$Paco_2$

- Assessed to evaluate effectiveness of ventilation
- Reflects changes in blood CO_2 levels
- Normal level: 35 to 45 mm Hg

The kidneys

The kidneys serve as yet another mechanism for maintaining acid-base balance in the body. They can reabsorb acids and bases or excrete them into urine. They can also produce HCO_3^- to replenish lost supplies. Such adjustments to pH can take the kidneys hours or days to complete.

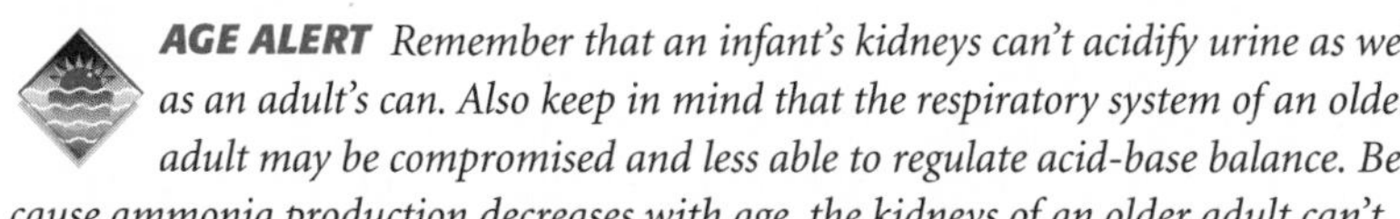

AGE ALERT *Remember that an infant's kidneys can't acidify urine as well as an adult's can. Also keep in mind that the respiratory system of an older adult may be compromised and less able to regulate acid-base balance. Because ammonia production decreases with age, the kidneys of an older adult can't handle excess acid as well as the kidneys of a younger adult.*

The kidneys also regulate the HCO_3^- level, which reflects the metabolic component of acid-base balance. Normally, the HCO_3^- level is reported with arterial blood gas results. The normal HCO_3^- level is 22 to 26 mEq/L. Also, HCO_3^- is reported with serum electrolyte levels as total serum CO_2 content.

If blood contains too much acid or not enough base, pH drops and the kidneys reabsorb sodium bicarbonate. The kidneys also excrete hydrogen along with phosphate or ammonia. Although urine tends to be acidic be-

The kidneys

- Reabsorb acids and bases or excrete them into urine
- Produce HCO_3^- to replenish lost supplies (can take hours or days)
- Regulate HCO_3^- level (normal, 22 to 26 mEq/L), reflecting metabolic component of acid-base balance

If pH drops

- Reabsorb HCO_3^- and excrete H^+, resulting in more acidic urine than normal

If pH rises

- Excrete HCO_3^- and retain more H^+, resulting in more alkaline urine than normal and lower blood HCO_3^- level

cause the body usually produces slightly more acids than bases, in such situations urine becomes more acidic than normal.

The reabsorption of HCO_3^- and the increased excretion of hydrogen causes more HCO_3^- to be formed in the renal tubules and eventually retained in the body. The HCO_3^- level in the blood then rises to a more normal level, increasing pH.

If blood contains more base and less acid, pH rises. The kidneys compensate by excreting HCO_3^- and retaining more H^+. As a result, urine becomes more alkaline and the blood HCO_3^- level drops. Conversely, if blood contains less HCO_3^- and more acid, pH drops.

Maintaining acid-base balance

- Body activates compensatory mechanisms that minimize pH changes
- Mainly involves metabolic or respiratory system adjustments

Metabolic disturbance

- When lack of HCO_3^- causes acidosis, lungs increase rate of breathing to lower CO_2 and raise pH to normal
- When excess HCO_3^- causes alkalosis, lungs decrease rate of breathing to retain CO_2 and lower pH to normal

Respiratory system disturbance

- Kidneys compensate by altering levels of HCO_3^- and H^+
- When $Paco_2$ is high (acidosis), kidneys retain HCO_3^- and excrete more acid to raise pH
- When $Paco_2$ is low (alkalosis), kidneys excrete HCO_3^- and retain acid to lower pH

MAINTAINING ACID-BASE BALANCE

The body responds to acid-base imbalances by activating compensatory mechanisms that minimize pH changes. Returning pH to a normal or near-normal level mainly involves changes in the component — metabolic or respiratory — not primarily affected by the imbalance.

If the body compensates only partially for an imbalance, pH remains outside the normal range. If the body compensates fully or completely, pH returns to normal.

If metabolic disturbance is the primary cause of an acid-base imbalance, the lungs compensate in one of two ways. When a lack of HCO_3^- causes acidosis, the lungs increase the rate of breathing, which blows off CO_2 and helps to raise pH to normal. When an excess of HCO_3^- causes alkalosis, the lungs decrease the rate of breathing, which retains CO_2 and helps lower pH.

If the respiratory system disturbs the acid-base balance, the kidneys compensate by altering levels of HCO_3^- and H^+. When $Paco_2$ is high (a state of acidosis), the kidneys retain HCO_3^- and excrete more acid to raise pH. When $Paco_2$ is low (a state of alkalosis), the kidneys excrete HCO_3^- and hold on to more acid to lower pH.

DIAGNOSING IMBALANCES

A number of tests are used to diagnose acid-base disturbances. Discussed here are the tests that are most commonly used to determine these imbalances.

Obtaining an ABG sample

When a needle puncture is needed to obtain an arterial blood gas (ABG) sample, the radial, brachial, or femoral arteries may be used. However, the angle of penetration varies.

For the radial artery—the artery most commonly used—the needle should enter bevel up at a 45-degree angle, as shown. For the brachial artery, the angle should be 60 degrees; for the femoral artery, 90 degrees.

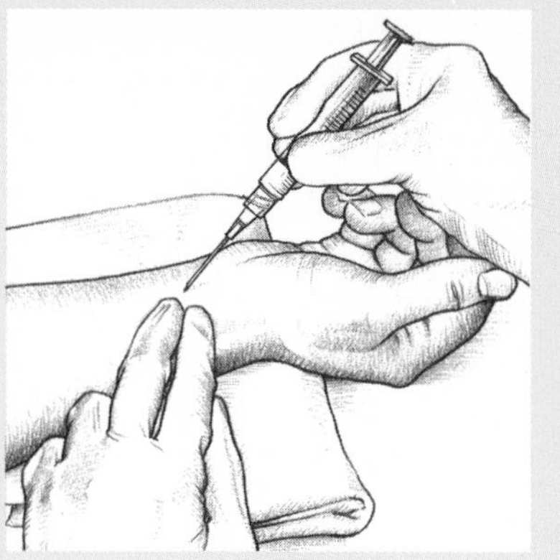

Obtaining ABG sample

- For radial artery, needle should enter bevel up at 45-degree angle
- For brachial artery, needle should enter at 60-degree angle, bevel up
- For femoral artery, needle should enter at 90-degree angle, bevel up

ABG analysis

An arterial blood gas (ABG) analysis is a diagnostic test in which a sample of blood obtained from an arterial puncture can be used to assess the effectiveness of a patient's breathing and overall acid-base balance. In addition to helping you identify problems with oxygenation and acid-base imbalances, the test can help you monitor a patient's response to treatment. (See *Obtaining an ABG sample.*)

Keep in mind that an ABG analysis should be used only in conjunction with a full patient assessment. You should assess all information about your patient so you can gain a clear picture of what's happening with his imbalances.

An ABG analysis involves several separate test results, only three of which relate to acid-base balance: pH, $Paco_2$, and HCO_3^- level. The normal ranges for adults are:

- pH—7.35 to 7.45
- $Paco_2$—35 to 45 mm Hg
- HCO_3^-—22 to 26 mEq/L.

Recall that pH is a measure of the H^+ concentration of blood and that $Paco_2$ is a measure of the partial pressure of carbon dioxide in arterial blood, which indicates the effectiveness of breathing. $Paco_2$ levels move in the opposite direction from pH. Moving in the same direction as pH, HCO_3^- represents the metabolic component of the body's acid-base balance.

ABG analysis

- Assesses effectiveness of breathing and overall acid-base balance
- Monitors response to treatment
- Normal test results: pH, 7.35 to 7.45; $Paco_2$, 35 to 45 mm Hg; HCO_3^-, 22 to 26 mEq/L

$Paco_2$

- Indicates effectiveness of breathing
- Level moves in opposite direction from pH

HCO_3^-

- Represents metabolic component of body's acid-base balance
- Level moves in same direction as pH

Pao_2

- Normal range: 80 to 100 mm Hg
- Varies with age; after age 60, may drop below 80 mm Hg without signs of hypoxia

Sao_2

- Normal range: 95% to 100%

Quick look at ABG results

Here's a quick look at how to interpret arterial blood gas (ABG) results and the questions you need to ask:

- ✦ Check the pH. Is it normal (7.35 to 7.45), acidotic (below 7.35), or alkalotic (above 7.45)?
- ✦ Determine the $Paco_2$ level. Is it normal (35 to 45 mm Hg), low, or high?
- ✦ Watch the HCO_3^- level. Is it normal (22 to 26 mEq/L), low, or high?
- ✦ Look for signs of compensation. Which value ($Paco_2$ or HCO_3^-) more closely corresponds to the change in pH?
- ✦ Determine the Pao_2 and Sao_2 levels. Is the Pao_2 normal (80 to 100 mm Hg), low, or high? Is the Sao_2 normal (95% to 100%), low, or high?

Interpreting ABG results

- ✦ Step 1: Check pH level
- ✦ Step 2: Determine $Paco_2$ level
- ✦ Step 3: Watch HCO_3^- level
- ✦ Step 4: Look for signs of compensation
- ✦ Step 5: Determine Pao_2 and Sao_2 levels

Check pH level

- ✦ If abnormal, determine if result reflects acidosis (<7.35) or alkalosis (>7.45)

Determine $Paco_2$ level

- ✦ Provides information about respiratory component of acid-base balance
- ✦ If abnormal, determine if low (< 35 mm Hg) or high (> 45 mm Hg)
- ✦ If abnormal, determine if it corresponds with change in pH (if pH is high, expect low $Paco_2$ [hypocapnia]; if pH is low, expect high $Paco_2$ [hypercapnia])

Other information routinely reported with ABG results include partial pressure of oxygen dissolved in arterial blood (Pao_2) and arterial oxygen saturation (Sao_2). The normal Pao_2 range is 80 to 100 mm Hg; however, Pao_2 varies with age. After age 60, the Pao_2 may drop below 80 mm Hg without signs of hypoxia. The normal Sao_2 range is 95% to 100%.

Interpreting ABG results

When interpreting results from an ABG analysis, be consistent in the sequence you use to analyze the information. (See *Quick look at ABG results* and *Inaccurate ABG results.*)

Check the pH level

First, check the pH level. This figure forms the basis for understanding most other figures.

If the pH level is abnormal, determine whether it reflects acidosis (below 7.35) or alkalosis (above 7.45). Then figure out whether the cause is respiratory or metabolic.

Determine the $Paco_2$ level

Remember that the $Paco_2$ level provides information about the respiratory component of acid-base balance.

If $Paco_2$ is abnormal, determine whether it's low (less than 35 mm Hg) or high (greater than 45 mm Hg). Then determine whether the abnormal result corresponds with a change in pH. For example, if the pH is high, you would expect the $Paco_2$ to be low (hypocapnia), indicating that the problem is primarily respiratory in origin. Conversely, if the

Inaccurate ABG results

To avoid altering arterial blood gas (ABG) results, be sure to use proper technique when drawing a sample of arterial blood. Remember:

- ✦ A delay in getting the sample to the laboratory or drawing blood for ABG analysis within 15 to 20 minutes of a procedure, such as suctioning or administering a respiratory treatment, could alter results.
- ✦ Air bubbles in the syringe could affect the oxygen level.
- ✦ Venous blood in the syringe could alter carbon dioxide and oxygen levels and pH.

pH is low, you would expect the $Paco_2$ to be high (hypercapnia), indicating that the problem is respiratory acidosis.

Watch the HCO_3^- level

Next, examine the HCO_3^- level. This value provides information about the metabolic aspect of acid-base balance.

If the HCO_3^- level is abnormal, determine whether it's low (less than 22 mEq/L) or high (greater than 26 mEq/L). Then determine whether the abnormal result corresponds with the change in pH. For example, if the pH is high, you would expect the HCO_3^- level to be high, indicating that the problem is metabolic alkalosis. Conversely, if the pH is low, you would expect the HCO_3^- level to be low, indicating that the problem is metabolic acidosis.

Look for compensation

Sometimes you'll see a change in both the $Paco_2$ and the HCO_3^- levels. One value indicates the primary source of the pH change; the other, the body's effort to compensate for the disturbance.

Complete compensation occurs when the body's ability to compensate is so effective that pH falls within the normal range. Partial compensation, on the other hand, occurs when pH remains outside the normal range.

Compensation involves opposites: If results indicate primary metabolic acidosis, compensation will come in the form of respiratory alkalosis. For example, the following ABG results indicate metabolic acidosis with compensatory respiratory alkalosis:

- ✦ pH — 7.27
- ✦ $Paco_2$ — 7 mm Hg

Interpreting ABG results *(continued)*

Watch HCO_3^- level

- ✦ Provides information about metabolic component of acid-base balance
- ✦ If abnormal, determine if low (< 22 mEq/L) or high (> 26 mEq/L)
- ✦ If abnormal, determine if it corresponds with change in pH (if pH is high, expect high HCO_3^-; if low, expect low HCO_3^-)

Look for compensation

- ✦ May see change in both $Paco_2$ and HCO_3^- levels (one indicates primary source of pH change; other indicates body's compensation effort)
- ✦ Complete compensation — occurs when compensation is so effective that pH falls within normal range
- ✦ Partial compensation — occurs when pH remains outside normal range

Interpreting ABG results *(continued)*

Determine Pao_2 and Sao_2

- Provide information about oxygenation status
- If abnormal, determine if values are low (Pao_2, < 80 mm Hg; Sao_2, < 95%) or high (Pao_2, > 100 mm Hg)

Anion gap result

- Arithmetical difference between concentrations of routinely measured cations and anions
- Helps differentiate among various acidotic conditions

- HCO_3^- — 10 mEq/L.

The low pH indicates acidosis. However, the $Paco_2$ is low, which normally leads to alkalosis, and the HCO_3^- level is low, which normally leads to acidosis. The HCO_3^- level, then, more closely corresponds with the pH, making the primary cause of the problem metabolic. The resultant decrease in $Paco_2$ reflects respiratory compensation.

Normal values for pH, $Paco_2$, and HCO_3^- would indicate that the patient's acid-base balance is normal.

Determine Pao_2 and Sao_2

Last, check Pao_2 and Sao_2, which yield information about the patient's oxygenation status. If the values are abnormal, determine whether they're high (Pao_2 greater than 100 mm Hg) or low (Pao_2 less than 80 mm Hg and Sao_2 less than 95%).

Remember that Pao_2 reflects the body's ability to pick up oxygen from the lungs. A low Pao_2 represents hypoxemia and can cause hyperventilation. The Pao_2 value also indicates when to make adjustments in the concentration of oxygen being administered to a patient.

ANION GAP RESULT

The anion gap is the arithmetical difference between the concentrations of routinely measured cations (sodium ions [Na^+] and potassium ions [K^+]) and of routinely measured anions (chloride [Cl^-] and HCO_3^-). Cations, positively charged ions, and anions, negatively charged ions, must be equal in the blood to maintain a proper balance of electrical charges. The anion gap result helps you differentiate among various acidotic conditions. (See *Calculating the anion gap*.)

Identifying the anion gap

The anion gap refers to the relationship among the body's cations and anions. Na^+ accounts for more than 90% of the circulating cations. Cl^- and HCO_3^- together account for 85% of the counterbalancing anions. K^+ is generally omitted because it occurs in such low, stable amounts.

The gap between the two measurements represents the anions not routinely measured, including sulfates, phosphates, proteins, and organic acids, such as lactic acid and ketone acids. Because these anions aren't measured in routine laboratory tests, the anion gap is a way of determining their presence.

Calculating the anion gap

This illustration depicts the normal anion gap. The gap is calculated by adding the chloride level and the bicarbonate level and then subtracting that total from the sodium level. The value normally ranges from 8 to 14 mEq/L and represents the level of unmeasured anions in extracellular fluid.

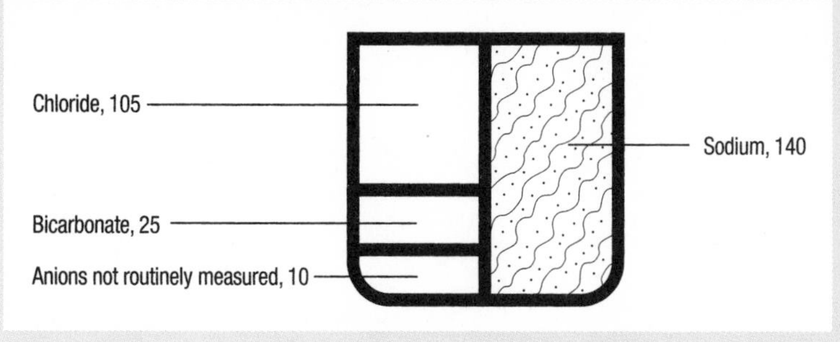

Calculating anion gap

- Add chloride level and bicarbonate level
- Subtract that total from sodium level
- Normal range: 8 to 14 mEq/L

Interpreting the anion gap

An increase in the anion gap that's greater than 14 mEq/L indicates an increase in the percentage of one or more unmeasured anions in the bloodstream. Increases can occur with acidotic conditions characterized by higher-than-normal amounts of organic acids, such as lactic acidosis and ketoacidosis.

The anion gap remains normal for certain other conditions, including hyperchloremic acidosis, renal tubular acidosis, and severe bicarbonate wasting conditions, such as biliary or pancreatic fistulas and poorly functioning ileal loops.

Interpreting anion gap

- Increase greater than 14 mEq/L can occur with lactic acidosis and ketoacidosis
- Normal for such conditions as hyperchloremic acidosis, renal tubular acidosis, and severe bicarbonate wasting conditions

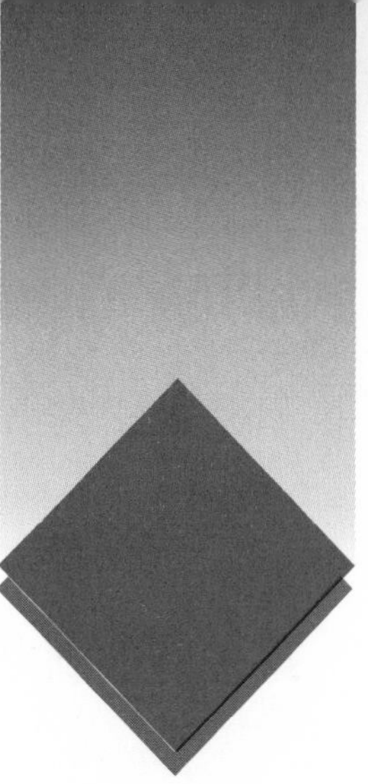

Part two

Imbalances

Fluid imbalances

Fluid volume

- Affects amount of blood heart pumps and extent of vasoconstriction present
- Assessed by blood pressure, PAP, and CVP

FLUID VOLUME

Blood pressure is related to the amount of blood the heart pumps and the extent of vasoconstriction present. Fluid volume affects these elements, making blood pressure measurement key in assessing a patient's fluid status. Certain types of pressure, such as pulmonary artery pressure (PAP) and central venous pressure (CVP), also help assess a patient's fluid volume status.

To maintain the accuracy of the blood pressure measurement system you use, periodically compare the readings of automated and direct measurement systems with manual readings.

Blood pressure cuff measurements

- Simple measurement with stethoscope still one of best methods for assessing fluid volume
- Make sure cuff is correct size
- Position patient's arm with brachial artery at heart level
- Wrap blood pressure cuff snugly around upper arm, above antecubital fossa

BLOOD PRESSURE CUFF MEASUREMENTS

A simple blood pressure measurement, taken with a stethoscope and a sphygmomanometer, is still one of the best tools for assessing a patient's fluid volume. It's quick and easy and carries little risk for the patient. Direct and indirect blood pressure measurements are generally related to the amount of blood flowing through the patient's circulatory system.

To measure blood pressure accurately, begin by making sure the cuff is the correct size. The bladder of the cuff should have a width of about 40% of the upper arm circumference. Position the patient's arm so that the brachial artery is at heart level. To position the blood pressure cuff

Positioning a blood pressure cuff

This illustration shows how to properly position a blood pressure cuff and stethoscope bell.

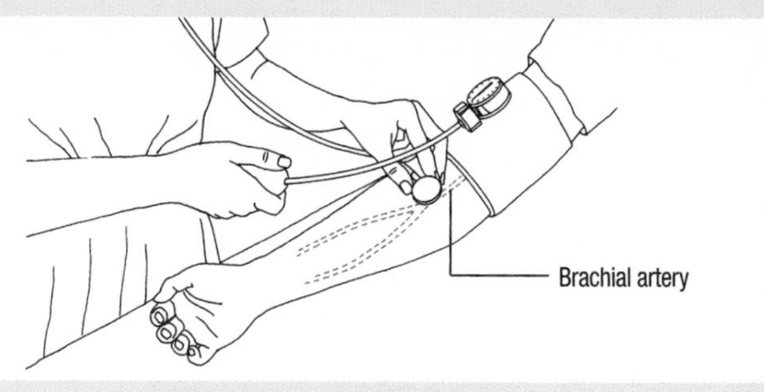

properly, wrap it snugly around the upper arm, above the antecubital fossa. For adults, place the lower border of the cuff about 1″ (2.5 cm) above the antecubital fossa. For children, place the lower border closer to the antecubital fossa.

Place the center of the cuff's bladder directly over the medial aspect of the arm, over the brachial artery. Most cuffs have a reference mark to help you position the bladder. After positioning the cuff, palpate the brachial artery, and place the bell of the stethoscope directly over the point where you can feel the strongest pulsations. (See *Positioning a blood pressure cuff.*)

If you have difficulty hearing the patient's blood pressure, which is common when a patient is hypotensive, palpate the blood pressure to estimate systolic pressure. To palpate blood pressure, place a cuff on the upper arm and palpate the brachial pulse or the radial pulse. Inflate the cuff until you no longer feel the pulse. Then slowly deflate the cuff, noting the point at which you feel the pulse again — the systolic pressure. If you palpate a patient's blood pressure at 90 mm Hg, for example, chart it as "90/P" (the P stands for palpable).

Automated blood pressure unit

You may also have access to an automated blood pressure unit. This unit is designed to take blood pressure measurements repeatedly, which is helpful when you're caring for a patient whose blood pressure is expected

Blood pressure cuff measurements *(continued)*

- Place center of cuff's bladder directly over arm's medial aspect, over brachial artery
- Palpate brachial artery
- Place stethoscope bell directly over strongest pulsations

Palpation

- Place cuff on upper arm
- Palpate brachial or radial pulse
- Inflate cuff until you detect no pulse
- Slowly deflate cuff, noting point you feel pulse again (systolic pressure)

Automated blood pressure unit

- Designed to take repeated blood pressure measurements
- Automatically detects and records blood pressure readings
- Cuff automatically inflates to check blood pressure and deflates immediately afterward

Doppler blood pressure

- ✦ For patient with undetectable blood pressure (swollen arm or low blood pressure)
- ✦ Place blood pressure cuff on arm as normal
- ✦ Apply lubricant to antetcubital area where brachial pulse expected
- ✦ Turn unit on and place probe lightly on arm over brachial artery
- ✦ Adjust volume control and placement of probe until pulse heard clearly
- ✦ Inflate blood pressure cuff until pulse sound disappears
- ✦ Slowly deflate cuff and note point when sound returns (systolic pressure)

Taking a Doppler blood pressure

When you can't hear or feel a patient's blood pressure, try using a Doppler ultrasound device, as shown here.

The Doppler probe uses ultrasound waves directed at the blood vessel to detect blood flow. Through the Doppler unit, you'll be able to hear the patient's blood flow with each pulse. To obtain a Doppler blood pressure:

- ✦ Place a blood pressure cuff on the arm as you normally would.
- ✦ Apply lubricant to the antecubital area where you would expect to find the brachial pulse.
- ✦ Turn the unit on and place the probe lightly on the arm over the brachial artery.
- ✦ Adjust the volume control and the placement of the probe until you hear the pulse clearly.

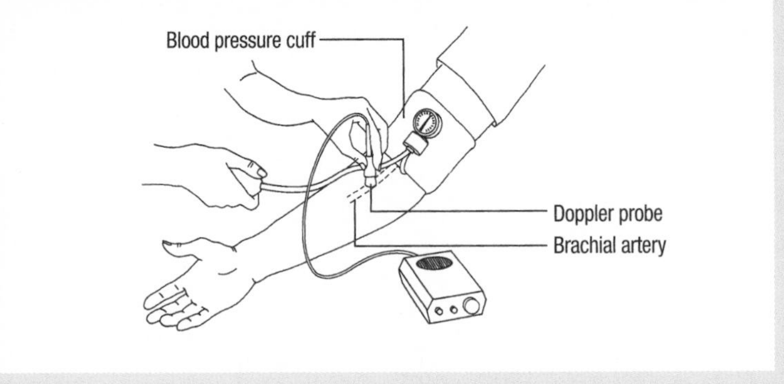

to change frequently (for example, a patient with a fluid imbalance). The unit automatically computes and digitally records blood pressure readings.

The blood pressure cuff automatically inflates to check the blood pressure and deflates immediately afterward. You can program the monitor to inflate the cuff as often as needed and set alarms for high, low, and mean blood pressures. Most monitors display each blood pressure reading until the next reading is taken.

Doppler device

If your patient's arm is swollen or his blood pressure is so low that you can't feel his pulse, you should first palpate his carotid artery to make sure he has a pulse. Then use a Doppler device to obtain a reading of his systolic pressure. (See *Taking a Doppler blood pressure.*)

Inflate the blood pressure cuff until the pulse sound disappears. Slowly deflate the cuff and note the point at which the pulse sound returns — the systolic pressure. If you hear the pulse at 80 mm Hg, for instance, record it as "80/D" (the D stands for Doppler). (See *Correcting blood pressure measurement problems,* page 46.)

Direct measurement

Direct measurement is an invasive method of obtaining blood pressure readings using arterial catheters. It's used when highly accurate or frequent blood pressure measurements are required, as with severe fluid imbalances.

Arterial lines

Arterial lines, or A-lines, are inserted into the radial or the brachial artery (or the femoral artery if needed). They continuously monitor blood pressure and can also be used to sample arterial blood for blood gas analysis or other laboratory tests. Because A-lines require a certain level of technology and staff training, patients who have them are usually placed in intermediate or intensive care units.

The catheter is connected to a continuous flush system — a bag of normal saline solution (which may contain heparin) inside a pressurized cuff or on an infusion pump. This system maintains the patency of the A-line. The A-line is connected to a transducer and then to a bedside monitor. The transducer converts fluid-pressure waves from the catheter into an electronic signal that can be analyzed and displayed on the monitor. Because the patient's blood pressure is displayed continuously, you can instantly note changes in the measurements and respond quickly.

Pulmonary artery catheters

An A-line directly measures blood pressure, whereas a pulmonary artery (PA) catheter directly measures other pressures. PA catheters are usually inserted into the subclavian vein or the internal jugular vein, although the catheters are sometimes inserted into a vein in the arm (brachial or axillary vein) or the leg (femoral vein).

The tip of the catheter is advanced through the vein into the right atrium, then into the right ventricle, and finally into the pulmonary artery. The hubs of the catheter are then connected to a pressurized transducer system that's similar to the system used for an A-line. (See *Pulmonary artery catheter ports,* page 47.)

Direct measurements

- Invasive method using arterial catheters
- Used when highly accurate or frequent blood pressure measurements required

Arterial lines

- Inserted into radial or brachial artery (femoral artery if needed)
- Continuously monitor blood pressure
- Sample arterial blood for blood gas analysis or other tests
- Connected to continuous flush system (maintains A-line patency)
- A-line connected to transducer and to bedside monitor
- Transducer converts fluid-pressure waves from catheter into electronic signal for analysis and display on monitor

Pulmonary artery catheters

- Usually inserted into subclavian vein or internal jugular vein
- Sometimes inserted into arm vein (brachial or axillary vein) or leg vein (femoral vein)
- Allow for measurement of PAP, PAWP, cardiac output, and CVP

False blood pressure readings: Possible causes

False-high readings

- Cuff too small
- Cuff wrapped too loosely
- Slow cuff deflation
- Tilted mercury column
- Poorly timed measurement
- Multiple attempts at reading in same arm

False-low readings

- Incorrect position of arm or leg
- Mercury column below eye level
- Failure to notice auscultatory gap
- Inaudible or low-volume sounds

Correcting blood pressure measurement problems

Use this chart to determine how to correct possible causes of a false-high or false-low blood pressure reading.

PROBLEM AND POSSIBLE CAUSE	INTERVENTIONS
False-high reading	
Cuff too small	Make sure the cuff bladder is long enough to completely encircle the extremity.
Cuff wrapped too loosely, reducing its effective width	Tighten the cuff.
Slow cuff deflation causing venous congestion in the arm or leg	Never deflate the cuff slower than 2 mm Hg/heartbeat.
Tilted mercury column	Read pressures with the mercury column vertical.
Poorly timed measurement (after the patient has eaten, ambulated, appeared anxious, or flexed his arm muscles)	Postpone blood pressure measurement, or help the patient relax before taking pressures.
Multiple attempts at reading blood pressure in the same arm, causing venous congestion	Don't attempt to measure blood pressure more than twice in the same arm; wait several minutes between attempts.
False-low reading	
Incorrect position of the arm or leg	Make sure the arm or leg is level with the patient's heart.
Mercury column below eye level	Read mercury column at eye level.
Failure to notice auscultatory gap (sound fades out for 10 to 15 mm Hg, then returns)	Estimate systolic pressure using palpation before actually measuring it. Then check the palpable pressure against the measured pressure.
Inaudible or low-volume sounds	Before reinflating the cuff, instruct the patient to raise his arm or leg to decrease venous pressure and amplify low-volume sounds. After inflating the cuff, tell the patient to lower his arm or leg. Then deflate the cuff and listen. If you still fail to detect low-volume sounds, chart the palpable systolic pressure.

Pulmonary artery catheter ports

The ports on a pulmonary artery catheter (shown here) can be used for pacing, infusing solutions, or monitoring oxygen saturation, body temperature, cardiac output, or various intraluminal pressures, such as central venous pressure (through the proximal lumen) or pulmonary artery wedge pressure (through the distal lumen).

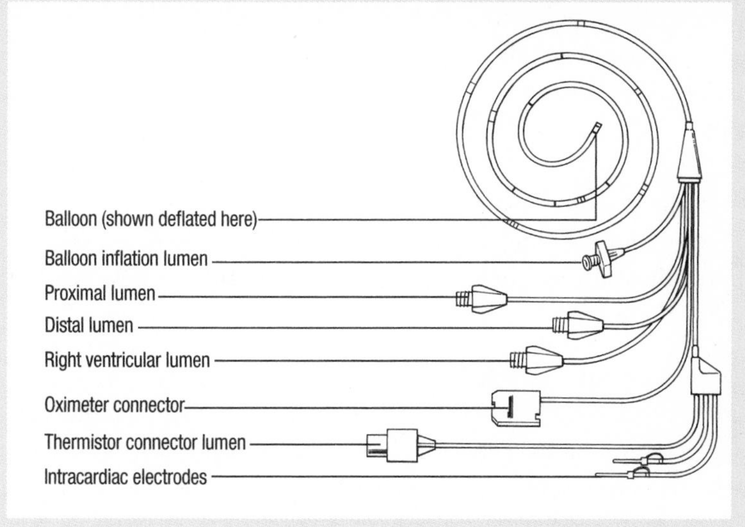

A PA catheter provides a clearer picture of the patient's fluid volume status than other measurement techniques. The catheter allows for measurement of PAP, pulmonary artery wedge pressure (PAWP), cardiac output, and CVP — all of which provide information about how the left side of the heart is functioning, including its pumping ability, filling pressures, and vascular volume.

PAP is the pressure routinely displayed on the monitor. A normal systolic PAP is 15 to 25 mm Hg and reflects pressure from contraction of the right atrium. A normal diastolic PAP is 8 to 15 mm Hg and reflects the lowest pressure in the pulmonary vessels. The mean PAP is 10 to 20 mm Hg.

When you inflate the small balloon at the catheter tip, blood carries the catheter tip farther into the pulmonary artery. The tip floats inside the artery until it stops — or becomes wedged — in a smaller branch. When the tip is wedged in a branch of the pulmonary artery, the catheter measures pressures coming from the left side of the heart, a measurement

Pulmonary artery catheters *(continued)*

PAP
- Normal systolic: 15 to 25 mm Hg (reflects pressure from contraction of right atrium)
- Normal diastolic: 8 to 15 mm Hg (reflects lowest pressure in pulmonary vessels)
- Mean: 10 to 20 mm Hg

PAWP
- Measures pressure from left side of heart when catheter tip is wedged in pulmonary artery branch
- Normal: 6 to 12 mm Hg

Cardiac output
- Amount of blood heart pumps in 1 minute
- Normal: 4 to 8 L/minute

Pulmonary artery catheters *(continued)*

Cardiac output
- Low if person lacks adequate blood volume; high if person overloaded with fluid
- Calculated by multiplying heart rate by stroke volume (monitor calculates)
- Stroke volume — amount of blood left ventricle pumps with each beat

that may prove useful in gauging changes in blood volume. A normal PAWP is 6 to 12 mm Hg.

PAP and PAWP are generally increased in cases of fluid overload and decreased in cases of fluid-volume deficit. That's why a PA catheter is useful when assessing and treating an acutely ill patient with a fluid imbalance.

PA catheters also measure cardiac output, either continuously or after injections of I.V. fluid through the proximal lumen. Cardiac output is the amount of blood that the heart pumps in 1 minute and is calculated by multiplying the heart rate by the stroke volume, which the monitor calculates.

The stroke volume is the amount of blood the left ventricle pumps out with each beat, and it's also calculated by the bedside monitor. Normal cardiac output is 4 to 8 L/minute. If a person lacks adequate blood volume, cardiac output is low (assuming the heart can pump normally otherwise). If the person is overloaded with fluid, cardiac output is high.

Central venous catheter
- Measures pressure of blood inside central venous circulation (CVP)
- Tip typically placed in jugular vein in neck or subclavian vein in chest
- Normal CVP: 0 to 7 mm Hg (5 to 10 cm H_2O)
- High if person is overloaded with fluid
- Low if person is low on fluid

Central venous catheter

A central venous catheter can measure CVP, another useful indication of a patient's fluid status. The term CVP refers to the pressure of the blood inside the central venous circulation. The tip of a CVP catheter is typically placed in one of the jugular veins in the neck or in a subclavian vein in the chest.

Normal CVP ranges from 0 to 7 mm Hg (5 to 10 cm H_2O). If CVP is high, it usually means the patient is overloaded with fluid. If it's low, it usually means the patient is low on fluid. (To calculate CVP, see *Estimating CVP.*)

Maintaining fluid balance
- If body can't compensate for fluid deficits or excesses, several problems may develop: dehydration, hypovolemia, hypervolemia, and water intoxication

MAINTAINING FLUID BALANCE

Most of the time, the body adequately compensates for minor fluid imbalances and keeps blood pressure readings and other measurements fairly normal. Sometimes, however, the body can't compensate for fluid deficits or excesses. When that happens, any of several problems may result, including dehydration, hypovolemia, hypervolemia, and water intoxication.

Dehydration
- Occurs when fluid isn't adequately replaced and body's cells lose water

DEHYDRATION

The body loses water all the time. A person responds to the thirst reflex by drinking fluids and eating foods that contain water. However, if water

Estimating CVP

To estimate a patient's central venous pressure (CVP), use the illustration below as a guide and take the following steps:

1. Place the patient at a 45- to 60-degree angle.
2. Use tangential lighting to observe the internal jugular vein.
3. Note the highest level of visible pulsation.
4. Locate the angle of Louis, or sternal notch, by palpating the point at which the clavicles join the sternum (the suprasternal notch).
5. Place two fingers on the patient's suprasternal notch and slide them down the sternum until they reach a bony protuberance—the angle of Louis. The right atrium lies about 2″ (5 cm) below this point.
6. Measure the distance between the angle of Louis and the highest level of visible pulsation. Normally, this distance is less than 1.2″ (3 cm).
7. Add 2″ to this figure to estimate the distance between the highest level of pulsation and the right atrium. A distance greater than 4″ (10 cm) may indicate elevated CVP.

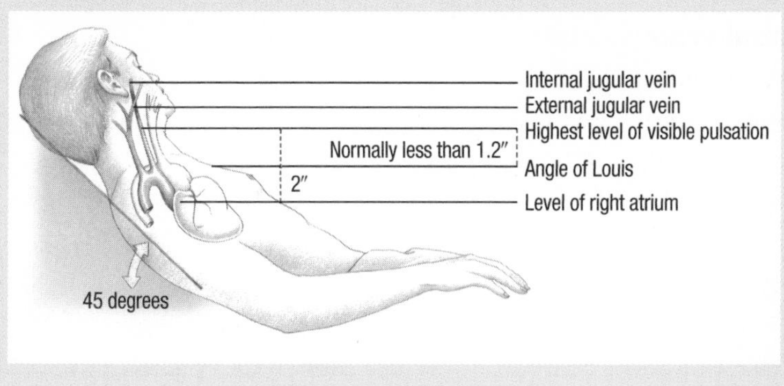

isn't adequately replaced, the body's cells can lose water, a condition called *dehydration.*

Causes and Pathophysiology

Loss of body fluids causes an increase in blood solute concentration (increased osmolality), and serum sodium levels rise. In an attempt to regain fluid balance between intracellular and extracellular spaces, water molecules shift out of cells into more concentrated blood. This process, combined with increased water intake and increased water retention in the kidneys, usually restores the body's fluid volume. (For more informa-

Pathophysiology

- Without adequate supply of water in extracellular space, fluid shifts out of cells into extracellular space

Pathophysiology *(continued)*

- As cells lose more fluid, they shrink and lose functionality
- Failure to respond to thirst stimulus increases risk
- Can result from syndromes that accelerate fluid loss

tion on dehydration, see the color pages on passive and active transport, between pages 54 and 55.)

Without an adequate supply of water in the extracellular space, fluid continues to shift out of the cells into the extracellular space. The cells begin to shrink as the process continues. Because water is essential for obtaining nutrients, expelling wastes, and maintaining cell shape, cells can't function properly without adequate fluid.

Causes

- Diabetes insipidus
- Prolonged fever
- Watery diarrhea
- Renal failure
- Hyperglycemia

Failure to respond adequately to the thirst stimulus increases the risk of dehydration. A patient who's confused, comatose, or bedridden is particularly vulnerable. A patient may also become dehydrated if he's receiving highly concentrated tube feedings without enough supplemental water.

AGE ALERT *Infants, who can't drink fluid on their own or express feelings of thirst and who have immature kidneys that can't concentrate urine efficiently, are at risk for dehydration. Older patients are also prone to dehydration because they have a lower body-water content, diminished kidney function, and a reduced ability to sense thirst, so they can't correct fluid-volume deficits as easily as younger adults.*

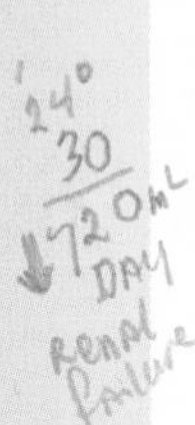

Any situation that accelerates fluid loss can lead to dehydration. For instance, in diabetes insipidus, the brain fails to secrete antidiuretic hormone (ADH). If the brain doesn't secrete enough ADH, the result is greater-than-normal diuresis. A patient with diabetes insipidus produces large amounts of highly dilute urine — as much as 30 L/day. The patient is also thirsty and tends to drink large amounts of fluids, although he generally can't keep up with the diuresis.

Other causes of dehydration include prolonged fever, watery diarrhea, renal failure, and hyperglycemia (which causes the person to produce large amounts of dilute urine).

Assessment findings

- Concentrated urine
- Decreased urine output
- Dry mucous membranes
- Extreme thirst
- Increased heart rate
- Low blood pressure
- Poor skin turgor
- Mental status changes

ASSESSMENT FINDINGS

As dehydration progresses, watch for changes in the patient's mental status. The patient may complain of dizziness, weakness, or extreme thirst. He may have a fever (because less fluid is available for perspiration, which lowers body temperature), dry skin, or dry mucous membranes. Skin turgor may be poor.

AGE ALERT *Because an older patient's skin may lack elasticity, checking skin turgor may be an unreliable indicator of dehydration.*

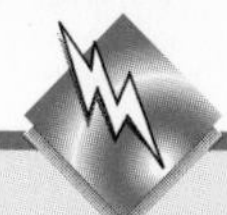

DANGER

Warning signs of dehydration

Begin emergency treatment for dehydration if your patient develops any of these conditions:

- ✦ impaired mental status
- ✦ seizure
- ✦ coma.

The patient's heart rate may increase, and his blood pressure may drop. In severe cases, seizures and coma may result. Also, urine output may fall because less fluid is circulating in the body. The patient's urine will be more concentrated unless he has diabetes insipidus, in which case the urine will probably be pale and produced in large volume. (See *Warning signs of dehydration.*)

Diagnostic test results

Typical laboratory findings for a patient who's dehydrated include:

- ✦ elevated hematocrit
- ✦ elevated serum osmolality (greater than 300 mOsm/kg)
- ✦ elevated serum sodium level (greater than 145 mEq/L)
- ✦ urine specific gravity greater than 1.030.

Because a patient with diabetes insipidus has more dilute urine, specific gravity is usually less than 1.005; osmolality, 50 to 200 mOsm/kg.

Diagnostic test results

- ✦ Elevated hematocrit
- ✦ Elevated serum sodium level
- ✦ Urine specific gravity > 1.030

Treatment

Treatment for dehydration aims to replace missing fluids. Because a dehydrated patient's blood is concentrated, avoid hypertonic solutions. If the patient can tolerate oral fluids, encourage them; however, because the serum sodium level is elevated, make sure the fluids given are salt-free.

A severely dehydrated patient should receive I.V. fluids to replace lost fluids. Most patients receive hypotonic, low-sodium fluids such as dextrose 5% in water.

DANGER *Remember, if you give a hypotonic solution too quickly, fluid moves from the veins into the cells, causing them to become edematous. Swelling of cells in the brain can create cerebral edema. To avoid such potentially devastating problems, give fluids gradually, over a period of about 48 hours.*

Treatment

- ✦ Replace missing fluids
- ✦ Avoid hypertonic solutions
- ✦ Encourage salt-free oral fluids
- ✦ Give I.V. fluids (for severely dehydrated patients)

Key nursing interventions

- ✦ Monitor symptoms and vital signs closely
- ✦ Accurately record intake and output
- ✦ Maintain I.V. access
- ✦ Watch for signs and symptoms of cerebral edema if patient is receiving hypotonic solutions
- ✦ Monitor serum sodium levels, urine osmolality, and urine specific gravity
- ✦ Obtain daily weight
- ✦ Provide skin and mouth care

Nursing interventions

Monitor at-risk patients closely to detect impending dehydration. If a patient becomes dehydrated, here are some steps you'll want to take:

✦ Monitor symptoms and vital signs closely so you can intervene quickly.

✦ Accurately record the patient's intake and output, including urine and stools.

✦ Maintain I.V. access as ordered. Monitor I.V. infusions. Watch for signs and symptoms of cerebral edema when your patient is receiving hypotonic solutions. Signs and symptoms include headache, confusion, irritability, lethargy, nausea, vomiting, widening pulse pressure, decreased pulse rate, and seizures.

✦ Keep in mind that vasopressin may be ordered for a patient with diabetes insipidus.

✦ Monitor serum sodium levels, urine osmolality, and urine specific gravity to assess fluid balance.

✦ Insert a urinary catheter, as ordered, to accurately monitor output.

✦ Provide a safe environment for any patient who's confused, dizzy, or at risk for a seizure, and teach his family to do the same.

✦ Obtain daily weight (same scale, same time of day) to evaluate treatment progress. (See *Documenting dehydration*.)

✦ Provide skin and mouth care to maintain the integrity of the skin surface and oral mucous membranes.

✦ Assess the patient for diaphoresis — it can be the source of major water loss.

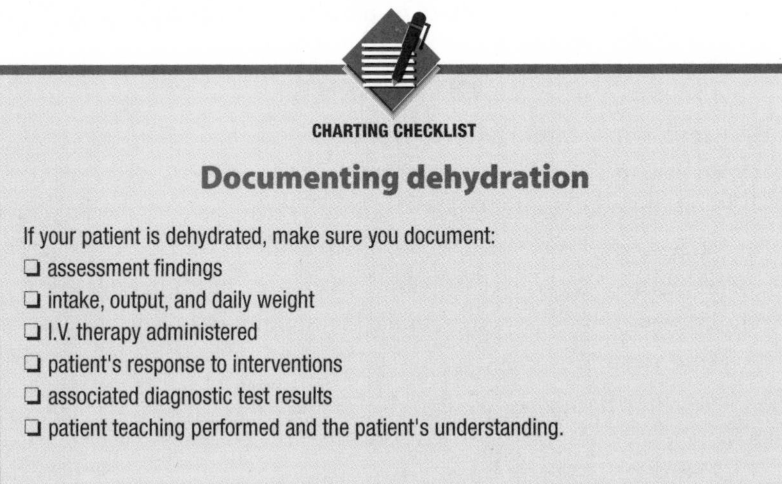

CHARTING CHECKLIST

Documenting dehydration

If your patient is dehydrated, make sure you document:

- ❑ assessment findings
- ❑ intake, output, and daily weight
- ❑ I.V. therapy administered
- ❑ patient's response to interventions
- ❑ associated diagnostic test results
- ❑ patient teaching performed and the patient's understanding.

Patient teaching

Be sure to cover these topics and then evaluate your patient's learning:
- ✦ explanation of dehydration and its treatment
- ✦ warning signs and symptoms
- ✦ prescribed medications
- ✦ importance of complying with therapy.

Patient teaching
- ✦ Description of disorder
- ✦ Warning signs and symptoms
- ✦ Medications
- ✦ Compliance

HYPOVOLEMIA

Hypovolemia refers to isotonic fluid loss, which includes loss of fluids and solutes, from the extracellular space. Children and older patients are especially vulnerable to hypovolemia. Some of the initial signs and symptoms of hypovolemia can be subtle as the body tries to compensate for the loss of circulating blood volume. Subtle signs can become more serious and, if not detected early and treated properly, can progress to hypovolemic shock, a common form of shock.

Hypovolemia
- ✦ Isotonic fluid loss (including loss of fluids and solutes) from extracellular space
- ✦ Children and older patients especially vulnerable
- ✦ Can progress to hypovolemic shock if not detected early and treated properly

Causes and pathophysiology

Excessive fluid loss, such as from bleeding, is a risk factor for hypovolemia, especially when combined with reduced fluid intake. Another risk factor is a third-space fluid shift, which occurs when fluid moves out of intravascular spaces but not into intracellular spaces. For instance, fluid may shift into the abdominal cavity (ascites), the pleural cavity, or the pericardial sac. These third-space fluid shifts may occur as a result of increased permeability of the capillary membrane or decreased plasma colloid osmotic pressure.

Fluid loss from the extracellular compartment can result from several causes, including:
- ✦ abdominal surgery
- ✦ diabetes mellitus (with increased urination)
- ✦ excessive diuretic therapy
- ✦ excessive laxative use
- ✦ excessive sweating
- ✦ fever
- ✦ fistulas
- ✦ hemorrhage (bleeding may be frank [obvious] or occult [hidden])
- ✦ nasogastric drainage
- ✦ renal failure with increased urination
- ✦ vomiting and diarrhea.

Causes
- ✦ Risk factors include excessive fluid loss (such as from bleeding) combined with reduced fluid intake, and third-space fluid shift

Fluid loss
- ✦ Diabetes mellitus (with increased urination)
- ✦ Excessive diuretic therapy
- ✦ Excessive sweating
- ✦ Hemorrhage
- ✦ Vomiting and diarrhea

Causes *(continued)*

Third-space fluid shift
- Burns
- Heart failure
- Liver failure

Assessment findings
- Vary depending if amount of blood loss is mild (10% to 15% of total circulating blood volume), moderate (about 25%), or severe (40% or more)
- Severe intravascular blood loss may progress to hypovolemic shock

Mild volume loss
- Cool, pale skin
- Delayed capillary refill time
- Increased heart rate
- Urine output > 30 ml/hour
- Weight loss (5% to 10 % of total body weight)

Moderate volume loss
- Cool, clammy skin
- Decreased blood pressure
- Decreased urine output (10 to 30 ml/hour)
- Extreme thirst
- Rapid, thready pulse
- Weight loss (5% to 10% of total body weight)

Severe volume loss
- Decreased cardiac output
- Decreased urine output (< 10 ml/hour)
- Deteriorated mental status (possibly unconsciousness)
- Marked tachycardia and hypertension
- Weak or absent peripheral pulses
- Weight loss (> 10% total body weight)

Third-space fluid shifts can result from various of conditions, including:
- acute intestinal obstruction
- acute peritonitis
- burns (during the initial phase)
- crush injuries
- heart failure
- hip fracture
- hypoalbuminemia
- liver failure
- pleural effusion.

Assessment findings

If volume loss is minimal (10% to 15% of an average of about 5 L of total circulating blood volume), the body tries to compensate for its lack of circulating volume by increasing its heart rate. You may also note orthostatic hypotension, restlessness, or anxiety. The patient will probably still produce more than 30 ml of urine per hour, but he may have delayed capillary refill and cool, pale skin over the arms and legs. (See *Warning signs of hypovolemia.*)

A patient with hypovolemia may also lose weight. Acute weight loss can indicate rapid fluid changes. A drop in weight of 5% to 10% can indicate mild to moderate loss; more than 10%, severe loss. As hypovolemia progresses, the patient's symptoms worsen. Central venous pressure (CVP) and pulmonary artery wedge pressure (PAWP) may fall as well. Monitor your patient for subtle signs, including orthostatic hypotension.

With moderate intravascular volume loss (about 25%), the patient may become more confused and irritable and complain of extreme thirst. The pulse usually becomes rapid and thready, and the blood pressure drops. The patient's skin may feel cool and clammy, and urine output may drop to 10 to 30 ml/hour.

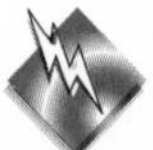

DANGER *Severe hypovolemia (40% or more of intravascular volume loss) may lead to hypovolemic shock. In a patient with this condition, cardiac output drops and mental status can deteriorate to unconsciousness. Signs and symptoms may progress to marked tachycardia and hypotension, with weak or absent peripheral pulses. The skin may become cool and mottled, or even cyanotic. Urine output drops to less than 10 ml/hour.*

Diagnostic test results

No single diagnostic finding can confirm hypovolemia. Laboratory test values can vary, depending on the underlying cause and other factors.

How electrolyte imbalances affect ECGs

Electrical impulses move through the heart's conduction system to create rhythmic contractions. Normal electrical activity in the heart depends on normal serum electrolyte concentrations.

The electrolytes sodium, potassium, and calcium, with the help of magnesium, shift back and forth across myocardial cell membranes. This shifting of electrolytes causes alternating periods of activity (depolarization) and rest (repolarization), which allow for normal myocardial function. Electrolyte imbalances cause trademark changes in electrocardiogram (ECG) readings and myocardial function. This special section details changes in two critical electrolytes: magnesium and potassium.

HYPERMAGNESEMIA

Hypermagnesemia (a serum magnesium level > 2.5 mEq/L) can be caused by excessive magnesium administration or renal failure. The condition can cause a prolonged PR interval and the ECG changes shown here. If left untreated, hypermagnesemia can lead to sinoatrial or atrioventricular (AV) heart block and, eventually, cardiac arrest.

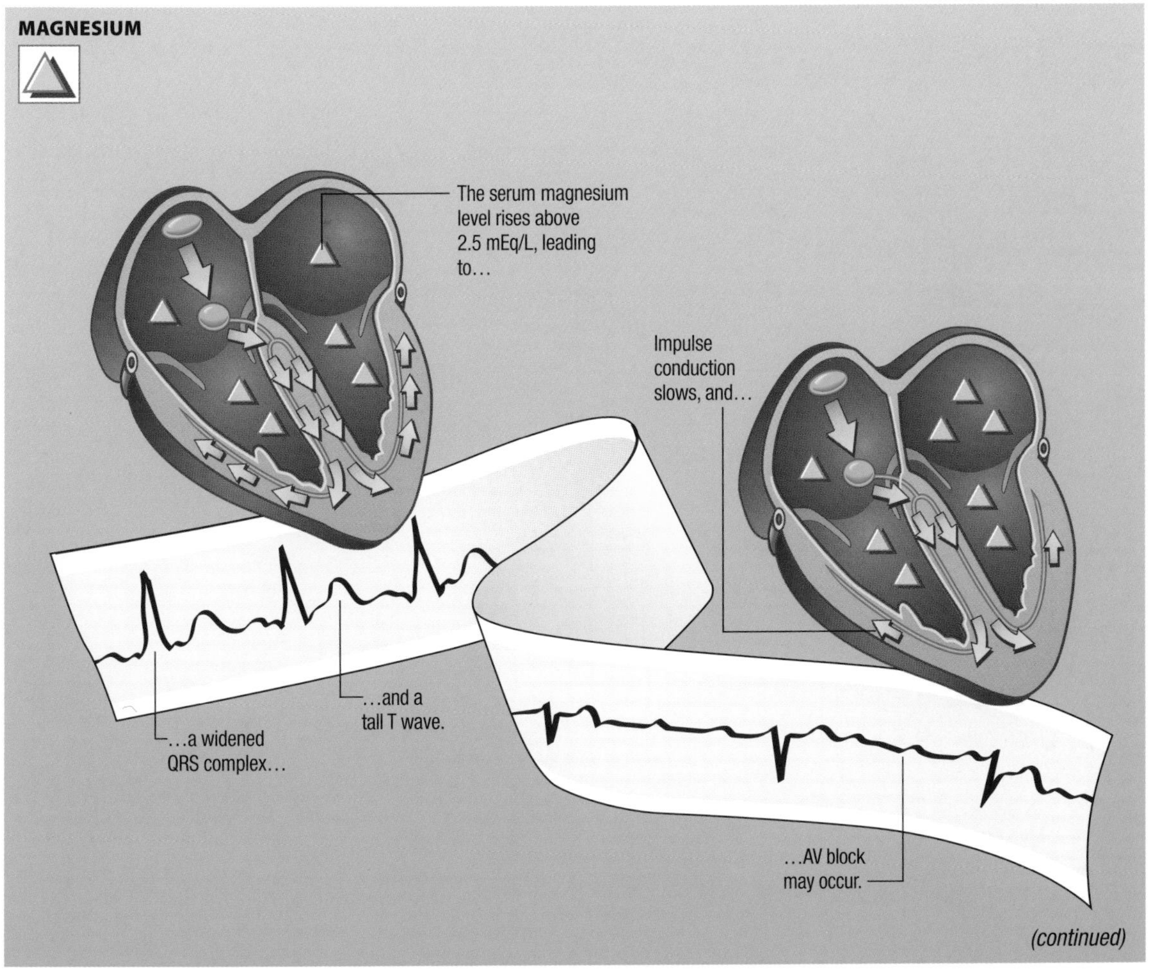
MAGNESIUM
The serum magnesium level rises above 2.5 mEq/L, leading to…
…a widened QRS complex…
…and a tall T wave.
Impulse conduction slows, and…
…AV block may occur.

(continued)

HYPERKALEMIA

Hyperkalemia (a serum potassium level > 5.5 mEq/L) can be caused by renal failure or excessive potassium administration. Excess potassium alters the heart's electrical activity and leads to depressed conduction. Among the earliest signs of hyperkalemia is a tall, tented T wave, as shown here. AV or ventricular block may develop. Other possible ECG abnormalities include a flattened P wave, a prolonged PR interval, a widened QRS complex as ventricular conduction slows, and a depressed ST segment.

If left untreated, severe hyperkalemia (serum potassium > 9 mEq/L) occurs, causing the P wave to disappear, the QRS complex to widen, and sine waves to form. Hyperkalemia may end in lethal arrhythmias.

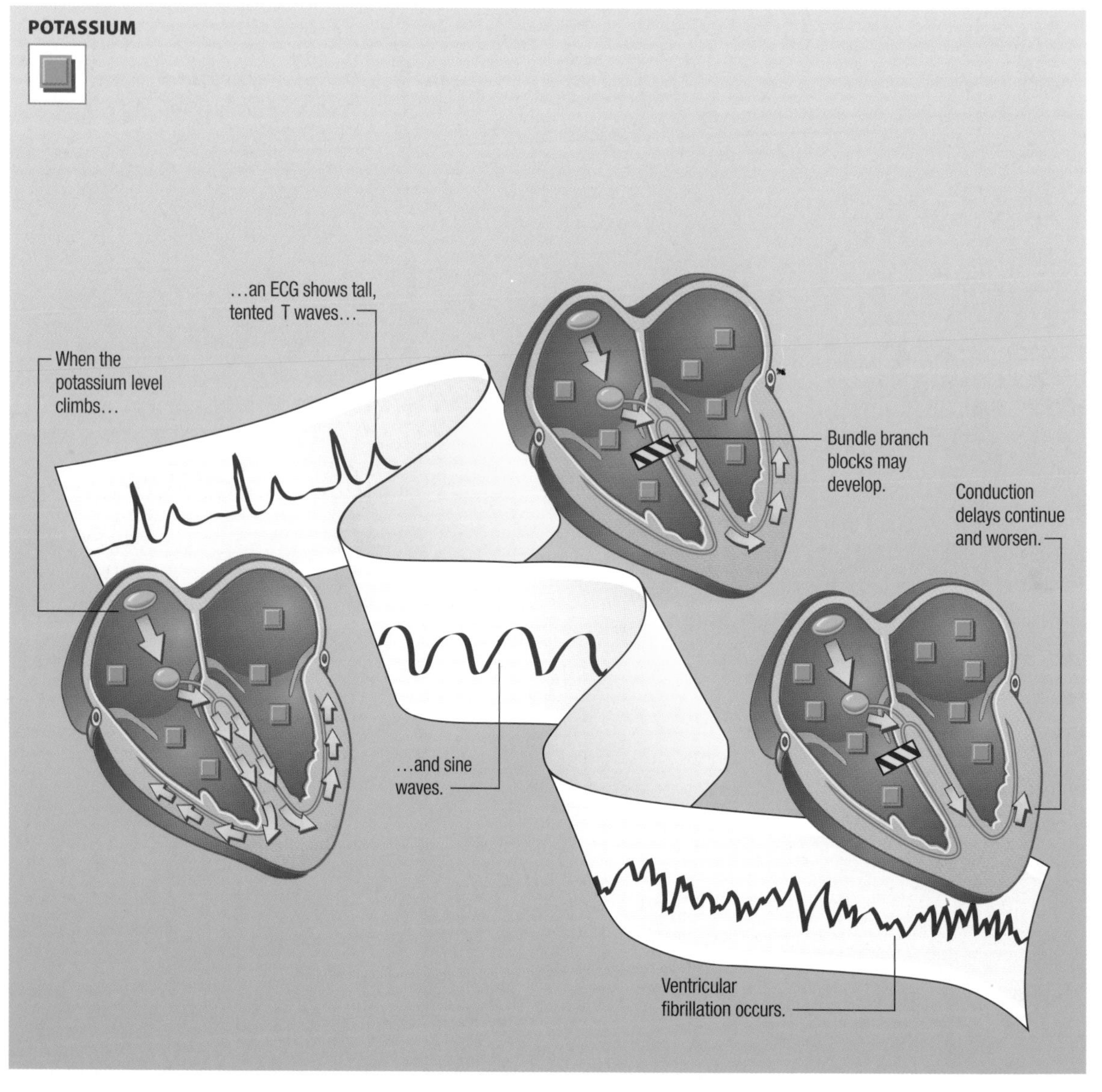
POTASSIUM
When the potassium level climbs…
…an ECG shows tall, tented T waves…
Bundle branch blocks may develop.
Conduction delays continue and worsen.
…and sine waves.
Ventricular fibrillation occurs.

HYPOKALEMIA

Hypokalemia (a serum potassium level < 3.5 mEq/L) can be caused by diuresis or loss of other body fluids. An abnormally low potassium level affects the heart's electrical activity, as shown here. Ventricular repolarization is prolonged. ECG changes include a prominent U wave—a hallmark of hypokalemia.

As the potassium level decreases, ectopic impulses form and conduction disturbances increase. Atrial and ventricular arrhythmias may develop. As ectopy becomes more frequent, the patient is at risk for potentially fatal arrhythmias. Examples of hypokalemic ECG changes are shown here.

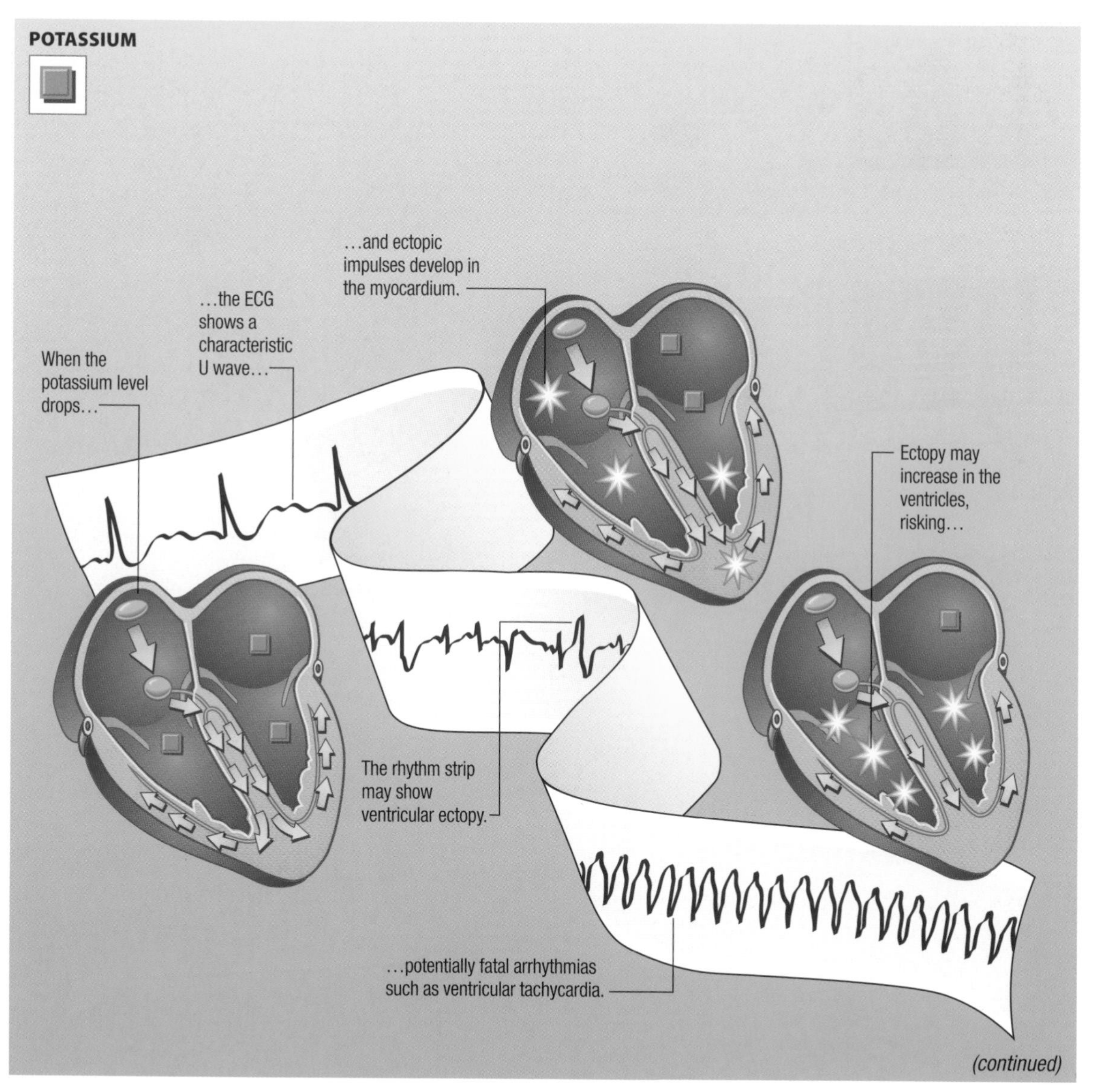
POTASSIUM
When the potassium level drops…
…the ECG shows a characteristic U wave…
…and ectopic impulses develop in the myocardium.
Ectopy may increase in the ventricles, risking…
The rhythm strip may show ventricular ectopy.
…potentially fatal arrhythmias such as ventricular tachycardia.

(continued)

HYPOMAGNESEMIA

Hypomagnesemia (a serum magnesium level < 1.5 mEq/L) can be caused by malnutrition or excessive loss of body fluids. Its effects on the electrical activity of the heart include ECG changes (shown here), such as a slightly widened QRS complex, a prolonged QT interval (which increases myocardial vulnerability to a stimulus), and a depressed ST segment.

Dangerously low magnesium levels make myocardial cells more excitable, which can trigger such life-threatening arrhythmias as ventricular tachycardia, torsades de pointes, and ventricular fibrillation.

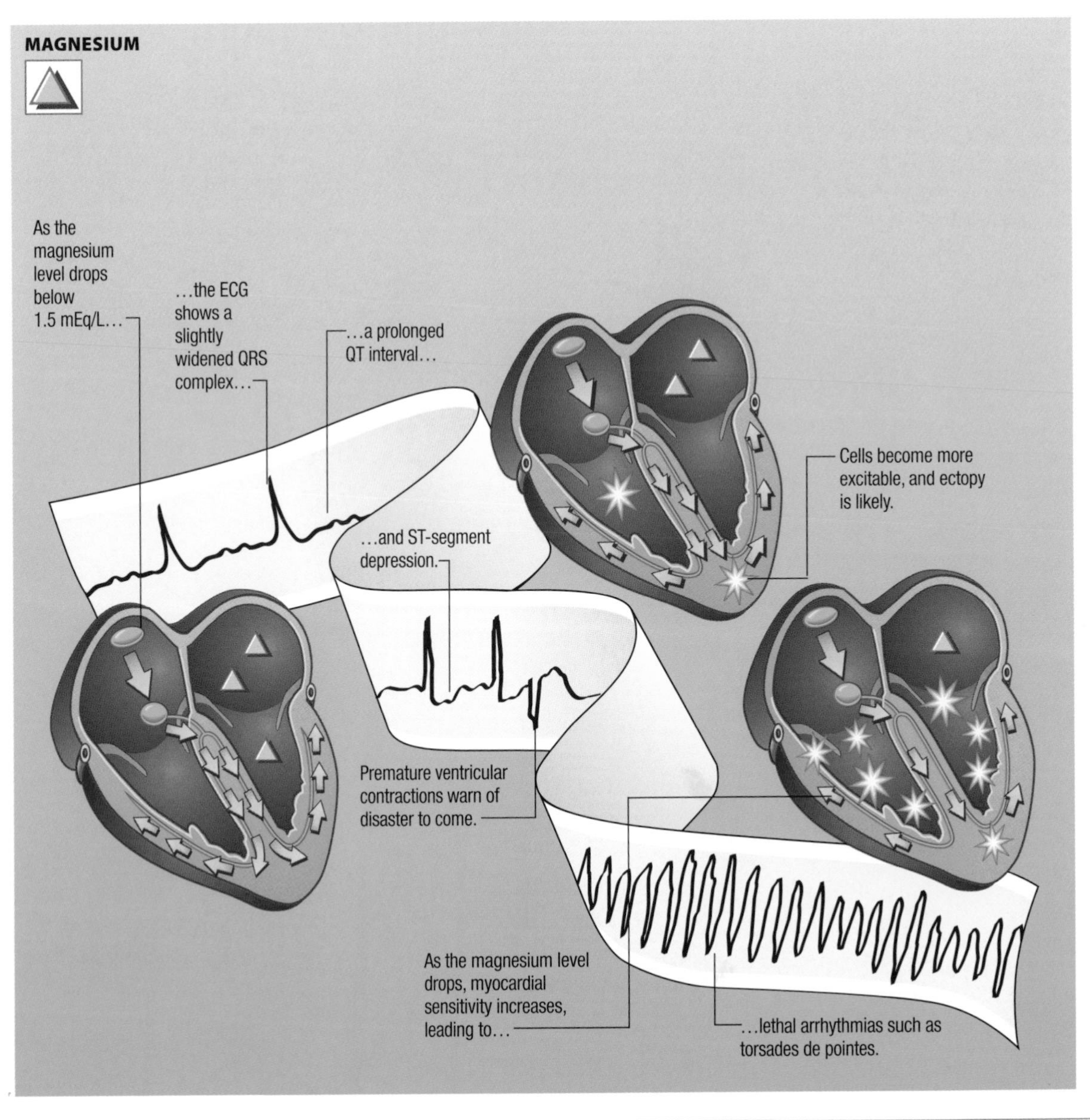

MAGNESIUM
As the magnesium level drops below 1.5 mEq/L…
…the ECG shows a slightly widened QRS complex…
…a prolonged QT interval…
…and ST-segment depression.
Cells become more excitable, and ectopy is likely.
Premature ventricular contractions warn of disaster to come.
As the magnesium level drops, myocardial sensitivity increases, leading to…
…lethal arrhythmias such as torsades de pointes.

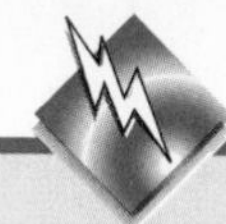

DANGER

Warning signs of hypovolemia

Begin emergency treatment for hypovolemia and impending shock if a patient shows any of these signs and symptoms:

- ✦ cool, pale skin over the arms and legs
- ✦ decreased central venous pressure
- ✦ delayed capillary refill
- ✦ deterioration in mental status (from restlessness and anxiety to unconsciousness)
- ✦ flat jugular veins
- ✦ orthostatic hypotension progressing to marked hypotension
- ✦ tachycardia
- ✦ thirst
- ✦ urine output initially more than 30 ml/minute, then dropping below 10 ml/hour
- ✦ weak or absent peripheral pulses
- ✦ weight loss.

Laboratory values usually suggest an increased concentration of blood. Typical laboratory test findings for a patient with hypovolemia include:

- ✦ normal or high serum sodium level (greater than 145 mEq/L), depending on the amount of fluid and sodium lost
- ✦ decreased hemoglobin levels and hematocrit, with hemorrhage
- ✦ elevated blood urea nitrogen and creatinine ratio
- ✦ increased urine specific gravity, as the kidneys try to conserve fluid
- ✦ increased serum osmolality.

Diagnostic test results

- ✦ Decreased hemoglobin levels and hematocrit, with hemorrhage
- ✦ Elevated blood urea nitrogen and creatinine ratio
- ✦ Increased urine specific gravity

Treatment

Treatment for hypovolemia includes replacing lost fluids with fluids of the same concentration. Such replacement helps normalize blood pressure and restore blood volume. Oral fluids generally aren't enough to adequately treat hypovolemia. Isotonic fluids, such as normal saline solution or lactated Ringer's solution, are given I.V. to expand circulating volume.

Fluids may initially be administered as a fluid challenge, in which the patient receives large amounts of I.V. fluids in a short amount of time. For hypovolemic shock, an emergency condition, multiple fluid chal-

Treatment

- ✦ Replacement of lost fluids with fluids of same concentration
- ✦ Isotonic fluids (normal saline solution or lactated Ringer's solution) to expand circulating volume
- ✦ Fluids possibly initially administered as fluid challenge (for hypovolemia, numerous fluid challenges essential)

Treatment *(continued)*

- I.V. infusions with shortest, largest catheters possible
- Rapid infusions of normal saline solution or lactated Ringer's solution, followed by plasma protein (albumin) infusion
- Blood transfusion and possibly vasopressor (dopamine), if patient hemorrhaging
- Oxygen therapy
- Surgery

Key nursing interventions

- Ensure patent airway
- Apply and adjust oxygen therapy
- Lower head of bed
- If patient is bleeding, apply direct continuous pressure to area and elevate it
- Maintain patent I.V. access
- Administer I.V. fluids, a vasopressor, and blood, as prescribed
- Closely monitor patient's mental status and vital signs

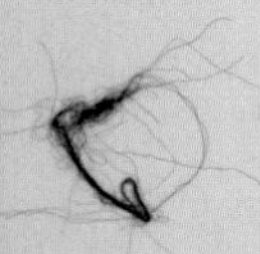

lenges are essential. Numerous I.V. infusions should be started with the shortest, largest-bore catheters possible, because they offer less resistance to fluid flow than long, thin catheters.

Infusions of normal saline solution or lactated Ringer's solution are given rapidly, commonly followed by an infusion of plasma proteins such as albumin. If a patient is hemorrhaging, he'll need a blood transfusion. He may also need a vasopressor, such as dopamine, to support his blood pressure until his fluid levels are back to normal.

Oxygen therapy should be initiated to ensure sufficient tissue perfusion. Surgery may be required to control bleeding.

Nursing interventions

Nursing responsibilities for a patient with hypovolemia include those listed here.

- Make sure the patient has a patent airway.
- Apply and adjust oxygen therapy as ordered.
- Lower the head of the bed to slow a declining blood pressure.
- If the patient is bleeding, apply direct continuous pressure to the area and elevate it, if possible. Assist with other interventions to stop bleeding.

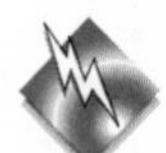

DANGER *If the patient's blood pressure doesn't respond to interventions as expected, recheck for a bleeding site that might have been missed. Remember, a patient can lose a large amount of blood internally from a fractured hip or pelvis. Furthermore, fluids alone may not be enough to correct hypotension associated with a hypovolemic condition. A vasopressor may be needed to raise blood pressure.*

- Maintain patent I.V. access. Use short, large-bore catheters to allow for faster infusion rates. Typically, this patient should have two large-bore I.V. catheters.
- Administer I.V. fluids, a vasopressor, and blood, as prescribed. An autotransfuser, which allows for reinfusion of the patient's own blood, may be required.
- Draw blood for typing and crossmatching, as ordered, to prepare for transfusion.
- Closely monitor the patient's mental status and vital signs, including orthostatic blood pressure measurements, when appropriate. Watch for arrhythmias.
- If available, monitor hemodynamics (cardiac output, CVP, pulmonary artery pressure, and PAWP) using arterial cannulation, to judge how well the patient is responding to treatment. (See *Hemodynamic values in hypovolemic shock.*)

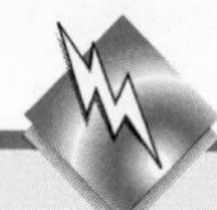

DANGER

Hemodynamic values in hypovolemic shock

Hemodynamic monitoring can help you evaluate your patient's cardiovascular status in hypovolemic shock. Look for these values:

- ✦ central venous pressure below the normal range of 5 to 10 cm H_2O
- ✦ pulmonary artery pressure below the normal mean of 10 to 20 mm Hg
- ✦ pulmonary artery wedge pressure below the normal mean of 6 to 12 mm Hg
- ✦ cardiac output below the normal range of 4 to 8 L/minute.

✦ Monitor the quality of peripheral pulses and skin temperature and appearance to assess for continued peripheral vascular constriction.

✦ Obtain and record results from diagnostic tests, such as a complete blood count, electrolyte levels, arterial blood gas values, a 12-lead electrocardiogram, and chest X-rays.

✦ Offer emotional support to the patient and his family.

✦ Encourage the patient to drink fluids as appropriate.

✦ Insert a urinary catheter, as ordered, and measure urine output hourly if indicated. (See *Documenting hypovolemia,* page 58.)

✦ Auscultate the patient for breath sounds to monitor for signs of fluid overload, a potential complication of I.V. therapy. Excess fluid in the lungs may cause a crackling sound on auscultation.

✦ Monitor the patient for increased oxygen requirements, a sign of fluid overload.

✦ Observe the patient for development of such complications as disseminated intravascular coagulation, myocardial infarction, or acute respiratory distress syndrome.

✦ Weigh the patient daily to monitor the progress of treatment.

✦ Provide effective skin care to prevent skin breakdown.

Key nursing interventions *(continued)*

- ✦ Monitor quality of peripheral pulses and skin temperature and appearance
- ✦ Auscultate for breath sounds
- ✦ Observe for complications (disseminated intravascular coagulation, myocardial infarction, acute respiratory distress syndrome)
- ✦ Weigh patient daily

Patient teaching

Be sure to cover these topics and then evaluate your patient's learning:

✦ nature of the condition and its causes

✦ warning signs and symptoms and when to report them

✦ treatment and the importance of compliance

✦ importance of changing positions slowly, especially when going from a supine position to a standing position, to avoid orthostatic hypotension

Patient teaching

- ✦ Description of disorder
- ✦ Warning signs and symptoms
- ✦ Treatment
- ✦ Self-care
- ✦ Medications

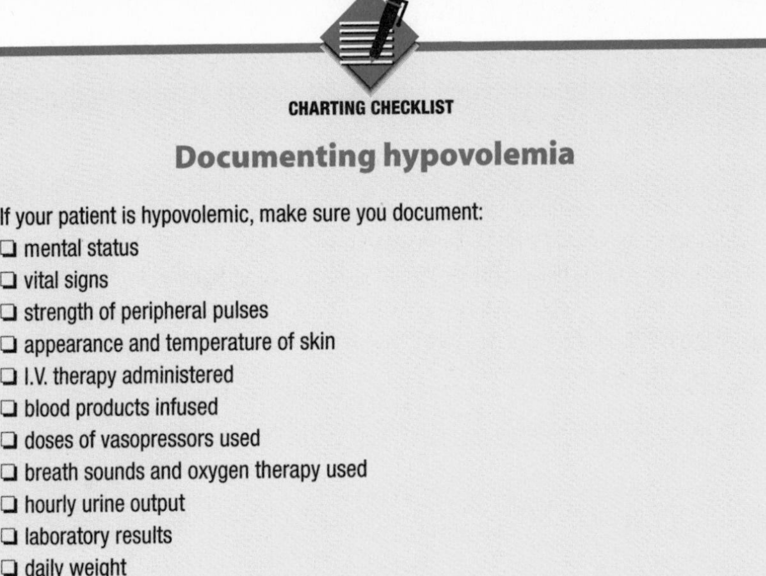

CHARTING CHECKLIST

Documenting hypovolemia

If your patient is hypovolemic, make sure you document:

- ❑ mental status
- ❑ vital signs
- ❑ strength of peripheral pulses
- ❑ appearance and temperature of skin
- ❑ I.V. therapy administered
- ❑ blood products infused
- ❑ doses of vasopressors used
- ❑ breath sounds and oxygen therapy used
- ❑ hourly urine output
- ❑ laboratory results
- ❑ daily weight
- ❑ interventions and the patient's response
- ❑ patient teaching.

✦ measuring blood pressure and pulse rate
✦ prescribed medications.

Hypervolemia

✦ Excess of isotonic fluid (water and sodium) in extracellular compartment

HYPERVOLEMIA

Hypervolemia is an excess of isotonic fluid (water and sodium) in the extracellular compartment. Osmolality is usually unaffected because fluid and solutes are gained in equal proportion. The body has compensatory mechanisms to deal with hypervolemia but, when they fail, the signs and symptoms of hypervolemia develop.

Pathophysiology

✦ Results from excessive sodium intake, fluid or sodium retention, or fluid shift from interstitial space into intravascular space
✦ May also result from acute or chronic renal failure with low urine output

CAUSES AND PATHOPHYSIOLOGY

Extracellular fluid volume may increase in either the interstitial or intravascular compartments. Usually, the body can compensate and restore fluid balance by fine-tuning circulating levels of aldosterone, antidiuretic hormone, and atrial natriuretic peptide — the hormone produced by the atrial muscle of the heart — causing the kidneys to release additional water and sodium.

However, if hypervolemia is prolonged or severe or the patient has poor heart function, the body can't compensate for the extra fluid volume. Heart failure and pulmonary edema may result. Fluid is forced out of the blood vessels and moves into the interstitial space, causing edema of the tissues.

Elderly patients and patients with impaired renal or cardiovascular function are especially prone to developing hypervolemia.

Hypervolemia results from excessive sodium or fluid intake, fluid or sodium retention, or a shift in fluid from the interstitial space into the intravascular space. It may also result from acute or chronic renal failure with low urine output.

Causes of excessive sodium or fluid intake include:

✦ I.V. replacement therapy using normal saline solution or lactated Ringer's solution
✦ blood or plasma replacement
✦ high intake of dietary sodium.

Causes of fluid and sodium retention include:

✦ heart failure
✦ cirrhosis of the liver
✦ nephrotic syndrome
✦ corticosteroid therapy
✦ hyperaldosteronism
✦ low intake of dietary protein.

Causes that make fluids shift into the intravascular space include:

✦ remobilization of fluids after burn treatment
✦ administration of hypertonic fluids, such as mannitol (Osmitrol) or hypertonic saline solution
✦ use of plasma proteins such as albumin.

Pathophysiology (continued)

✦ If prolonged or severe or if patient has poor heart function, body can't compensate for excess fluid
✦ Heart failure or pulmonary edema possibly develops
✦ Fluid forced out of blood vessels and into interstitial spaces causes tissue edema
✦ Elderly patients and patients with impaired renal or cardiovascular function especially prone

ASSESSMENT FINDINGS

Because no single diagnostic test confirms hypervolemia, signs and symptoms are key to diagnosis. Cardiac output increases as the body tries to compensate for the excess volume. The pulse becomes rapid and bounding. Blood pressure, central venous pressure, pulmonary artery pressure, and pulmonary artery wedge pressure rise. As the heart fails, blood pressure and cardiac output drop. A third heart sound (S_3) gallop develops with heart failure. You'll see distended veins, especially in the hands and neck. When the patient raises his hand above the level of his heart, his hand veins remain distended for more than 5 seconds.

Assessment findings

✦ Distended veins (especially in head and neck)

Evaluating pitting edema

- Use a scale of +1 to +4
- +1: slight imprint
- +4: deep imprint, with skin slow to return to original contour
- Brawny edema — skin resists pressure and appears distended

Evaluating pitting edema

Edema can be evaluated using a scale of +1 to +4. Press your fingertip firmly into the patient's skin over a bony surface for a few seconds. Then note the depth of the imprint your finger leaves on the skin.

A slight imprint indicates +1 pitting edema.

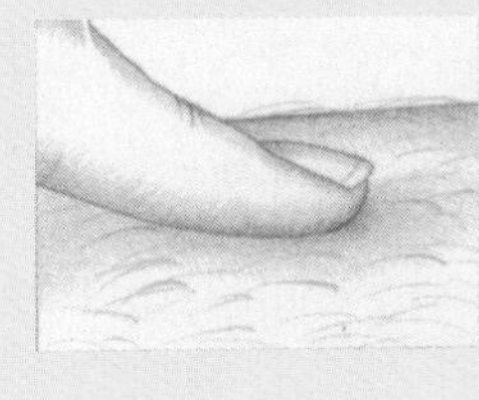

A deep imprint, with the skin slow to return to its original contour, indicates +4 pitting edema.

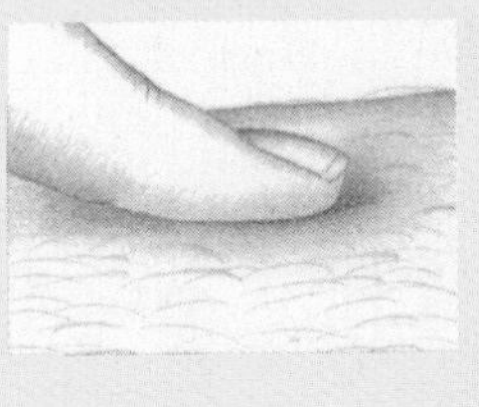

When the skin resists pressure and appears distended, the condition is called *brawny edema,* which causes the skin to swell so much that fluid can't be displaced.

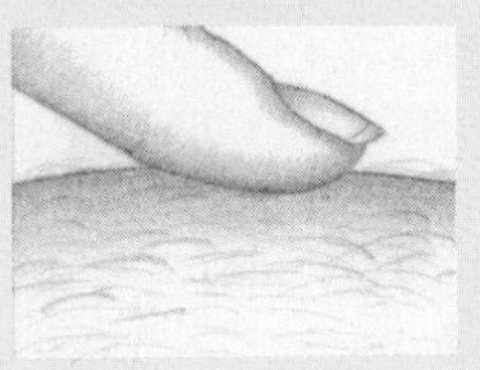

Assessment findings *(continued)*

- Edema (first visible only in dependent areas, later becoming generalized)
- Pulmonary edema (crackles on auscultation, shortness of breath, tachypnea, and pink, frothy sputum)
- Rapid, bounding pulse
- Weight gain (mild to moderate fluid gain, 5% to 10% of total body weight; severe fluid gain, > 10% of total body weight)

Edema results as hydrostatic pressure builds in the vessels, and fluid is forced into the tissues. Edema may first be visible only in dependent areas, such as the sacrum and buttocks when the patient is lying down, or in the legs and feet when the patient is standing. (See *Evaluating pitting edema.*) Later, the edema may become generalized. *Anasarca* is the term used to describe severe, generalized edema. Edematous skin looks puffy, even around the eyes, and feels cool and pits when touched. The patient gains weight as a result of fluid retention (each 17 oz [502.7 ml] of fluid gained translates to a 1-lb [0.5-kg] weight gain). An increase in weight of 5% to 10% indicates mild to moderate fluid gain; an increase of more than 10%, a more severe fluid gain.

Edema may also occur in the lungs. As the left side of the heart becomes overloaded and pump efficiency declines, fluid backs up into the lungs. Hydrostatic pressure forces fluid out of the pulmonary blood vessels (just as in other blood vessels) and into the interstitial and alveolar areas, causing pulmonary edema. In a patient with this condition, you'll hear crackles on auscultation. The patient becomes short of breath and tachypneic with a frequent, sometimes frothy, cough. Pink frothy sputum is a hallmark of pulmonary edema. Arterial blood gas (ABG) results will reflect pulmonary edema. (See *How pulmonary edema develops.*)

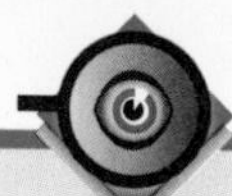

CLOSER LOOK

How pulmonary edema develops

Excess fluid volume in the extravascular spaces of the lung can cause pulmonary edema. It may occur as a chronic condition or develop quickly and rapidly become fatal. These illustrations show how pulmonary edema develops.

Normal
Normal pulmonary fluid movement depends on the equal force of two opposing pressures—hydrostatic pressure and plasma osmotic pressure from protein molecules in the blood.

Congestion
Abnormally high pulmonary hydrostatic pressure (indicated by increased pulmonary artery wedge pressure) forces fluid out of the capillaries and into the interstitial space, causing pulmonary congestion.

Edema
When the amount of interstitial fluid becomes excessive, fluid is forced into the alveoli. Pulmonary edema results. Fluid fills the alveoli and prevents the exchange of gases.

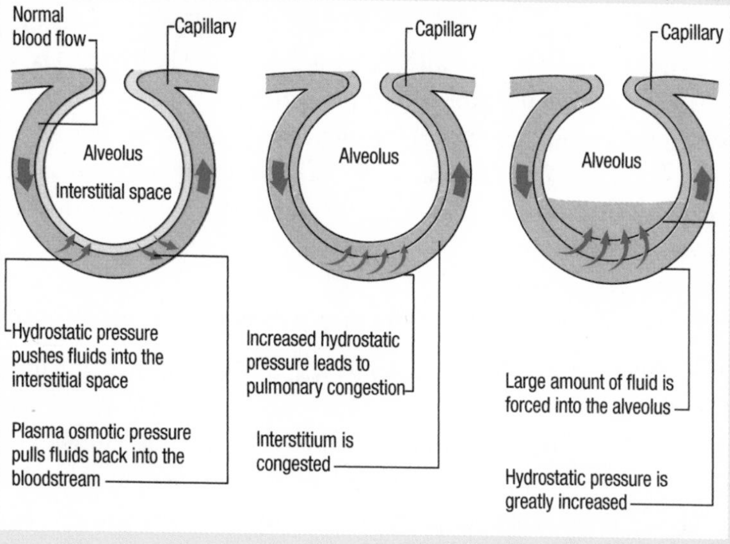

Pulmonary edema development

- ✦ Normal movement—depends on equal force of hydrostatic pressure and plasma osmotic pressure
- ✦ Congestion—develops when abnormally high hydrostatic pressure forces fluid out of capillaries and into interstitial space
- ✦ Edema— develops when fluid forced into interstitial space fills alveoli and prevents exchange of gases

Diagnostic test results

Typical laboratory findings for a patient with hypervolemia include:

- ✦ low hematocrit (HCT) due to hemodilution
- ✦ normal serum sodium level

Diagnostic test results

- ✦ Low HCT
- ✦ Low serum potassium and blood urea nitrogen levels
- ✦ Normal serum sodium level
- ✦ Pulmonary congestion (on chest X-rays)

✦ low serum potassium and blood urea nitrogen levels due to hemodilution (higher levels may indicate renal failure or impaired renal perfusion)
✦ decreased serum osmolality
✦ low oxygen level (with early tachypnea, partial pressure of arterial carbon dioxide may be low, causing a drop in pH and respiratory alkalosis)
✦ pulmonary congestion on chest X-rays.

Treatment

Treatment for hypervolemia includes restriction of sodium and fluid intake and administration of medications to prevent such complications as heart failure and pulmonary edema. The cause of the hypervolemia should also be treated. Diuretics are given to promote the loss of excess fluid.

If the patient has pulmonary edema, additional drugs, such as morphine and nitroglycerin (Nitro-Dur), may be given to dilate blood vessels, which in turn reduces pulmonary congestion and the amount of blood returning to the heart. Heart failure is treated with digoxin (Lanoxin), which strengthens cardiac contractions and slows the heart rate. Oxygen and bed rest are also used to support the patient.

When the kidneys aren't working properly, diuretics may not be enough to rid the body of extra fluid. The patient may require hemodialysis or continuous renal replacement therapy. (See *Continuous venovenous hemofiltration.*)

Treatment

✦ Sodium and fluid intake restrictions to prevent complications (heart failure and pulmonary edema)
✦ Digoxin (heart failure)
✦ Diuretics (promote excess fluid loss)
✦ Morphine and nitroglycerin to dilate blood vessels (pulmonary edema)
✦ Oxygen and bed rest (pulmonary edema)
✦ Hemodialysis or continuous renal replacement therapy (improperly working kidneys

Nursing interventions

Caring for a patient with hypervolemia requires a number of nursing actions:

✦ Assess the patient's vital signs and hemodynamic status, noting his response to therapy. Watch for signs of hypovolemia caused by overcorrection. Remember that elderly, pediatric, and otherwise compromised patients are at higher risk for complications with therapy.
✦ Monitor respiratory patterns for worsening distress, such as increased tachypnea or dyspnea.
✦ Watch for distended veins in the hands or neck.
✦ Record intake and output hourly.
✦ Listen to breath sounds regularly to assess for pulmonary edema. Note crackles or rhonchi.
✦ Follow ABG results and watch for a drop in oxygen level or changes in acid-base balance.

Key nursing interventions

✦ Assess vital signs and hemodynamic status
✦ Monitor respiratory patterns for worsening distress
✦ Watch for distended veins in hands or neck
✦ Record intake and output hourly
✦ Listen to breath sounds regularly

Continuous venovenous hemofiltration

This illustration shows the standard setup for one type of continuous renal replacement therapy (CRRT) called *continuous venovenous hemofiltration.* In the standard setup for CRRT, a dual-lumen venous catheter provides access to the patient's blood. A pulsatile pump propels the blood through the tubing circuit.

In continuous venovenous hemofiltration (as shown), the patient's blood enters the hemofilter from a line connected to one lumen of the venous catheter, flows through the hemofilter, and returns to the patient through the second lumen of the catheter.

At the first pump, an anticoagulant may be added to the blood. A second pump moves dialysate through the hemofilter. A third pump adds replacement fluid if needed. Finally, the ultrafiltrate (plasma water and toxins) that's removed from the blood drains into a collection bag.

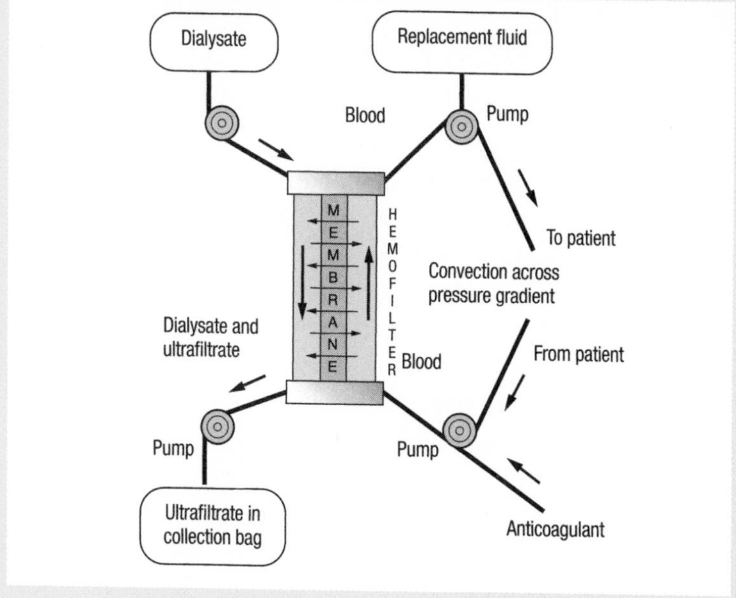

✦ Monitor other laboratory test results for changes, including potassium levels (decreased with use of most diuretics) and HCT.

✦ Raise the head of the bed (if blood pressure allows) to facilitate breathing, and administer oxygen as ordered.

✦ Make sure the patient restricts fluids if necessary. Alert the family and staff to ensure compliance.

✦ Insert a urinary catheter, as ordered, to more accurately monitor output before starting diuretic therapy.

Key nursing interventions
(continued)

✦ Raise head of bed

✦ Make sure patient restricts fluids if necessary

CHARTING CHECKLIST

Documenting hypervolemia

If your patient is hypervolemic, make sure you document:

- ❑ your assessment findings, including vital signs, hemodynamic status, pulmonary status, and edema
- ❑ oxygen therapy in use
- ❑ intake and output
- ❑ interventions, such as administration of a diuretic, and the patient's response
- ❑ daily weight and the type of scale used
- ❑ pertinent laboratory results
- ❑ dietary or fluid restrictions
- ❑ safety measures implemented
- ❑ patient teaching.

Key nursing interventions *(continued)*

- ✦ Maintain I.V. access for administration of medications
- ✦ Watch for edema, especially in dependent areas
- ✦ Obtain daily weight
- ✦ Provide skin care

✦ Maintain I.V. access, as ordered, for the administration of medications such as diuretics. If the patient is prone to hypervolemia, use an infusion pump with any infusions to prevent administering too much fluid.

✦ Give prescribed diuretics and other medications and monitor the patient for effectiveness and adverse reactions.

✦ Watch for edema, especially in dependent areas.

✦ Check for S_3, which can be heard when the ventricles are volume overloaded. S_3 is best heard over the heart's apex over the mitral area.

✦ Provide frequent mouth care.

✦ Obtain daily weight and evaluate trends.

✦ Provide skin care because edematous skin is prone to breakdown.

✦ Offer emotional support to the patient and his family.

✦ Document your assessment and interventions. (See *Documenting hypervolemia*.)

Patient teaching

- ✦ Description of disorder
- ✦ Warning signs and symptoms
- ✦ Treatment
- ✦ Self-care
- ✦ Diet
- ✦ Weight monitoring
- ✦ Medications
- ✦ Referrals

Patient teaching

If your patient has hypervolemia, teach him about the following points and then evaluate his learning:

- ✦ nature of the condition and its causes
- ✦ warning signs and symptoms and when to report them
- ✦ treatment and the importance of compliance
- ✦ measuring blood pressure and pulse rate
- ✦ restricting intake of sodium and fluids

- importance of being weighed regularly
- prescribed medications
- referral to dietitian, if appropriate.

WATER INTOXICATION

Water intoxication occurs when excess fluid moves from the extracellular space to the intracellular space.

CAUSES AND PATHOPHYSIOLOGY

Excessive low-sodium fluid in the extracellular space is hypotonic to the cells; the cells are hypertonic to the fluid. Because of this imbalance, fluid shifts — by osmosis — into the cells, which have comparatively less fluid and more solutes. That fluid shift, which causes the cells to swell, occurs as a means of balancing the concentration of fluid between the two spaces.

By causing the body to hold on to electrolyte-free water (despite low plasma osmolality [dilute plasma] and high fluid volume) syndrome of inappropriate antidiuretic hormone (SIADH) can cause water intoxication. SIADH can result from central nervous system or pulmonary disorders, head trauma, certain medications, tumors, and some surgeries.

Water intoxication can also occur with rapid infusions of hypotonic solutions such as dextrose 5% in water (D_5W). Excessive use of tap water as a nasogastric tube irrigant or enema also increases water intake.

Psychogenic polydipsia, a psychological condition, is another cause. It occurs when a person continues to drink water or other fluids in large amounts, even when they aren't needed. The condition is especially dangerous if the person's kidneys don't function well.

ASSESSMENT FINDINGS

Signs and symptoms of water intoxication are indicative of low sodium levels and increased intracranial pressure (ICP), which occurs as brain cells swell. Although headache and personality changes are the first indications, be suspicious of any change in behavior or level of consciousness (LOC), such as confusion, irritability, or lethargy. The patient may also experience nausea, vomiting, cramping, muscle weakness, twitching, thirst, dyspnea on exertion, and dulled sensorium.

Water intoxication

- Occurs when excess fluid moves from extracellular space to intracellular space

Causes

- SIADH
- Rapid infusions of hypotonic solutions (D_5W)
- Excessive use of tap water as a nasogastric tube irrigant or enema
- Psychogenic polydipsia

Assessment findings

- Signs and symptoms indicative of low sodium levels and increased ICP (as brain cells swell)

Early

- Changes in LOC
- Dyspnea on exertion
- Headache
- Nausea
- Personality changes
- Thirst
- Vomiting

Assessment findings *(continued)*

Late
- ✦ Bradycardia
- ✦ Pupillary changes
- ✦ Weight gain
- ✦ Widened pulse pressure

Treatment
- ✦ Correction of underlying cause
- ✦ Oral and parenteral fluid intake restrictions
- ✦ Avoiding use of hypotonic solutions until serum sodium levels rise

Key nursing interventions
- ✦ Closely assess patient's neurologic status
- ✦ Monitor vital signs and intake and output
- ✦ Maintain oral and I.V. fluid restrictions
- ✦ Insert and maintain I.V. catheter
- ✦ Weigh patient daily

Late signs of increased ICP include pupillary and vital sign changes, such as bradycardia and widened pulse pressure. A patient with water intoxication may develop seizures and coma. Any weight gain reflects additional cellular fluid.

Diagnostic test results

Typical laboratory findings for a patient with water intoxication include:
- ✦ serum sodium level less than 125 mEq/L
- ✦ serum osmolality less than 280 mOsm/kg.

Treatment

Treatment for water intoxication includes correcting the underlying cause, restricting both oral and parenteral fluid intake, and avoiding the use of hypotonic I.V. solutions, such as D_5W, until serum sodium levels rise. Hypertonic solutions are used only in severe situations to draw fluid out of the cells and must be accompanied by close patient monitoring. The original cause of the water intoxication should also be addressed.

Nursing interventions

Prevention is the best intervention for water intoxication. However, if your patient develops this condition, you'll want to implement these nursing actions:
- ✦ Closely assess his neurologic status; watch for deterioration, especially changes in personality or LOC.
- ✦ Monitor vital signs and intake and output to evaluate the patient's progress.
- ✦ Maintain oral and I.V. fluid restrictions, as prescribed.
- ✦ Alert the dietitian and the patient's family to the restrictions.
- ✦ Post a sign in the patient's room to alert staff to fluid restrictions.
- ✦ Insert an I.V. catheter and maintain it, as ordered; infuse hypertonic solutions with care, using an infusion pump.
- ✦ Closely observe the patient's response to therapy.
- ✦ Weigh the patient daily to detect water retention.
- ✦ Monitor laboratory test results such as serum sodium levels.
- ✦ Provide a safe environment for the patient who has an alteration in neurologic status and teach his family to do the same.
- ✦ Institute seizure precautions in severe cases.
- ✦ Document your assessment and interventions. (See *Documenting water intoxication.*)

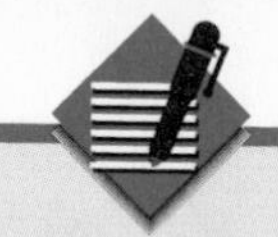

CHARTING CHECKLIST

Documenting water intoxication

If your patient has water intoxication, make sure you document:

- ❑ all assessment findings
- ❑ intake and output, noting fluid restrictions
- ❑ safety measures
- ❑ types of seizure activity and treatment
- ❑ laboratory results
- ❑ daily weight
- ❑ nursing interventions and the patient's response
- ❑ patient teaching.

Patient teaching

Be sure to cover these topics and then evaluate your patient's learning:

- ✦ nature of the condition and its causes
- ✦ need for fluid restriction
- ✦ warning signs and symptoms and when to report them
- ✦ prescribed medications
- ✦ importance of being weighed regularly.

Patient teaching

- ✦ Description of disorder
- ✦ Fluid restrictions
- ✦ Warning signs and symptoms
- ✦ Medications
- ✦ Weight monitoring

Sodium imbalances

Sodium

- Most abundant solute in extracellular fluid
- Attracts fluid and preserves extracellular fluid volume and fluid distribution in the body
- Transmits impulses in nerve and muscle fibers
- Combines with chloride and bicarbonate to regulate acid-base balance
- Normal serum sodium level: 135 to 145 mEq/L

Maintaining sodium balance

- Minimum daily requirement: 0.5 to 2.7 g
- Excreted by kidneys, GI tract, and sweat
- Directly linked to water

SODIUM

Sodium is one of the most important elements in the body. It accounts for 90% of extracellular fluid cations (positively charged ions) and is the most abundant solute in extracellular fluid. In fact, almost all sodium in the body is found in extracellular fluid.

The body needs sodium to maintain proper extracellular fluid osmolality (concentration). It attracts fluid and helps preserve the extracellular fluid volume and fluid distribution in the body. It also helps transmit impulses in nerve and muscle fibers and combines with chloride and bicarbonate to regulate acid-base balance. Because the electrolyte compositions of serum and interstitial fluid are essentially equal, sodium concentration in extracellular fluid is measured in serum levels. The normal range for the serum sodium level is 135 to 145 mEq/L. As a comparison, the amount of sodium inside a cell is 10 mEq/L.

MAINTAINING SODIUM BALANCE

Sodium requirements vary according to a person's size and age. The minimum daily requirement is 0.5 to 2.7 g; however, the salty American diet provides at least 6 g/day. Even so, sodium levels stay fairly constant because the more sodium a person takes in, the more sodium the kidneys excrete. (See *Dietary sources of sodium.*)

Dietary sources of sodium

Major dietary sources of sodium include:
- ✦ canned soups and vegetables
- ✦ cheese
- ✦ ketchup
- ✦ processed meats
- ✦ seafood
- ✦ snack foods
- ✦ table salt.

Sodium is also excreted through the GI tract and in sweat through the skin, and it's directly linked to water. The normal range of serum sodium levels reflects this close relationship. If sodium intake suddenly increases, extracellular fluid concentration also rises, and vice versa.

The body makes adjustments when the sodium level rises. Increased levels cause a person to feel thirsty and the posterior pituitary gland to release antidiuretic hormone (ADH). ADH causes the kidneys to retain water, which dilutes the blood and normalizes serum osmolality.

When sodium levels decrease and serum osmolality decreases, the body suppresses thirst and ADH secretion, and the kidneys excrete more water to restore normal osmolality. (See *Regulating sodium and water,* page 70.)

Aldosterone also regulates extracellular sodium balance via a feedback loop. The adrenal cortex secretes aldosterone, which stimulates the renal tubules to conserve water and sodium when the body's sodium level is low, thus helping to normalize extracellular fluid sodium levels.

Sodium-potassium pump

Normally, extracellular sodium levels are extremely high compared to intracellular sodium levels. The body contains an active transport mechanism, called the *sodium-potassium pump,* which helps maintain normal sodium levels.

The sodium-potassium pump works against diffusion, a passive form of transport in which a substance moves from an area of higher concentration to one of lower concentration. Sodium ions, normally most abundant outside the cells, tend to diffuse inward; potassium ions, normally most abundant inside the cells, tend to diffuse outward. To combat this

Sodium-potassium pump
- ✦ Active transport mechanism
- ✦ Helps maintain normal sodium levels
- ✦ Constantly works against ionic diffusion (sodium ions, most abundant outside cells, diffuse inward; potassium ions, most abundant inside cells, diffuse outward)
- ✦ Requires adenosine triphosphate to move sodium from cell and return potassium to cell

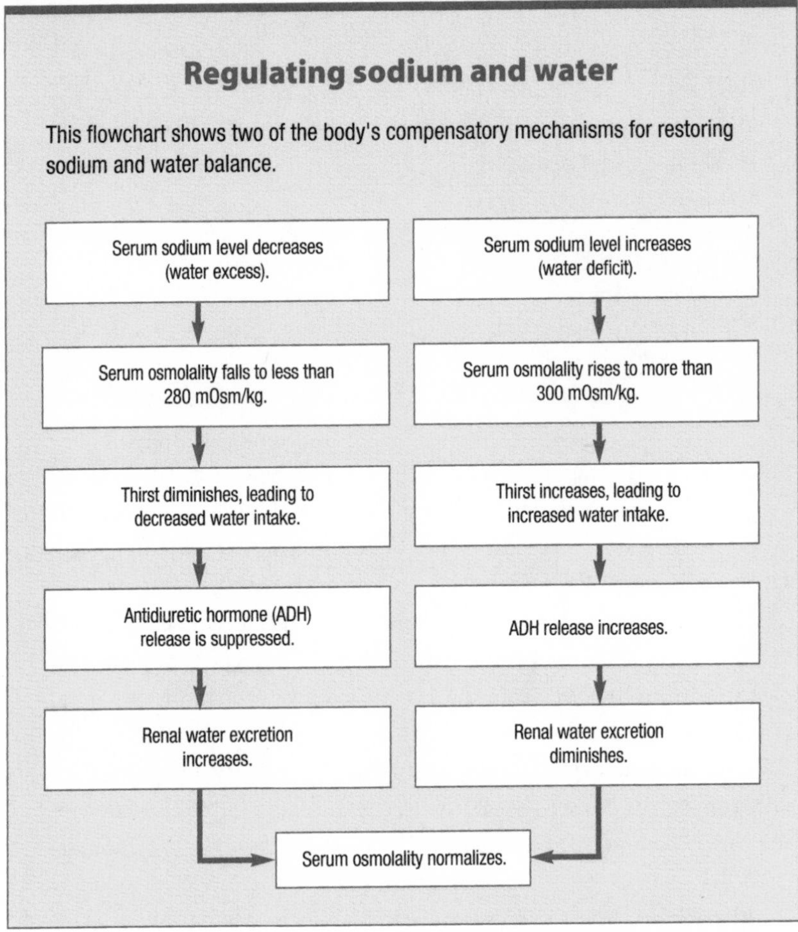

Regulating sodium and water
This flowchart shows two of the body's compensatory mechanisms for restoring sodium and water balance.
Serum sodium level decreases (water excess).
Serum osmolality falls to less than 280 mOsm/kg.
Thirst diminishes, leading to decreased water intake.
Antidiuretic hormone (ADH) release is suppressed.
Renal water excretion increases.
Serum sodium level increases (water deficit).
Serum osmolality rises to more than 300 mOsm/kg.
Thirst increases, leading to increased water intake.
ADH release increases.
Renal water excretion diminishes.
Serum osmolality normalizes.

Sodium-potassium pump *(continued)*

- Allows body to carry out essential functions
- Helps prevent cellular swelling
- Creates an electrical charge in cell, permitting transmission of neuromuscular impulses

ionic diffusion and maintain normal sodium and potassium levels, the sodium-potassium pump is constantly working in every body cell.

However, moving sodium out of the cell and potassium back in can't happen without the help of a carrier. Each sodium ion links with a carrier because it can't get through the cell wall alone. This movement requires energy (a form of active transport), which comes from adenosine triphosphate — made up of phosphorus, magnesium, and an enzyme. These substances help move sodium from the cell and return potassium to the cell.

The sodium-potassium pump allows the body to carry out its essential functions and helps prevent cellular swelling caused by too many ions inside the cell attracting excessive amounts of water. The pump also creates

Understanding the sodium-potassium pump

This illustration shows how the sodium-potassium pump carries ions when their concentrations change.

Normal placement
Normally, more sodium (Na) ions exist outside the cells than inside. More potassium (K) ions exist inside the cells than outside.

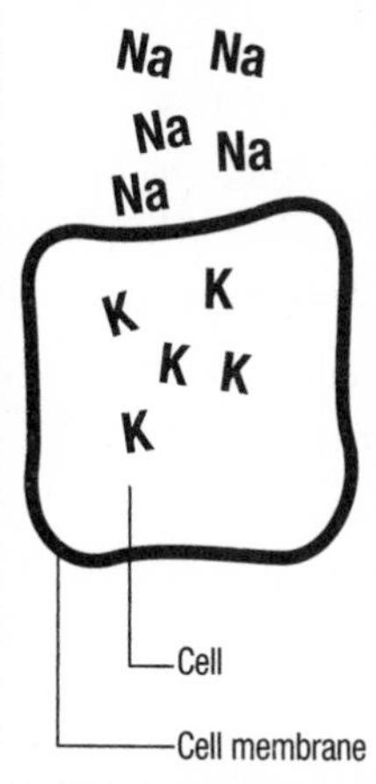

Increased permeability
Certain stimuli increase the membrane's permeability. Sodium ions diffuse inward; potassium ions diffuse outward.

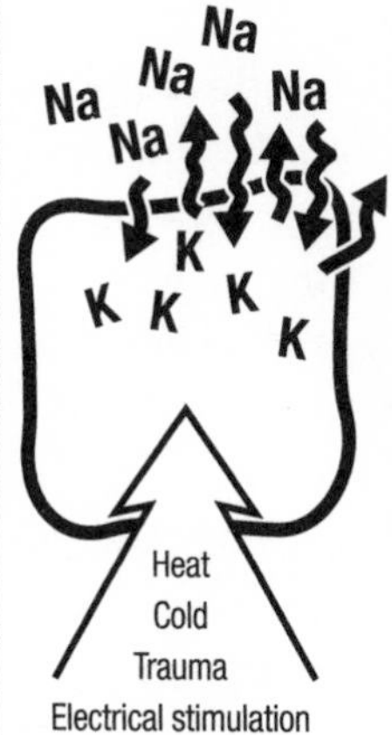

Energy source
The cell links each ion with a carrier molecule that returns the ion through the cell wall. Adenosine triphosphate (ATP), magnesium (Mg), and an enzyme commonly found in cells create the energy that returns the ion to the cell.

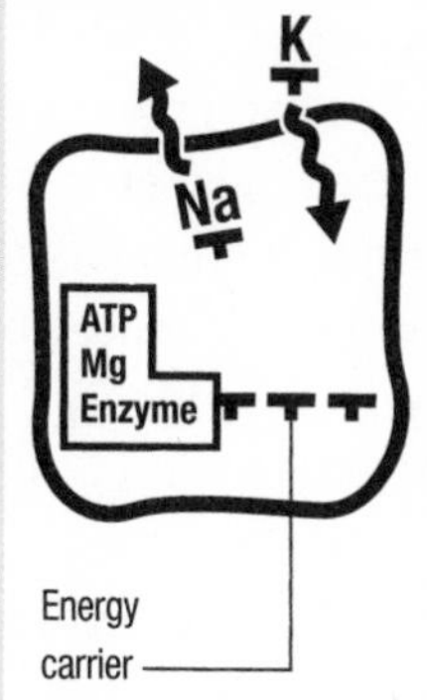

an electrical charge in the cell from the movement of ions, permitting transmission of neuromuscular impulses. (See *Understanding the sodium-potassium pump.*)

Maintaining sodium balance

To maintain proper extracellular fluid osmolality, the body needs sodium. When the body can't maintain adequate levels of sodium and water the result is either sodium deficit (less than 135 mEq/L) or sodium excess (greater than 145 mEq/L). When this happens, hyponatremia or hypernatremia occurs, resulting in severe problems for the patient.

Sodium balance

- Sodium deficit: < 135 mEq/L (hyponatremia)
- Sodium excess: > 145 mEq/L (hypernatremia)

Hyponatremia
- Causes diluted body fluids and swollen cells
- If severe, can lead to seizures, coma, and permanent neurologic damage

HYPONATREMIA

Hyponatremia, a common electrolyte imbalance, refers to a sodium deficiency (less than 135 mEq/L) in relation to the amount of water in the body. It causes diluted body fluids and swollen cells from decreased extracellular fluid osmolality. Severe hyponatremia can lead to seizures, coma, and permanent neurologic damage.

Pathophysiology
- Body eliminates excess water by secreting less ADH, causing diuresis; without this regulatory function, hyponatremia occurs

CAUSES AND PATHOPHYSIOLOGY

Normally, the body gets rid of excess water by secreting less antidiuretic hormone (ADH); less ADH causes diuresis. For that to happen, the nephrons must be functioning normally, receiving and excreting excess water and reabsorbing sodium.

Hyponatremia develops when this regulatory function goes awry. Serum sodium levels decrease, and fluid shifts occur. When the blood vessels contain more water and less sodium, fluid moves by osmosis from the extracellular area into the more concentrated intracellular area. With more fluid in the cells and less in the blood vessels, cerebral edema and hypovolemia (causing fluid-volume deficit) can occur. (See *Fluid movement in hyponatremia.*)

Causes
- Inadequate sodium intake
- Sodium loss
- Water gain

Hyponatremia occurs from sodium loss, water gain (dilutional hyponatremia), or inadequate sodium intake (depletional hyponatremia). It may be classified according to whether extracellular fluid volume is abnormally decreased (hypovolemic hyponatremia), abnormally increased (hypervolemic hyponatremia), or equal to intracellular fluid volume (isovolumic hyponatremia).

Hypovolemic hyponatremia
- Extracellular sodium and water levels both decrease, but sodium loss is greater
- Renal causes: Diuretics, osmotic diuresis
- Nonrenal causes: Diarrhea, excessive sweating, gastric suctioning, vomiting

Hypovolemic hyponatremia

In hypovolemic hyponatremia, both sodium and water levels decrease in the extracellular area, but sodium loss is greater than water loss. Causes may be nonrenal or renal. Nonrenal causes include vomiting, diarrhea, fistulas, gastric suctioning, excessive sweating, cystic fibrosis, burns, and wound drainage. Renal causes include osmotic diuresis, salt-losing nephritis, adrenal insufficiency, and diuretics.

Diuretics cause sodium loss and volume depletion from the blood vessels, causing the patient to feel thirsty and his kidneys to retain water. Drinking large quantities of water can worsen hyponatremia. Sodium deficits can also become more pronounced if the patient is on a sodium-restricted diet. Diuretics can also cause potassium loss (hypokalemia),

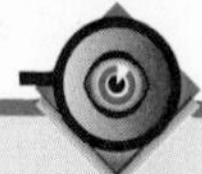

CLOSER LOOK

Fluid movement in hyponatremia

This illustration shows fluid movement in hyponatremia. When serum osmolality decreases because of decreased sodium concentration, fluid moves by osmosis from the extracellular area to the intracellular area.

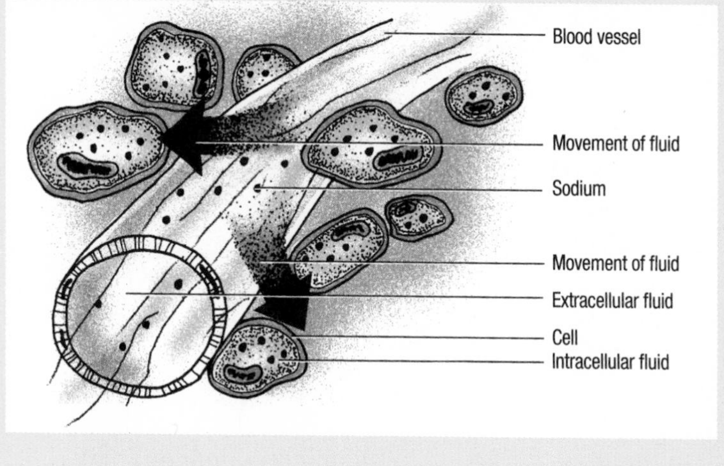

which is also linked to hyponatremia. (See *Drugs causing hyponatremia,* page 74.)

Hypervolemic hyponatremia

In hypervolemic hyponatremia, both water and sodium levels increase in the extracellular area, but the water gain is more impressive. Serum sodium levels are diluted and edema occurs. Causes include heart failure, liver failure, nephrotic syndrome, excessive administration of hypotonic I.V. fluids, and hyperaldosteronism.

Isovolumic hyponatremia

In isovolumic hyponatremia, sodium levels may appear low because too much fluid is in the body. However, a patient with isovolumic hyponatremia has no physical signs of fluid volume excess, and total body sodium remains stable. Causes include glucocorticoid deficiency (causing inadequate fluid filtration by the kidneys), hypothyroidism (causing limited water excretion), and renal failure.

Hypervolemic hyponatremia

- Extracellular water and sodium levels both increase, but water increase is greater
- Results in diluted serum sodium levels and edema
- Causes include excessive administration of hypotonic I.V. fluids, heart failure, liver failure

Isovolumic hyponatremia

- Sodium levels may appear low because of too much body fluid
- No physical signs of fluid volume excess
- Total body sodium remains stable
- Causes include glucocorticoid deficiency, hypothyroidism, renal failure, SIADH

Drugs causing hyponatremia

Drugs can cause hyponatremia by potentiating the action of antidiuretic hormone or by causing syndrome of inappropriate antidiuretic hormone. Diuretics may also cause hyponatremia by inhibiting sodium reabsorption in the kidney.

Anticonvulsants
- Carbamazepine (Tegretol)

Antidiabetics
- Chlorpropamide (Diabinese)
- Tolbutamide (Orinase) (rarely)

Antineoplastics
- Cyclophosphamide (Cytoxan)
- Vincristine (Oncovin)

Antipsychotics
- Fluphenazine (Prolixin Decanoate)
- Thioridazine (Mellaril)
- Thiothixene (Navane)

Diuretics
- Loop (such as bumetanide [Bumex], furosemide [Lasix], ethacrynic acid [Edecrin])
- Thiazides (such as hydrochlorothiazide [HydroDIURIL)

Sedatives
- Barbiturates
- Morphine

SIADH
- Causes excessive release of ADH, causing inappropriate and excessive water retention and low sodium levels
- Patient treated for underlying cause and hyponatremia

SIADH

Another cause of isovolumic hyponatremia is syndrome of inappropriate antidiuretic hormone (SIADH). This secretion causes excessive release of ADH, which causes inappropriate and excessive water retention and, in turn, disturbs the fluid and electrolyte balance, causing low sodium levels. (See *What happens in SIADH.*)

SIADH occurs with:
- cancers, especially of the duodenum and pancreas and oat cell carcinoma of the lung
- central nervous system disorders, such as trauma, tumors, and stroke
- pulmonary disorders, such as tumors, asthma, and chronic obstructive pulmonary disease

CLOSER LOOK

What happens in SIADH

This flowchart shows the events that occur in the development of syndrome of inappropriate antidiuretic hormone (SIADH).

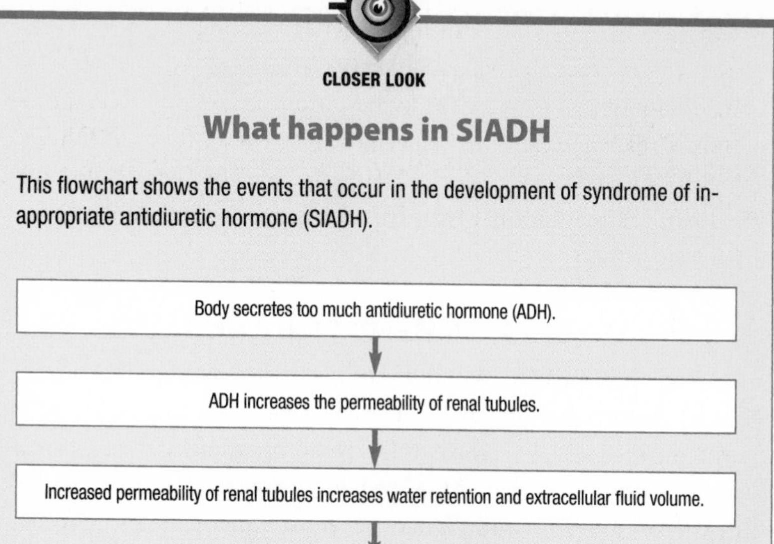
Body secretes too much antidiuretic hormone (ADH).
ADH increases the permeability of renal tubules.
Increased permeability of renal tubules increases water retention and extracellular fluid volume.
Increased extracellular fluid volume leads to:
Reduced plasma osmolality
Dilutional hyponatremia
Diminished aldosterone secretion
Elevated glomerular filtration rate
These factors lead to increased sodium excretion and a shifting of fluid into cells.
Patient develops thirst, dyspnea on exertion, vomiting, abdominal cramps, confusion, lethargy, and hyponatremia.

✦ medications, such as certain oral antidiabetics, chemotherapeutic drugs, psychoactive drugs, diuretics, synthetic hormones, and barbiturates.

The patient is treated for the underlying cause of SIADH and for hyponatremia. For instance, if a tumor caused the syndrome, the patient would receive cancer treatment; if a medication caused it, the drug would be stopped. Low sodium levels are treated with fluid restrictions (about 1 qt [1 L]/day) and diuretics such as furosemide.

The patient is placed on fluid restriction to lower water intake to match the low volume of urine caused by the increased ADH. Serum os-

SIADH
(continued)

Treatment

- ✦ Fluid restriction; if inadequate, oral urea or high-sodium diet
- ✦ Medications (demeclocycline or lithium) to block ADH in renal tubule
- ✦ Hypertonic saline solution (if fluid restriction doesn't raise sodium levels)

molality will then increase, causing the ADH level to balance it. If this treatment is inadequate, the patient may receive oral urea or follow a high-sodium diet to increase the kidneys' excretion of solutes (water will follow). Medications, such as demeclocycline (Declomycin) or lithium (Eskalith), may be used to block ADH in the renal tubule. If fluid restriction doesn't raise sodium levels, a hypertonic saline solution may be given.

Assessment findings
- ✦ Acute signs and symptoms (nausea, vomiting, anorexia) begin when serum sodium levels fall between 115 and 120 mEq/L
- ✦ Primarily neurologic changes (headache, irritability, muscle twitching, tremors, weakness, LOC changes)
- ✦ If serum sodium levels drop to 110 mEq/L, neurologic status deteriorates further (stupor, delirium, psychosis, ataxia, seizures, coma)

Hypovolemic patient
- ✦ Dry, cracked mucous membranes
- ✦ Low blood pressure
- ✦ Poor skin turgor
- ✦ Weak, rapid pulse

Hypervolemic patient
- ✦ Edema
- ✦ Hypertension
- ✦ Rapid, bounding pulse
- ✦ Weight gain

Assessment findings

As you look for signs and symptoms of hyponatremia, remember that they vary from patient to patient. They also vary depending on how quickly the sodium level drops. If the level drops quickly, the patient will be more symptomatic than if the level drops slowly. The patient with a sodium level above 125 mEq/L may not show signs or symptoms of hyponatremia at all — but, again, this depends on how quickly sodium levels drop. Usually, acute initial signs and symptoms of nausea, vomiting, and anorexia begin when the serum sodium levels fall between 115 and 120 mEq/L.

When signs and symptoms occur, they're primarily neurologic. The patient may complain of a headache or irritability or he may become disoriented. He may experience muscle twitching, tremors, or weakness. Changes in level of consciousness (LOC) may start as a shortened attention span and progress to lethargy or confusion.

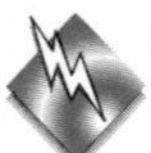

DANGER *If sodium levels drop to 110 mEq/L, the patient's neurologic status will deteriorate further (usually due to brain edema), leading to stupor, delirium, psychosis, ataxia, and even coma. He may also develop seizures.*

A patient with hypovolemic hyponatremia may have poor skin turgor and dry, cracked mucous membranes. Assessment of vital signs shows a weak, rapid pulse and low blood pressure or orthostatic hypotension. Central venous pressure (CVP), pulmonary artery pressure (PAP), and pulmonary artery wedge pressure may be decreased.

A patient with hypervolemic hyponatremia (fluid volume excess) may have edema, hypertension, weight gain, and rapid, bounding pulse, and CVP and PAP may be elevated.

Diagnostic test results
- ✦ Serum sodium level <135 mEq/L
- ✦ In patient with SIADH, increased urine specific gravity and elevated urine sodium levels

Diagnostic test results

Typical laboratory findings for a patient with hyponatremia include:
- ✦ serum osmolality less than 280 mOsm/kg (dilute blood)
- ✦ serum sodium level less than 135 mEq/L (low sodium level in blood)
- ✦ urine specific gravity less than 1.010

✦ increased urine specific gravity and elevated urine sodium levels (above 20 mEq/L) in a patient with SIADH
✦ elevated hematocrit and plasma protein levels.

Treatment

Generally, treatment varies with the cause and severity of hyponatremia. For example, hormone therapy may be needed to treat underlying endocrine disorders.

Therapy for mild hyponatremia associated with hypervolemia or isovolemia usually consists of restricted fluid intake and, possibly, oral sodium supplements. If hypovolemia is related to hyponatremia, isotonic I.V. fluids such as normal saline solution may be given to restore volume. High-sodium foods may also be offered to the patient.

When serum sodium levels fall below 120 mEq/L, treatment in the intensive care unit may include infusion of a hypertonic saline solution (such as 3% or 5% saline). If the patient is symptomatic (seizures, coma), monitor him carefully during the infusion for signs of circulatory overload or worsening neurologic status. A hypertonic saline solution causes water to shift out of cells, which may lead to intravascular volume overload and serious brain damage (osmotic demyelination), especially in the pons.

Fluid-volume overload can be fatal if untreated. To prevent fluid overload, a hypertonic sodium chloride solution is infused slowly and in small volumes. Furosemide is usually administered simultaneously.

A patient who's hypervolemic shouldn't receive hypertonic sodium chloride solutions, except in rare instances of severe symptomatic hyponatremia. During treatment, monitor serum sodium levels and related diagnostic tests to follow the patient's progress.

Treatment

✦ For mild hyponatremia associated with hypervolemia or isovolemia, fluid restriction and oral sodium supplements
✦ For hyponatremia associated with hypovolemia, isotonic I.V. fluid (normal saline solution) and high-sodium diet
✦ For serum sodium level < 120 mEq/L, infusion of hypertonic saline solution
✦ Monitoring serum sodium levels and related diagnostic tests

Nursing interventions

Closely watch patients at risk for hyponatremia, including those with heart failure, cancer, or GI disorders with fluid losses. Review your patient's medications, noting those that are associated with hyponatremia. If he develops hyponatremia, take these actions:

✦ Monitor and record vital signs, especially blood pressure and pulse, and watch for orthostatic hypertension and tachycardia.
✦ Monitor neurologic status frequently. Report deterioration in LOC. Assess the patient for lethargy, muscle twitching, seizures, and coma.
✦ Accurately measure and record intake and output.

Key nursing interventions

✦ Monitor and record vital signs, especially blood pressure and pulse
✦ Monitor neurologic status frequently
✦ Measure and record intake and output

Key nursing interventions *(continued)*

- ✦ Weigh patient daily
- ✦ Watch for and report extreme changes in serum sodium levels and accompanying serum chloride levels
- ✦ Restrict fluid intake as ordered
- ✦ Administer oral sodium supplements if prescribed
- ✦ For severe hyponatremia, administer prescribed I.V. isotonic or hypertonic saline solutions

✦ Weigh the patient daily to monitor the success of fluid restriction.

✦ Assess skin turgor at least every 8 hours for signs of dehydration.

✦ Watch for and report extreme changes in serum sodium levels and accompanying serum chloride levels. Also monitor other test results, such as urine specific gravity and serum osmolality.

✦ Restrict fluid intake as ordered. (Fluid restriction is the primary treatment for dilutional hyponatremia.) Post a sign about fluid restriction in the patient's room and make sure the staff, the patient, and his family are aware of the restrictions.

✦ Administer oral sodium supplements, if prescribed, to treat mild hyponatremia. If the physician has instructed the patient to increase his intake of dietary sodium, teach him about foods high in sodium.

✦ For severe hyponatremia, make sure a patent I.V. line is in place. Then administer prescribed I.V. isotonic or hypertonic saline solutions cautiously to avoid inducing hypernatremia, brain injury, or fluid-volume overload from an excessive or too rapid infusion. Watch closely for signs of hypervolemia (dyspnea, crackles, engorged neck or hand veins), and report them immediately. Use an infusion pump to ensure that the patient receives only the prescribed volume of fluid.

✦ Keep the patient safe while he undergoes treatment. Provide a safe environment for a patient who has altered thought processes and reorient him as needed. If seizures are likely, pad the bed's side rails and keep suction equipment and an artificial airway handy. (See *Documenting hyponatremia.*)

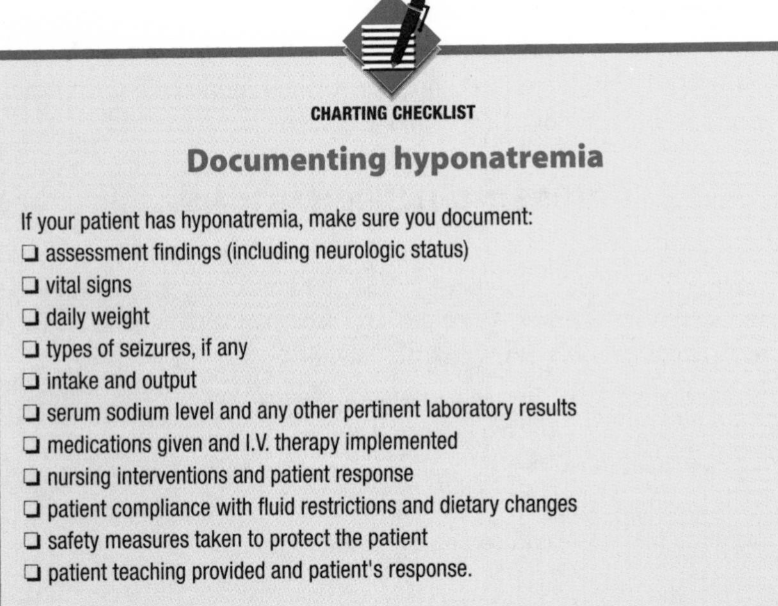

CHARTING CHECKLIST

Documenting hyponatremia

If your patient has hyponatremia, make sure you document:

- ❑ assessment findings (including neurologic status)
- ❑ vital signs
- ❑ daily weight
- ❑ types of seizures, if any
- ❑ intake and output
- ❑ serum sodium level and any other pertinent laboratory results
- ❑ medications given and I.V. therapy implemented
- ❑ nursing interventions and patient response
- ❑ patient compliance with fluid restrictions and dietary changes
- ❑ safety measures taken to protect the patient
- ❑ patient teaching provided and patient's response.

Patient teaching

Be sure to cover these topics and then evaluate your patient's learning:

- ✦ explanation of hyponatremia, including its causes and treatment
- ✦ medication therapy and possible adverse effects
- ✦ dietary changes and fluid restrictions (if any)
- ✦ warning signs and symptoms and when to report them
- ✦ importance of monitoring weight daily.

Patient teaching
- ✦ Description of disorder
- ✦ Medications
- ✦ Diet
- ✦ Warning signs and symptoms
- ✦ Weight monitoring

HYPERNATREMIA

Hypernatremia, which is less common than hyponatremia, refers to an excess of sodium relative to the amount of water in the body. It's indicated by a serum sodium level greater than 145 mEq/L. Severe hypernatremia can lead to seizures, coma, and permanent neurologic damage.

Hypernatremia
- ✦ An excess of sodium relative to amount of water in body
- ✦ Less common than hyponatremia
- ✦ Indicated by serum sodium level > 145 mEq/L
- ✦ If severe, can lead to seizures, coma, and permanent neurologic damage

Causes and pathophysiology

Thirst is the body's main defense against hypernatremia. The hypothalamus, with its osmoreceptors, is the brain's thirst center. High serum osmolality (increased solute concentrations in the blood) stimulates the hypothalamus and initiates the sensation of thirst.

The drive to respond to thirst is so strong that severe, persistent hypernatremia usually occurs only in people who can't drink voluntarily, such as infants, confused elderly patients, or patients who are immobile or unconscious. Hypothalamic disorders, such as a lesion on the hypothalamus, may cause a disturbance of the thirst mechanism, but this condition is rare. However, when hypernatremia occurs, it usually has a high mortality (greater than 50%).

The body strives to maintain a normal sodium level by secreting antidiuretic hormone (ADH) from the posterior pituitary gland. This hormone causes water to be retained, which helps to lower serum sodium levels.

The body's cells also play a role in maintaining sodium balance. When serum osmolality increases because of hypernatremia, fluid moves by osmosis from inside the cells to outside the cells, to balance the concentrations in the two compartments. As fluid leaves the cells, they become dehydrated and shrink — especially those of the central nervous system. When this occurs, the patient may show signs of neurologic impairment. He may also show signs of hypervolemia (fluid overload) from increased

Pathophysiology
- ✦ Thirst — main defense against hypernatremia; drive to quench so strong that severe, persistent hypernatremia usually occurs only in those who can't drink voluntarily
- ✦ Hypothalamic disorders may cause disturbance in thirst mechanism

Cellular role
- ✦ When serum osmolality increases due to hypernatremia, fluid moves by osmosis from inside cells to outside cells to balance compartment concentrations
- ✦ Cells become dehydrated and shrink (patient may show signs of neurologic impairment)

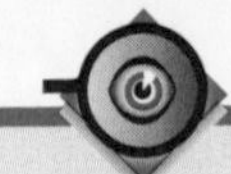

CLOSER LOOK

Fluid movement in hypernatremia

With hypernatremia, the body tries to maintain balance by shifting fluid from the inside of the cells to the outside of the cells. This illustration shows fluid movement in hypernatremia.

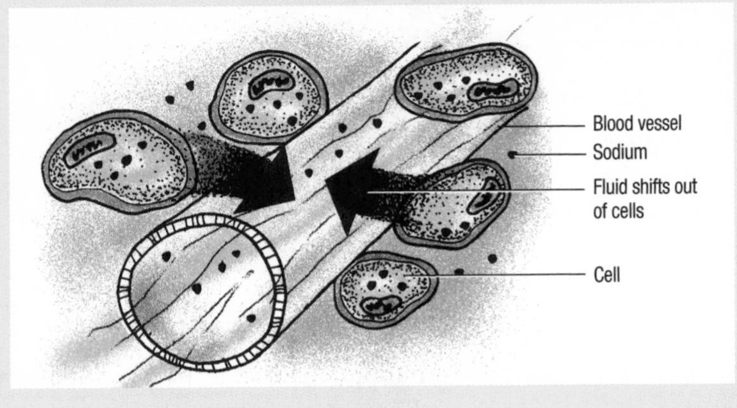

Causes

- ✦ Water deficit
- ✦ Excessive sodium intake

extracellular fluid volume in the blood vessels. (See *Fluid movement in hypernatremia.*) If the overload is severe enough, subarachnoid hemorrhage may occur.

Water deficit and excessive sodium intake can cause hypernatremia. Regardless of the cause, body fluids become hypertonic or more concentrated.

Water deficit

- ✦ Occurs when more water than sodium is lost, resulting in elevated serum sodium levels
- ✦ Can also result from fever, vomiting, watery diarrhea, osmotic diuresis, diabetes insipidus

Water deficit

A water deficit may occur alone or with a sodium loss — as long as more water than sodium is lost, elevated serum sodium levels will occur. This elevation is more dangerous in patients who are debilitated and those with a deficient water intake.

Insensible water losses of several liters per day can result from fever and heatstroke, with older adults and athletes being equally susceptible. Significant water losses also occur in patients with pulmonary infections (who lose water vapor from the lungs through hyperventilation) and in patients with extensive burns. Vomiting or severe watery diarrhea are sensible causes of water loss and subsequent hypernatremia; either can be especially dangerous in children. Patients with hyperosmolar hyperglycemic nonketotic syndrome can also develop hypernatremia due to severe water losses from osmotic diuresis. Urea diuresis occurs with administration of high-protein feedings or high-protein diets without adequate water supplementation, and can lead to hypernatremia.

AGE ALERT *Hypernatremia is more common in infants and children for two key reasons: Patients in this age-group tend to lose more water as a result of diarrhea, vomiting, inadequate fluid intake, and fever. Their intake of water is generally inadequate because they have difficulty swallowing, limited communication of needs, and lack proper access.*

Patients with diabetes insipidus have extreme thirst and enormous urinary losses, in many cases more than 4 gal (15.1 L)/day. Usually, they can drink enough fluids to match the urinary losses; otherwise, severe dehydration and hypernatremia occur. Diabetes insipidus may result from a lack of ADH from the brain causing central diabetes insipidus or a lack of response from the kidneys to ADH causing nephrogenic diabetes insipidus.

Central diabetes insipidus may result from a tumor or head trauma (such as injury or surgery) or be idiopathic. It responds well to vasopressin (Pitressin). Nephrogenic diabetes insipidus doesn't respond well to vasopressin and is more likely to occur with electrolyte imbalance, such as hypokalemia, or with certain medications such as lithium (Eskalith).

Excessive sodium intake

In addition to water losses from the body, sodium gains can also cause hypernatremia. Several factors can contribute to a high sodium intake, including salt tablets, food, and medications such as sodium polystyrene sulfonate (Kayexalate).

Excessive parenteral administration of sodium solutions, such as hypertonic saline solutions, sodium bicarbonate preparations, and gastric or enteral tube feedings, can also cause hypernatremia. Other causes of increased sodium levels include inadvertent introduction of hypertonic saline solution into maternal circulation during therapeutic abortion, near drowning in salt water, and excessive amounts of adrenocortical hormones, as in Cushing's syndrome and hyperaldosteronism, which affect water and sodium balance. (See *Drugs associated with hypernatremia,* page 82.)

Excessive sodium intake

- ✦ Can result from salt tablets, food, medications (sodium polystyrene sulfonate), excessive parenteral administration of sodium solutions, gastric or enteral tube feedings

Assessment findings

The most important signs and symptoms of hypernatremia are neurologic because fluid shifts have a significant effect on brain cells. Remember,

Drugs associated with hypernatremia

The drugs listed here can cause high sodium levels. Ask your patient if any of these are a part of his drug therapy:

- ✦ antacids with sodium bicarbonate
- ✦ antibiotics such as ticarcillin disodium-clavulanate potassium (Timentin)
- ✦ salt tablets
- ✦ sodium bicarbonate injections (such as those given during cardiac arrest)
- ✦ I.V. sodium chloride preparations
- ✦ sodium polystyrene sulfonate (Kayexalate).

Assessment findings

Early

- ✦ Anorexia
- ✦ Nausea
- ✦ Restlessness or agitation
- ✦ Vomiting

Later

- ✦ Ataxia
- ✦ Coma
- ✦ Confusion
- ✦ Flushed skin
- ✦ Hyperreflexia
- ✦ Intense thirst
- ✦ Lethargy
- ✦ Low-grade fever
- ✦ Seizures
- ✦ Stupor
- ✦ Tremors
- ✦ Twitching
- ✦ Weakness

Diagnostic test results

- ✦ Serum osmolality > 300 mOsm/kg
- ✦ Serum sodium level > 145 mEq/L
- ✦ Urine specific gravity > 1.03

the body can tolerate a high sodium level that develops over time better than one that occurs rapidly. Early signs and symptoms of hypernatremia may include restlessness or agitation, anorexia, nausea, and vomiting. These may be followed by weakness, lethargy, confusion, stupor, seizures, and coma. Neuromuscular signs and symptoms also commonly occur, including twitching, hyperreflexia, ataxia, and tremors.

You may also observe a low-grade fever and flushed skin. In addition, the patient may complain of intense thirst from stimulation of the hypothalamus from increased osmolality. Other signs vary depending on the cause of the high sodium levels. If a sodium gain has occurred, fluid may be drawn into the blood vessels and the patient will appear hypervolemic, with an elevated blood pressure, bounding pulse, and dyspnea. If water loss occurs, fluid will leave the blood vessels and you'll notice signs of hypovolemia, such as dry mucous membranes, oliguria, and orthostatic hypotension (blood pressure drop and heart rate increase with position changes).

Diagnostic test results

Typical laboratory findings for a patient with hypernatremia include:

- ✦ serum sodium level greater than 145 mEq/L
- ✦ urine specific gravity greater than 1.03 (except in diabetes insipidus, where urine specific gravity is decreased)
- ✦ serum osmolality greater than 300 mOsm/kg.

Treatment

Treatment for hypernatremia varies with the cause. The underlying disorder must be corrected, and serum sodium levels and related diagnostic tests must be monitored. If too little water in the body is causing the hypernatremia, treatment may include oral fluid replacement. Note that the fluids should be given gradually over 48 hours to avoid shifting water into brain cells.

Remember, as sodium levels rise in the blood vessels, fluid shifts out of the cells — including the brain cells — to dilute the blood and equalize concentrations. If too much water is introduced into the body too quickly, water moves into brain cells and they get bigger, causing cerebral edema.

The patient may receive salt-free solutions (such as dextrose 5% in water) to return serum sodium levels to normal, followed by infusion of half-normal saline solution to prevent hyponatremia and cerebral edema. If the patient can't drink enough fluids, he'll need I.V. fluid replacement. Other treatments include restricting sodium intake and administering diuretics along with oral or I.V. fluid replacement to increase sodium loss.

Treatment for diabetes insipidus may include vasopressin, hypotonic I.V. fluids, and thiazide diuretics to decrease free water loss from the kidneys. The underlying cause should also be treated.

Treatment

- ✦ Underlying disorder must be corrected
- ✦ Serum sodium levels and related diagnostic tests must be monitored
- ✦ Oral fluid replacement if caused by too little water in body
- ✦ Salt-free solutions followed by infusion of half-normal saline solution
- ✦ I.V. fluid replacement if patient can't drink enough salt-free solutions
- ✦ Restricted sodium intake
- ✦ Diuretics to increase sodium loss
- ✦ Vasopressin, hypotonic I.V. fluids, and thiazide diuretics for diabetes insipidus

Nursing interventions

Closely observe high-risk patients, such as those recovering from surgery near the pituitary gland, to prevent hypernatremia. Also find out if they're taking medications that may cause hypernatremia. If your patient does develop hypernatremia, take these measures:

✦ Monitor and record vital signs, especially blood pressure and pulse.

✦ If the patient needs I.V. fluid replacement, monitor fluid delivery and his response to the therapy. Watch for signs of cerebral edema and check his neurologic status frequently. Report deterioration in level of consciousness.

✦ Carefully measure and record intake and output. Weigh the patient daily to check for body-fluid loss.

✦ Assess skin and mucous membranes for signs of breakdown and infection as well as water loss from perspiration.

✦ Monitor the patient's serum sodium level and report an increase. Monitor urine specific gravity and other laboratory test results.

✦ If the patient can't take oral fluids, recommend the I.V. route to the physician. If the patient can drink and is alert and responsible, involve him in his treatment. Give him a target amount of fluid to drink each shift, mark cups with the volume they hold, leave fluids within easy reach, and provide paper and pen to record amounts. If family members will be helping the patient drink, give them specific instructions as well.

Key nursing interventions

- ✦ Monitor and record vital signs, especially blood pressure and pulse
- ✦ Monitor fluid delivery and patient's response to therapy; watch for signs of cerebral edema
- ✦ Carefully measure intake and output
- ✦ Monitor patient's serum sodium level and report increase
- ✦ Assist with oral hygiene

CHARTING CHECKLIST

Documenting hypernatremia

If your patient has hypernatremia, make sure you document:

- ❑ assessment findings (including neurologic status)
- ❑ vital signs
- ❑ types of seizures, if any
- ❑ daily weight
- ❑ serum sodium level and other pertinent laboratory test results
- ❑ intake and output
- ❑ medications given and I.V. therapy implemented
- ❑ notification of the physician when the patient's condition changes
- ❑ nursing interventions and the patient's response
- ❑ patient compliance with fluid restrictions and dietary changes
- ❑ safety measures taken to protect the patient (seizure precautions)
- ❑ patient teaching provided and the patient's response.

✦ Insert and maintain a patent I.V. line as ordered. Use an infusion pump to control delivery of I.V. fluids to prevent cerebral edema.

✦ Assist with oral hygiene. Lubricate the patient's lips frequently with a water-based lubricant and provide mouthwash or gargle if he's alert. Good mouth care helps keep mucous membranes moist and decreases mouth odor.

✦ Provide a safe environment for a patient who's confused or agitated. If seizures are likely, pad the bed's side rails and keep an artificial airway and suction equipment handy. Reorient the patient as needed, and reduce environmental stimuli. (See *Documenting hypernatremia.*)

Patient teaching

- ✦ Description of disorder
- ✦ Diet
- ✦ Medications
- ✦ Warning signs and symptoms

Patient teaching

Be sure to cover these topics and then evaluate your patient's learning:

✦ explanation of hypernatremia, including its causes and treatment

✦ importance of restricting sodium intake, including both dietary sources and over-the-counter medications that contain sodium

✦ medication therapy given and possible adverse effects

✦ warning signs and symptoms and when to report them.

Potassium imbalances

POTASSIUM

Potassium, which plays a critical role in many metabolic cell functions, is the major cation in intracellular fluid, where it's most abundant. Almost all of it (98%) is in intracellular fluid, whereas only 2% is found in extracellular fluid. That difference affects nerve impulse transmission.

Diseases, injuries, medications, and therapies can all disturb potassium levels. Small, untreated alterations in serum potassium levels can seriously affect a person's neuromuscular and cardiac functioning.

Potassium directly affects how well the body's cells, nerves, and muscles function by:

✦ maintaining cells' electrical neutrality and osmolality
✦ aiding neuromuscular transmission of nerve impulses
✦ assisting skeletal and cardiac muscle contraction and electrical conductivity
✦ affecting acid-base balance in relationship to the hydrogen ion. (See *Potassium's role in acid-base balance,* page 86.)

Potassium

✦ Major cation in intracellular fluid
✦ Most abundant in intracellular fluid
✦ Maintains cells' electrical neutrality and osmolality
✦ Aids neuromuscular transmission of nerve impulses
✦ Assists skeletal and cardiac muscle contraction and electrical conductivity
✦ Affects acid-base balance in relationship to hydrogen ion

MAINTAINING POTASSIUM BALANCE

Normal serum potassium levels range from 3.5 to 5 mEq/L. In the cell, the potassium level (usually not measured) is much higher, at 140 mEq/L. Because the body can't conserve it, it must be ingested daily.

Maintaining potassium balance

✦ Normal serum potassium level: 3.5 to 5 mEq/L
✦ Recommended daily requirement: 40 mEq/L; average daily intake: 60 to 100 mEq/L

Potassium's role in acid-base balance

The illustrations below show the movement of potassium ions (K) in response to changes in extracellular hydrogen ion (H^+) concentration. H^+ concentration changes with acidosis and alkalosis.

NORMAL BALANCE
Under normal conditions, the K content in intracellular fluid is much greater than in extracellular fluid. H^+ concentration is low in both compartments.

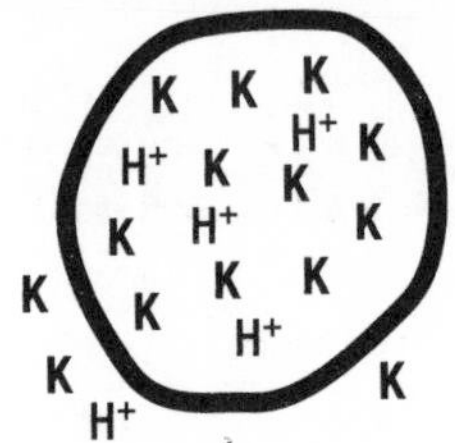

ACIDOSIS
In acidosis, H^+ content in extracellular fluid increases and the ions move into the intracellular fluid. To keep the intracellular fluid electrically neutral, an equal number of K leave the cell, which causes hyperkalemia.

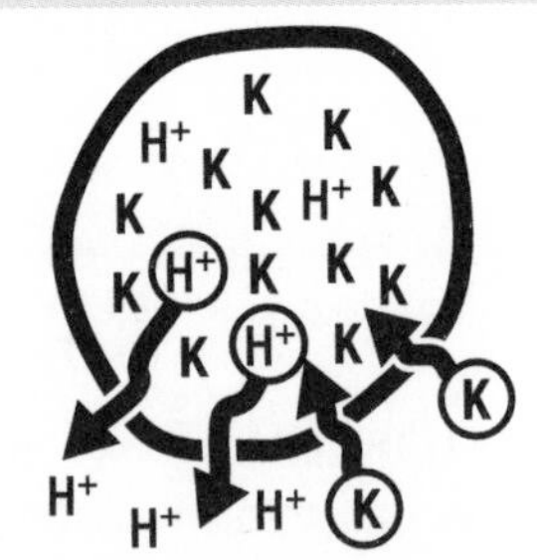

ALKALOSIS
In alkalosis, more H^+ are present in intracellular fluid than in the extracellular fluid. Therefore, H^+ move from the intracellular fluid into the extracellular fluid. To keep the intracellular fluid electrically neutral, K ions move from the extracellular fluid into the intracellular fluid, causing hypokalemia.

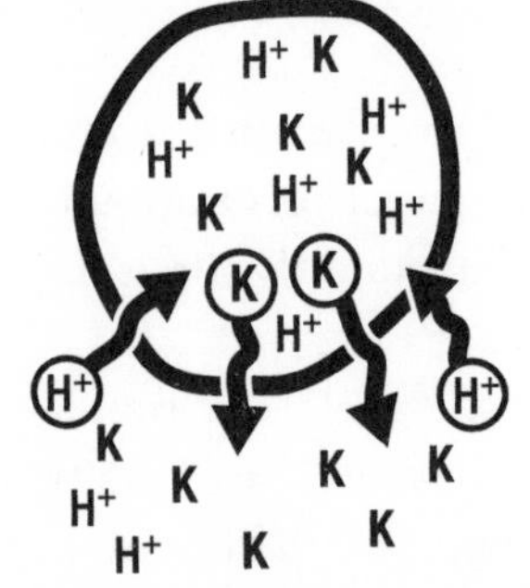

The recommended daily requirement for adults is about 40 mEq; the average daily intake is 60 to 100 mEq. (See *Dietary sources of potassium.*)

Extracellular fluid also gains potassium when cells are destroyed, thus, releasing intracellular potassium. It also gains potassium when the potassium shifts out of intracellular fluid.

Dietary sources of potassium

Major dietary sources of potassium include:

- ✦ chocolate
- ✦ dried fruit, nuts, and seeds
- ✦ fruits, such as oranges, bananas, apricots, and cantaloupe
- ✦ meats
- ✦ vegetables, especially beans, potatoes, mushrooms, tomatoes, and carrots.

About 80% of the potassium taken in is excreted in urine, with each liter of urine containing 20 to 40 mEq of the electrolyte. Any remaining potassium is excreted in feces and sweat. Extracellular potassium loss also occurs when potassium moves from the extracellular fluid to the intracellular fluid and when cells undergo anabolism. Three additional factors that affect potassium levels include the sodium-potassium pump, the kidneys, and pH level.

Sodium-potassium pump

The sodium-potassium pump is an active transport mechanism that moves ions across the cell membrane against a concentration gradient. Specifically, the pump moves sodium from the cell into the extracellular fluid and maintains high intracellular potassium levels by pumping potassium into the cell.

The kidneys

The body also rids itself of excess potassium through the kidneys. As serum potassium levels rise, the renal tubules excrete more potassium, leading to increased potassium loss in urine.

Sodium and potassium have a reciprocal relationship. The kidneys reabsorb sodium and excrete potassium when the hormone aldosterone is secreted. The kidneys, however, have no effective mechanism to combat loss of potassium and may excrete it even when the serum potassium level is low. Even when potassium intake is zero, the kidneys will excrete 10 to 15 mEq/day.

pH level

A change in pH may affect serum potassium levels because hydrogen ions (H^+) and potassium ions (K) freely exchange across plasma cell mem-

Maintaining potassium balance *(continued)*

- ✦ About 80% of potassium taken in excreted in urine (remaining potassium excreted in feces and sweat)
- ✦ Levels affected by sodium-potassium pump, kidneys, and pH level

Sodium potassium pump

- ✦ Active transport mechanism
- ✦ Moves sodium from cell into intracellular fluid
- ✦ Maintains high intracellular potassium levels by pumping potassium into cell

Kidneys

- ✦ Eliminate excess potassium by excreting more via renal tubules (causing increased potassium loss in urine) as levels rise

pH level

- ✦ Change in level may affect serum potassium levels because H^+ and K freely exchange across plasma cell membranes
- ✦ Acidosis can cause hyperkalemia
- ✦ Alkalosis can cause hypokalemia

branes. For example, in acidosis, excess H^+ move into cells and push K into the extracellular fluid. Thus, acidosis can cause hyperkalemia as potassium moves out of the cell to maintain balance. Likewise, alkalosis can cause hypokalemia by increasing potassium movement into the cell to maintain balance.

Hypokalemia
- Indicated by serum potassium level < 3.5 mEq/L
- Moderate hypokalemia: 2.5 to 3 mEq/L
- Severe hypokalemia: < 2.5 mEq/L

Pathophysiology
- Body can't conserve potassium, allowing inadequate intake and excessive output of potassium to create moderate deficit
- Makes potassium levels vulnerable to prolonged intestinal suctioning and ileostomy

Causes

Inadequate potassium intake
- Diet deficient in potassium-rich foods
- Potassium-deficient I.V. fluids
- Total parenteral nutrition that lacks adequate potassium supplementation

Excessive potassium output
- Intestinal fluids contain large amounts of potassium
- Levels can be depleted by severe GI fluid losses from suctioning, prolonged vomiting, diarrhea, or laxative abuse
- In elderly patients, most common causes include diuretic therapy, diarrhea, and chronic laxative abuse

HYPOKALEMIA

In hypokalemia, the serum potassium level drops below 3.5 mEq/L. Because the normal range for a serum potassium level is narrow (3.5 to 5 mEq/L), a slight decrease has profound effects. Moderate hypokalemia is a serum potassium level of 2.5 to 3 mEq/L. Severe hypokalemia is a serum potassium level less than 2.5 mEq/L.

Causes and pathophysiology

Because the body can't conserve potassium, inadequate intake and excessive output of potassium can cause a moderate drop in its level, upsetting the balance and causing a potassium deficiency in the body.

Conditions, such as prolonged intestinal suction, recent ileostomy, and villous adenoma can cause a decrease in the body's overall potassium level. In certain situations, potassium shifts from the extracellular space to the intracellular space and hides in the cells. Because the cells contain more potassium than usual, less can be measured in the blood.

Inadequate potassium intake

Inadequate potassium intake causes a drop in the body's overall potassium level. That could mean a person isn't eating enough potassium-rich foods, is receiving potassium-deficient I.V. fluids, or is getting total parenteral nutrition that lacks adequate potassium supplementation.

Excessive potassium output

Intestinal fluids contain large amounts of potassium. Severe GI fluid losses from suction, lavage, or prolonged vomiting can deplete the body's potassium supply, thereby dropping the body's potassium level. Diarrhea, fistulas, laxative abuse, and severe diaphoresis also contribute to potassium loss.

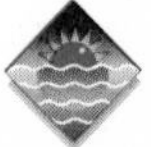

AGE ALERT *In elderly patients, the most common causes of hypokalemia are diuretic therapy, diarrhea, and chronic laxative abuse. Elderly patients who can't cook for themselves or can't chew and swallow may also have poor potassium intake.*

Drugs associated with hypokalemia

The drugs listed below can deplete potassium and cause hypokalemia:

- ✦ adrenergics, such as albuterol (Proventil) and epinephrine (Bronkaid)
- ✦ antibiotics, such as amphotericin B (Fungizone) and gentamicin (Garamycin)
- ✦ cisplatin (Platinol-AQ)
- ✦ corticosteroids
- ✦ diuretics, such as furosemide (Lasix) and thiazides
- ✦ insulin
- ✦ laxatives (when used excessively).

Potassium can also be depleted through the kidneys. Diuresis that occurs with a newly functioning transplanted kidney can lead to hypokalemia. High urine glucose levels cause osmotic diuresis, and potassium is lost through urine. Other potassium losses are seen in renal tubular acidosis, magnesium depletion, Cushing's syndrome, and during periods of high stress.

Other causes

Drugs, such as diuretics (especially thiazide and furosemide [Lasix]), corticosteroids, insulin, cisplatin (Platinol-AQ), and certain antibiotics (gentamicin [Garamycin] and amphotericin B [Fungizone], for instance), also cause potassium loss. (See *Drugs associated with hypokalemia.*)

Excessive secretion of insulin, whether endogenous or exogenous, may shift potassium into the cells. Insulin can be released from the body and cause hypokalemia in patients receiving large amounts of dextrose solutions. Potassium levels also drop when adrenergics, such as epinephrine (Bronkaid) or albuterol (Proventil), are used to treat asthma.

Conditions such as vomiting that lead to the loss of gastric acids can cause alkalosis and hypokalemia. Alkalosis moves K into the cell as H^+ move out. Other disorders associated with hypokalemia are hepatic disease, hyperaldosteronism, acute alcoholism, heart failure, malabsorption syndrome, nephritis, Bartter's syndrome, and acute leukemias.

Assessment findings

The signs and symptoms of a low potassium level reflect how important the electrolyte is to normal body functions. Neuromuscular problems — such as skeletal muscle weakness, especially in the legs — are signs of a

Causes *(continued)*

- ✦ Excessive potassium output
- ✦ Potassium can deplete through kidneys; factors include diuresis that occurs with newly functioning transplanted kidney and osmotic diuresis

Other causes

- ✦ Excessive insulin secretion (endogenous or exogenous) may shift potassium into cells
- ✦ Conditions such as vomiting that lead to loss of gastric acids

Assessment findings

- ✦ Skeletal muscle weakness (especially in legs)
- ✦ Leg cramps
- ✦ Decreased or absent deep tendon reflexes

Assessment findings *(continued)*

Cardiac abnormalities
- Weak, irregular pulse
- Orthostatic hypotension
- In moderate to severe hypokalemia: ventricular arrhythmias, ectopic beats, bradycardia, tachycardia, cardiac arrest

ECG changes
- Flattened or inverted T wave
- Depressed ST segment
- Characteristic U wave

moderate potassium loss. Weakness progresses, and paresthesia develops and leg cramps occur. Deep tendon reflexes may be decreased or absent. Rarely, paralysis could involve the respiratory muscles. If respiratory muscles become weak, the patient may also be tachycardic and tachypneic. Because potassium affects cell function, hypokalemia can lead to rhabdomyolysis, a breakdown of muscle fibers leading to myoglobin in the urine. As hypokalemia affects smooth muscle, the patient may develop anorexia, nausea, and vomiting.

Intestinal problems include decreased bowel sounds, constipation, and paralytic ileus. The patient may also have difficulty concentrating urine (when hypokalemia is prolonged) and pass large volumes of urine.

Cardiac problems can result from a low potassium level. The patient's pulse may be weak and irregular and he may have orthostatic hypotension or experience palpitations. The electrocardiogram (ECG) may show a flattened or inverted T wave, a depressed ST segment, and a characteristic U wave. In moderate to severe hypokalemia, ventricular arrhythmias, ectopic beats, bradycardia, tachycardia, and full cardiac arrest may occur.

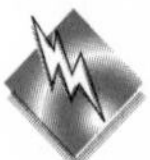

DANGER *A patient taking digoxin (Lanoxin), especially if he's also taking a diuretic, should be closely watched for hypokalemia, which can potentiate the action of digoxin and cause a toxic reaction. (See* Warning signs of hypokalemia.*)*

Diagnostic test results

- Serum potassium level < 3.5 mEq/L
- Characteristic ECG changes
- Decreased serum magnesium level

Diagnostic test results

Typical laboratory findings for a patient with hypokalemia include:
- serum potassium level less than 3.5 mEq/L
- increased 24-hour urine level
- elevated pH and bicarbonate levels
- slightly elevated serum glucose level
- characteristic ECG changes
- decreased serum magnesium level
- increased digoxin level (if patient is taking the drug).

Treatment

- Focuses on restoring potassium balance, preventing serious complications, and removing or treating underlying causes
- High-potassium, low-sodium diet

TREATMENT

Treatment for hypokalemia focuses on restoring a normal potassium balance, preventing serious complications, and removing or treating the underlying causes. Treatment varies depending on the severity of the imbalance and the underlying cause:
- Place the patient on a high-potassium, low-sodium diet. (Increasing the intake of dietary potassium may be insufficient to treat less acute hy-

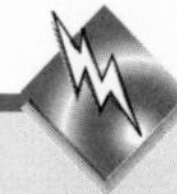

DANGER

Warning signs of hypokalemia

Begin emergency treatment for hypokalemia if a patient shows any of these signs and symptoms:

- ✦ arrhythmias
- ✦ cardiac arrest
- ✦ digoxin toxicity
- ✦ muscle paralysis
- ✦ paralytic ileus
- ✦ respiratory arrest.

pokalemia. The patient may need oral potassium supplementation using potassium salts, in which case potassium chloride is preferred.)

✦ Treat the patient who has severe hypokalemia or who can't take oral supplements with I.V. potassium replacement therapy. Oral and parenteral potassium can be safely given at the same time. Whether through a peripheral or a central catheter, administer I.V. potassium with care to prevent serious complications.

After the serum potassium level returns to normal, the patient may receive a sustained-release oral potassium supplement and may need to increase his dietary intake of potassium. Also, after the underlying cause of the hypokalemia has been determined and treated, make sure the treatment plan is adequate and implemented. A patient taking a diuretic may be switched to a potassium-sparing diuretic to prevent excessive loss of potassium in the urine.

Treatment *(continued)*

- ✦ I.V. potassium replacement therapy (for patient with severe hypokalemia or who can't take oral supplements)
- ✦ Potassium-sparing diuretic (for patient taking diuretic)

Nursing interventions

Careful monitoring and skilled interventions can help prevent hypokalemia and spare your patient from its associated complications. For a patient who's at risk for developing hypokalemia or who already has hypokalemia, you'll want to perform these actions:

✦ Monitor vital signs, especially pulse and blood pressure, because hypokalemia is commonly associated with hypovolemia, which can cause orthostatic hypotension.

✦ Check heart rate and rhythm and ECG tracings in a patient with a serum potassium level less than 3 mEq/L (severe hypokalemia) because

Key nursing interventions

- ✦ Monitor vital signs, especially pulse and blood pressure
- ✦ Check heart rate and rhythm and ECG tracings

Raising potassium levels

If you're having difficulty raising a patient's potassium level, reevaluate his fluid and electrolyte status and ask yourself these questions:

- Is the patient still experiencing diuresis or suffering losses from the GI tract or the skin? If so, he's losing fluid and potassium.
- Is the patient's magnesium level normal, or does he need supplementation? Keep in mind that low magnesium levels make it difficult for the kidneys to conserve potassium.

Key nursing interventions *(continued)*

- Assess respiratory rate, depth, and pattern
- Monitor serum potassium levels
- Monitor and document fluid intake and output
- Administer I.V. potassium replacement solutions as prescribed
- Administer I.V. potassium infusions cautiously
- Administer oral potassium supplements with fluid or food to prevent gastric irritation

hypokalemia is commonly associated with hypovolemia, which may create tachyarrhythmias.

✦ Assess the patient's respiratory rate, depth, and pattern. Hypokalemia may weaken or paralyze respiratory muscles. Notify the physician immediately if respirations become shallow and rapid. Keep a handheld resuscitation bag at the bedside of a patient with severe hypokalemia. (See *Raising potassium levels.*)

✦ Monitor serum potassium levels. Changes in serum potassium levels can lead to serious cardiac complications.

✦ Assess the patient for clinical evidence of hypokalemia, especially if he's receiving a diuretic or digoxin. A patient who has hypokalemia and takes digoxin is at increased risk for digoxin toxicity because the body has less potassium with which to work (potassium is needed to balance the level of digoxin in the blood).

✦ Monitor and document fluid intake and output. About 40 mEq of potassium is lost in each liter of urine. Diuresis can put the patient at risk for potassium loss.

✦ Check for signs of hypokalemia-related metabolic alkalosis, including irritability and paresthesia.

✦ Insert and maintain patent I.V. access as ordered. When choosing a vein, remember that I.V. potassium preparations can irritate peripheral veins and cause discomfort.

✦ Administer I.V. potassium replacement solutions as prescribed. (See *Guidelines for I.V. potassium administration.*)

✦ Monitor heart rate and rhythm and ECG tracings of the patient receiving a potassium infusion of more than 5 mEq/hour or a concentration of more than 40 mEq/L of fluid.

Guidelines for I.V. potassium administration

When administering I.V. potassium, there are several guidelines and monitoring points you should follow. Remember, potassium only needs to be replaced using an I.V. line if hypokalemia is severe or if the patient can't take oral potassium supplements.

Administration

- When adding the potassium preparation to an I.V. solution, mix well. Don't add it to a hanging container; the potassium will pool, and the patient will receive a highly concentrated bolus. Use premixed potassium when possible.
- To prevent or reduce toxic effects, I.V. infusion concentrations shouldn't exceed 60 mEq/L. Rates are usually 10 mEq/hour. More rapid infusions may be used in severe cases; however, rapid infusion requires closer monitoring of cardiac status. A rapid rise in serum potassium levels can lead to hyperkalemia, resulting in cardiac complications. The maximum adult dose generally shouldn't exceed 200 mEq/24 hours unless prescribed.
- Use infusion devices when administering potassium solutions to control flow rate.
- Never administer potassium by I.V. push or bolus; doing so can cause arrhythmias and cardiac arrest.

Patient monitoring

- Monitor the patient's cardiac rhythm during rapid I.V. potassium administration to prevent toxic effects from hyperkalemia. Report irregularities immediately.
- Evaluate the results of treatment by checking serum potassium levels and assessing the patient for signs and symptoms of toxic reaction, such as muscle weakness and paralysis.
- Watch the I.V. site for signs and symptoms of infiltration, phlebitis, or tissue necrosis.
- Monitor the patient's urine output and notify the physician if volume is inadequate. Urine output should exceed 30 ml/hour to avoid hyperkalemia.
- Repeat potassium level measurements every 1 to 3 hours.

- Administer I.V. potassium infusions cautiously. Make sure that infusions are diluted and mixed thoroughly in adequate amounts of fluid. Use premixed potassium solutions when possible.
- Watch the I.V. infusion site for infiltration.

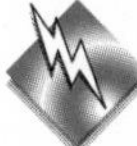

DANGER *Never give potassium by I.V. push or as a bolus. Instead, give it slowly as a dilute solution. Too rapid an infusion may result in potentially fatal hyperkalemia.*

Administering I.V. potassium

Administration

- Mix potassium preparation and I.V. solution well
- To reduce toxic effects, make sure I.V infusion concentrations don't exceed 60 mEq/L
- Use infusion devices
- Never administer by I.V. push or bolus

Patient monitoring

- Cardiac rhythm
- Serum potassium levels
- Signs and symptoms of toxic reaction
- Signs and symptoms of infiltration, phlebitis, and tissue necrosis
- Urine output

CHARTING CHECKLIST

Documenting hypokalemia

If your patient has hypokalemia, make sure you document:

- ❑ assessment findings
- ❑ vital signs (including arrhythmias)
- ❑ serum potassium level and other pertinent laboratory data
- ❑ intake and output
- ❑ notification of the physician
- ❑ potassium supplements given and method of administration
- ❑ nursing interventions and the patient's response
- ❑ safety measures implemented
- ❑ patient teaching provided and the patient's response.

✦ To prevent gastric irritation from oral potassium supplements, administer the supplements in at least 4 oz (118.3 ml) of fluid or with food.
✦ To prevent a quick load of potassium from entering the body, don't crush slow-release tablets.
✦ Use the same care when giving an oral supplement as you would when administering an I.V. supplement.
✦ Provide a safe environment for the patient who's weak from hypokalemia. Explain imposed activity restrictions.
✦ Check for signs of constipation, such as abdominal distention and decreased bowel sounds. Although medication may be prescribed to combat constipation, don't use laxatives that promote potassium loss. (See *Documenting hypokalemia.*)
✦ Emphasize the importance of taking potassium supplements as prescribed, especially when the patient is also taking digoxin or a diuretic. If appropriate, teach the patient to recognize and report signs and symptoms of digoxin toxicity, such as pulse irregularities, anorexia, nausea, and vomiting.

Patient teaching

- ✦ Description of disorder
- ✦ Causes and risk factors
- ✦ Prevention
- ✦ Medications
- ✦ Diet
- ✦ Warning signs and symptoms

Patient teaching

Be sure to cover these topics and then evaluate your patient's learning:
✦ explanation of hypokalemia, including its signs, symptoms, and complications
✦ causes and risk factors
✦ prevention of future episodes

- medication, including dosages and possible adverse effects
- need for a potassium-rich diet
- warning signs and symptoms and when to report them.

HYPERKALEMIA

Hyperkalemia occurs when the serum potassium level rises above 5 mEq/L. Because the normal serum potassium range is so narrow (3.5 to 5 mEq/L), a slight increase can have profound effects. Moderate hyperkalemia occurs when the potassium level ranges from 6.1 to 7 mEq/L. Severe hyperkalemia occurs when the level is greater than 7 mEq/L. Although less common than hypokalemia, hyperkalemia is more serious. Treatments for other conditions are commonly the cause of hyperkalemia.

CAUSES AND PATHOPHYSIOLOGY

Potassium is gained through intake and lost by excretion; if either is altered, hyperkalemia can result. The kidneys, which excrete potassium, are vital in preventing a toxic buildup of this electrolyte. Acid-base imbalances can alter potassium balance as well. Acidosis moves potassium outside the cell as hydrogen ions shift into the cell and inhibits potassium movement into the cell. Cell injury results in release, or spilling, of potassium into the serum, which is reflected in the patient's laboratory test results.

Excessive intake

Increased dietary intake of potassium, especially with decreased urine output, can cause the potassium level to rise. Excessive use of salt substitutes, most of which use potassium as a substitute for sodium, further compounds the situation. Potassium supplements, whether oral or I.V., raise the potassium level. Excessive doses can lead to hyperkalemia.

Transfusions and drugs

The serum potassium level of donated blood increases the longer the blood is stored. Therefore, a patient's potassium level may rise if he's given a large volume of donated blood that's nearing its expiration date.

Certain medications are associated with high potassium levels, such as beta-adrenergic blockers, which inhibit potassium shifts into cells, potassium-sparing diuretics such as spironolactone (Aldactone), and

Hyperkalemia

- Indicated by serum potassium level > 5 mEq/L
- Moderate hyperkalemia: 6.1 to 7 mEq/L
- Severe hyperkalemia: > 7 mEq/L

Pathophysiology

- Acidosis moves potassium outside cell as hydrogen ions shift into cell, inhibiting potassium movement into cell
- Cell injury results in release (spilling) of potassium into serum

Causes

Excessive intake

- Increased dietary intake of sodium
- Excessive use of salt substitutes (most substitute potassium for sodium)
- Potassium supplements (oral and I.V.)

Transfusions and drugs

- Potassium level of donated blood high as it nears its expiration date
- Beta-adrenergic blockers
- Potassium-sparing diuretics
- Certain antibiotics
- ACE inhibitors
- NSAIDs

Drugs associated with hyperkalemia

The drugs listed below can cause increased potassium levels. Ask your patient if any of these are a part of his drug therapy:

- ✦ angiotensin-converting enzyme inhibitors
- ✦ antibiotics
- ✦ beta-adrenergic blockers
- ✦ chemotherapeutic drugs
- ✦ digoxin
- ✦ heparin
- ✦ nonsteroidal anti-inflammatory drugs
- ✦ potassium (in excessive amounts)
- ✦ potassium-sparing diuretics (such as spironolactone).

some antibiotics such as penicillin G potassium. Chemotherapy, which causes cell death and sometimes renal injury, can lead to hyperkalemia.

Angiotensin-converting enzyme (ACE) inhibitors, nonsteroidal anti-inflammatory drugs (NSAIDs), and heparin are thought to cause hyperkalemia by influencing aldosterone secretion, which promotes potassium excretion in the kidneys. When administering any medication that can cause renal injury, such as an aminoglycoside, monitor the patient for hyperkalemia. (See *Drugs associated with hyperkalemia.*)

Causes *(continued)*

Inadequate output

- ✦ Acute or chronic renal failure (diminishes potassium excretion)
- ✦ Diabetes or sickle cell disease (can cause kidney damage)

Inadequate output

Potassium excretion is diminished with acute or chronic renal failure. Any disease that can cause kidney damage, including diabetes, sickle cell disease, or systemic lupus erythematosus, can lead to hyperkalemia. Addison's disease and hypoaldosteronism can also decrease potassium excretion from the body.

AGE ALERT *Premature neonates and elderly patients are at greatest risk for hyperkalemia. Premature neonates are at risk because of their immature renal function; they commonly experience hyperkalemia within the first 48 hours of life. People older than age 60 are at high risk because their renal function deteriorates with age, renal blood flow decreases, and oral fluid intake decreases, thereby decreasing urine flow rates. Their plasma renin activity and aldosterone levels also decrease with age, thus decreasing their ability to excrete potassium. In addition, they're more likely to take medications, such as NSAIDs, ACE inhibitors, and potassium-sparing diuretics that interfere with potassium excretion. Those who are bedridden may be placed on subcutaneous heparin, which also decreases aldosterone production.*

Verifying potassium test results

When a laboratory test result indicates that your patient has a high serum potassium level, and the result just doesn't seem to make sense, verify that it's a true result. If the sample was drawn using poor technique, the results may be falsely high. Some of the causes of high potassium levels that don't truly reflect the patient's serum potassium level include:

- drawing the sample above an I.V. infusion containing potassium
- using a recently exercised extremity for the venipuncture site
- causing hemolysis (cell damage) as the sample is obtained.

Cell injury

When a burn, severe infection, trauma, crush injury, or intravascular hemolysis has injured a cell, potassium may leave the cell. Chemotherapy causes cell lysis and the release of potassium. Metabolic acidosis and insulin deficiency decrease the movement of potassium into cells. (See *Verifying potassium test results.*)

Causes *(continued)*

Cell injury

- Burn
- Severe infection
- Chemotherapy

Assessment findings

Signs and symptoms of hyperkalemia reflect its effects on neuromuscular and cardiac functioning in the body. Paresthesia, an early symptom, and irritability signal hyperkalemia.

Neuromuscular problems include skeletal muscle weakness that, in turn, may lead to flaccid paralysis. Deep tendon reflexes may be decreased. Muscle weakness tends to spread from the legs to the trunk and involves respiratory muscles. Hyperkalemia also causes smooth-muscle hyperactivity, particularly in the GI tract, which can result in nausea, abdominal cramping, and diarrhea, an early sign.

Cardiac complications include a decreased heart rate, irregular pulse, decreased cardiac output, hypotension and, possibly, cardiac arrest. The tall, tented T wave is a prominent electrocardiogram (ECG) characteristic of the patient with hyperkalemia. Other ECG changes include a flattened P wave, prolonged PR interval, bundle-branch blocks causing widened QRS complex, and depressed ST segment. In the late phase, seen in prolonged hyperkalemic states, the QRS complex and T wave may combine to form a biphasic or "sine" wave, which precedes ventricular standstill. The condition can also lead to heart block, ventricular arrhythmias, and

Assessment findings

- Paresthesia
- Irritability

Neuromuscular

- Skeletal muscle weakness
- Decreased deep tendon reflexes

Cardiac

- Decreased heart rate
- Irregular pulse
- Decreased cardiac output
- Hypotension
- Cardiac arrest

ECG

- Tall, tented T wave
- Biphasic (sine) wave preceding ventricular standstill (formed by QRS complex and T wave)

asystole. The more serious arrhythmias become especially dangerous when serum potassium levels reach 7 mEq/L or more.

Diagnostic test results
- Serum potassium level > 5 mEq/L
- ECG abnormalities

Diagnostic test results

Typical laboratory findings for a patient with hyperkalemia include:
- serum potassium level greater than 5 mEq/L
- decreased arterial pH, indicating acidosis
- ECG abnormalities.

Treatment
- Aimed at lowering potassium level, treating its cause, stabilizing myocardium, and promoting renal and GI potassium excretion

Sodium polystyrene sulfonate
- Common treatment
- Can be administered orally, through nasogastric tube, or through retention enema
- 4-to-6–hour duration of action
- Causes potassium excretion in loose stools

Mild hyperkalemia
- Loop diuretic
- Dietary potassium restriction
- Readjustment or restriction of medications associated with high potassium levels

Moderate to severe hyperkalemia
- Hemodialysis

Emergency treatment
- For more severe hyperkalemia
- ECGs to monitor progress
- 10% calcium gluconate or 10% calcium chloride to counteract myocardial effects of hyperkalemia
- Patient must be connected to cardiac monitor
- I.V. sodium bicarbonate for patient with acidosis

TREATMENT

Treatment for hyperkalemia is aimed at lowering the potassium level, treating its cause, stabilizing the myocardium, and promoting renal and GI excretion of potassium. The severity of hyperkalemia dictates how it will be treated.

Sodium polystyrene sulfonate (Kayexalate), a cation-exchange resin, is a common treatment for hyperkalemia. Sorbitol, or another osmotic substance, should be given with this medication to promote its excretion. Kayexalate can be given orally, through a nasogastric tube, or as a retention enema (may require repeated treatments). The onset of action may take several hours; the duration of action is 4 to 6 hours. As the medication sits in the intestines, sodium moves across the bowel wall into the blood, and potassium moves out of the blood into the intestines. Loose stools remove potassium from the body.

Mild hyperkalemia may be treated with a loop diuretic to increase potassium loss from the body or to resolve any acidosis present. Dietary potassium is restricted. Medications associated with high potassium level should be readjusted or stopped. Underlying disorders leading to the high potassium level are treated.

With moderate to severe hyperkalemia, other measures may be undertaken. If the patient has renal failure, a diuretic may not be effective. For acute symptom-producing hyperkalemia, hemodialysis may be required.

More severe hyperkalemia is treated as an emergency. Closely monitor the patient's cardiac status. ECGs are obtained to follow progress. To counteract the myocardial effects of hyperkalemia, administer 10% calcium gluconate or 10% calcium chloride I.V. over 2 minutes. The patient must be connected to a cardiac monitor. However, calcium gluconate isn't a treatment for hyperkalemia itself, and the hyperkalemia must still be treated because the effects of calcium last only a short time. (See *Comparing calcium chloride and calcium gluconate.*)

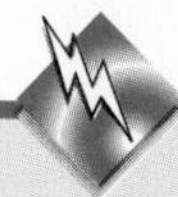

DANGER

Comparing calcium chloride and calcium gluconate

Either calcium chloride or calcium gluconate may be ordered to counteract the myocardial effects of hyperkalemia. However, there's a distinct difference between the two: One ampule of calcium chloride has three times more calcium than calcium gluconate. Therefore, when preparing a dose for administration, check the order and carefully read the label. If bradycardia develops during administration, stop either type of infusion.

A patient with acidosis may receive sodium bicarbonate I.V., which helps decrease the serum potassium level by temporarily shifting potassium into the cells. The drug becomes effective within 15 to 30 minutes and lasts 1 to 3 hours. These alkalinizing agents may be given with insulin to enhance the insulin's effects, raising blood pH.

Another method of moving potassium into the cells and lowering the serum level in patients with severe hyperkalemia is to administer 10 units of regular insulin I.V. The drug becomes active within 15 to 60 minutes and lasts 4 to 6 hours. It's given with I.V. hypertonic dextrose (10% to 50% glucose).

Nursing interventions

Patients at risk for hyperkalemia require frequent monitoring of serum potassium and other electrolyte levels. Those at risk include patients with acidosis or renal failure and those receiving a potassium-sparing diuretic, an oral potassium supplement, or an I.V. potassium preparation. If a patient develops hyperkalemia, take these nursing actions:

✦ Assess vital signs. Anticipate cardiac monitoring if the patient's serum potassium level exceeds 6 mEq/L. A patient with ECG changes may need aggressive treatment to prevent cardiac arrest.

✦ Monitor the patient's intake and output. Report an output of less than 30 ml/hour. An inability to excrete potassium adequately may lead to dangerously high potassium levels. (See *Lowering potassium levels,* page 100.)

✦ Prepare to administer a slow calcium chloride or calcium gluconate I.V. infusion in a patient with acute hyperkalemia to counteract its myocardial depressant effects.

Key nursing interventions

✦ Monitor patients with hyperkalemia (and those at risk for developing it)
✦ Assess vital signs
✦ Monitor intake and output
✦ Administer slow calcium chloride or calcium gluconate I.V. infusion in patient with acute hyperkalemia

Lowering potassium levels

If you can't bring down your patient's potassium level as expected, ask yourself these questions:

- ✦ Is the patient taking an antacid? Antacids containing magnesium or calcium can interfere with ion exchange resins.
- ✦ Is the patient's renal status worsening?
- ✦ Is the patient taking a medication that could raise the potassium level?
- ✦ Is the patient receiving old donated blood during transfusions?

Key nursing interventions *(continued)*

- ✦ Monitor for signs and symptoms of hypoglycemia in patient receiving repeated insulin and glucose treatment
- ✦ Monitor serum potassium level
- ✦ Monitor digoxin level if appropriate
- ✦ Prepare patient with acute hyperkalemia for dialysis if unresponsive to other treatments
- ✦ Implement safety measures if patient has muscle weakness
- ✦ Help patient select low-potassium foods

✦ For a patient receiving repeated insulin and glucose treatment, check for clinical signs and symptoms of hypoglycemia, including muscle weakness, syncope, hunger, and diaphoresis.

✦ Keep in mind when giving Kayexalate that serum sodium levels may rise. Watch for signs of heart failure.

✦ Monitor bowel sounds and the number and character of bowel movements. Hyperactive bowel sounds result from the body's attempt to maintain homeostasis by causing significant potassium excretion through the bowels.

✦ Monitor the serum potassium level and related laboratory test results. A patient with a serum potassium level exceeding 6 mEq/L requires cardiac monitoring because asystole may occur as hyperkalemia makes depolarization of cardiac muscle easier and shortens repolarization times.

✦ Monitor the patient's digoxin level if he's taking this medication. The patient may be at risk for digoxin toxicity.

✦ Administer prescribed medications and monitor the patient for their effectiveness and for adverse effects.

✦ Encourage the patient to retain Kayexalate enemas for 30 to 60 minutes. Monitor the patient for hypokalemia when administering this drug on 2 or more consecutive days.

✦ If the patient has acute hyperkalemia that doesn't respond to other treatments, prepare him for dialysis.

✦ If the patient has muscle weakness, implement safety measures. Advise him to ask for help before attempting to get out of bed and walk. Continue to evaluate muscle strength.

✦ Administer prescribed antidiarrheals and monitor the patient's response.

✦ Help the patient select foods low in potassium.

CHARTING CHECKLIST

Documenting hyperkalemia

If your patient has hyperkalemia, make sure you document:

- ❑ assessment findings
- ❑ vital signs (including arrhythmias)
- ❑ serum potassium level and other pertinent laboratory test results
- ❑ intake and output
- ❑ notification of physician
- ❑ medications administered
- ❑ nursing interventions and the patient's response
- ❑ safety measures implemented
- ❑ patient teaching provided and the patient's response.

✦ If the patient has hyperkalemia and needs a transfusion, obtain fresh blood.

✦ Watch for signs of hypokalemia after treatment.

✦ Document all care given and the patient's response. (See *Documenting hyperkalemia.*)

✦ Explain the signs and symptoms of hyperkalemia, including muscle weakness, diarrhea, and pulse irregularities. Urge the patient to report such signs and symptoms to the physician.

✦ Describe the signs and symptoms of hypokalemia to the patient if he's taking medication to lower his serum potassium level.

Key nursing interventions ***(continued)***

✦ Describe signs and symptoms of hypokalemia if patient is taking medication to lower serum potassium level

Patient teaching

Be sure to cover these topics and then evaluate your patient's learning:

✦ explanation of hyperkalemia, including its signs, symptoms, and complications

✦ medication, including dosage and potential for hypokalemia

✦ need for a potassium-restricted diet and importance of avoiding salt substitutes

✦ prevention of future episodes of hyperkalemia

✦ warning signs and symptoms and when to report them.

Patient teaching

✦ Description of disorder
✦ Medications
✦ Diet
✦ Prevention
✦ Warning signs and symptoms

Magnesium imbalances

MAGNESIUM

After potassium, magnesium is the most abundant cation in the intracellular fluid. The bones contain about 60% of the body's magnesium, extracellular fluid contains less than 1%, and intracellular fluid holds the rest.

Magnesium

- Second most abundant cation in intracellular fluid

Functions of magnesium

Magnesium performs many important functions in the body. For example, it:

- promotes enzyme reactions within the cell during carbohydrate metabolism
- helps the body produce and use adenosine triphosphate for energy
- takes part in deoxyribonucleic acid and protein synthesis
- influences vasodilation, and irritability and contractility of the cardiac muscles, thereby helping the cardiovascular system function normally
- aids in neurotransmission and hormone-receptor binding
- makes the production of parathyroid hormone (PTH) possible
- helps sodium and potassium ions cross the cell membrane (this is why magnesium affects sodium and potassium ion levels both inside and outside the cell).

Functions

- Produces and uses adenosine triphosphate for energy
- Influences vasodilation and irritability and contractility of cardiac muscles
- Aids in neurotransmission and hormone-receptor binding
- Makes production of PTH possible
- Helps sodium and potassium ions cross cell membrane

Regulating muscle movements

Magnesium also regulates muscle contractions, making it especially vital to the neuromuscular system. By acting on the myoneural junctions — the sites where nerve and muscle fibers meet — magnesium affects the irritability and contractility of cardiac and skeletal muscle. A recent study, in fact, concluded that patients with vascular disease and low magnesium levels are at greater risk for neuromuscular problems.

Influencing calcium levels

Magnesium influences the body's calcium level through its effect on PTH, which maintains a constant calcium level in extracellular fluid.

Interpreting magnesium levels

Keep the magnesium-calcium connection in mind when assessing a patient's laboratory values. However, your patient's serum magnesium level itself may be misleading. Normally, the body's total serum magnesium level is 1.8 to 2.5 mEq/L.

AGE ALERT *Don't forget that magnesium levels in neonates and children are different from those of adults. In neonates, magnesium levels range from 1.4 to 2.9 mEq/L; in children, 1.6 to 2.6 mEq/L.*

The magnesium level may not accurately reflect your patient's actual magnesium stores. That's because most magnesium is found within cells, where it measures about 40 mEq/L. In serum, magnesium levels are relatively low.

Interpreting a patient's serum magnesium level can be a challenge. More than half of circulating magnesium moves in a free, ionized form. Another 30% binds with a protein — mostly albumin — and the remainder binds with other substances. Ionized magnesium is physiologically active and must be regulated to maintain homeostasis. However, this form alone can't be measured, so a patient's measured levels reflect the total amount of circulating magnesium.

To complicate matters, magnesium levels are linked to albumin levels. A patient with a low serum albumin level will have a low total serum magnesium level — even if the level of ionized magnesium remains unchanged. That's why serum albumin levels need to be measured with serum magnesium levels.

Serum calcium and certain other laboratory values also come into play when assessing and treating magnesium imbalances. Because magnesium is mainly an intracellular electrolyte, changes in the levels of other intra-

Interpreting magnesium levels

- Normal total serum magnesium level in adults: 1.8 to 2.5 mEq/L; in neonates, 1.4 to 2.9 mEq/L; in children, 1.6 to 2.6 mEq/L
- Affected by serum albumin, calcium, potassium, and phosphorus levels

Dietary sources of magnesium

Most healthy people can get all the magnesium they need by eating a well-balanced diet that includes such magnesium-rich foods as:
- chocolate
- dry beans and peas
- green, leafy vegetables
- meats
- nuts
- seafood
- whole grains.

cellular electrolytes, such as potassium and phosphorus, can also affect serum magnesium levels.

Regulating magnesium

Regulating magnesium
- Well-balanced diet should provide 25 mEq/L of magnesium daily
- If serum magnesium levels rise, GI tract and kidneys excrete more
- If serum magnesium levels drop, GI tract absorbs more and kidneys conserve supplies

The body's GI and urinary systems regulate magnesium through absorption, excretion, and retention — that is, through dietary intake and output in urine and stools. A well-balanced diet should provide roughly 25 mEq (or 300 to 350 mg) of magnesium daily. (See *Dietary sources of magnesium.*) Of this amount, about 40% is absorbed in the small intestine.

The body tries to adjust to any change in the magnesium level. For instance, if the serum magnesium level drops, the GI tract may absorb more magnesium and, if the magnesium level rises, the GI tract excretes more in stools.

The kidneys balance magnesium by altering its reabsorption at the proximal tubule and loop of Henle. So, if serum magnesium levels climb, the kidneys excrete the excess in the urine. Diuretics heighten this effect. Likewise, if serum magnesium levels fall, the kidneys conserve magnesium. That conservation is so efficient that the daily loss of circulating ionized magnesium can be restricted to just 1 mEq.

HYPOMAGNESEMIA

Hypomagnesemia
- Serum magnesium level < 1.8 mEq/L
- Most common in patients who are critically ill

Hypomagnesemia occurs when the body's serum magnesium level falls below 1.8 mEq/L. Although sometimes overlooked, this imbalance is relatively common, affecting about 10% of all hospitalized patients. It's

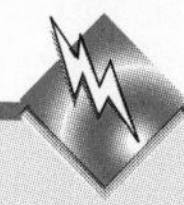

DANGER

Critical signs of low magnesium levels

Your patient with hypomagnesemia is in imminent danger if he has any of these late-developing signs or symptoms:
- ✦ cardiac arrhythmias
- ✦ digoxin (Lanoxin) toxicity
- ✦ laryngeal stridor
- ✦ respiratory muscle weakness
- ✦ seizures.

most common among critically ill patients. (See *Critical signs of low magnesium levels.*)

Most symptoms of hypomagnesemia occur when the magnesium level drops below 1 mEq/L. Symptoms tend to be nonspecific but may include hyperactive deep tendon reflexes (DTRs), weakness, muscle cramping, rapid heartbeats, tremors, vertigo, ataxia, and depression.

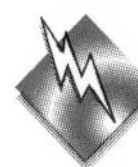

DANGER *At its worst, hypomagnesemia can lead to respiratory muscle paralysis, complete heart block, altered mental status, or coma.*

Causes and pathophysiology

Any condition that impairs either of the body's magnesium regulators — the GI system or the urinary system — can lead to a magnesium shortage. These conditions fall into four main categories:
- ✦ poor dietary intake of magnesium
- ✦ poor magnesium absorption by the GI tract
- ✦ excessive magnesium loss from the GI tract
- ✦ excessive magnesium loss from the urinary tract.

Chronic alcoholics are at risk for hypomagnesemia because they tend to eat a poor diet. What's worse, alcohol overuse causes the urinary system to excrete more magnesium than normal. Alcoholics can also lose magnesium through poor intestinal absorption or from frequent or prolonged vomiting.

Patients who can't take magnesium orally are at high risk for developing a magnesium deficiency unless they get adequate supplementation. These include patients receiving prolonged I.V. fluid therapy, total par-

Hypomagnesemia *(continued)*

- ✦ Hypomagnesemia can lead to respiratory muscle paralysis, complete heart block, altered mental status, and coma

Causes

Poor dietary intake of magnesium
- ✦ Chronic alcoholics
- ✦ Patients unable to take magnesium orally
- ✦ Patients with diabetes mellitus

Causes *(continued)*

Poor GI absorption of magnesium
- ✦ Malabsorption syndromes
- ✦ Steatorrhea
- ✦ Ulcerative colitis
- ✦ Crohn's disease
- ✦ Bowel resection

Excessive GI loss of magnesium
- ✦ Prolonged diarrhea
- ✦ Fistula drainage
- ✦ Laxative abuse
- ✦ Nasogastric suctioning

Excessive urinary loss of magnesium
- ✦ Primary aldosteronism
- ✦ Hyperparathyroidism
- ✦ Diabetic ketoacidosis
- ✦ Use of amphotericin B, cisplatin, cyclosporine, pentamidine, or aminoglycoside antibiotics
- ✦ Prolonged administration of loop or thiazide diuretics
- ✦ Impaired renal absorption

enteral nutrition, or enteral feeding formulas that contain insufficient magnesium.

Patients who have diabetes mellitus are also at risk for magnesium loss due to osmotic diuresis. A recent study concluded that increased consumption of magnesium-rich foods may help prevent the development of type 2 diabetes mellitus.

Poor GI absorption can occur if a patient's dietary intake seems adequate but his serum magnesium level remains low. Malabsorption syndromes, steatorrhea, ulcerative colitis, and Crohn's disease can diminish magnesium absorption. Surgery to treat these disorders can also reduce absorption. Bowel resection, for example, reduces potential absorption sites by decreasing the surface area within the GI tract. Other conditions that can cause hypomagnesemia from poor GI absorption include cancer, pancreatic insufficiency, and excessive calcium or phosphorus in the GI tract.

GI problems occur because fluids in the GI tract (especially the lower part) contain magnesium. A person who loses a great deal of these fluids — from prolonged diarrhea or fistula drainage, for example — can have a magnesium deficiency. A patient who abuses laxatives or who has a nasogastric tube connected to suction is also at risk. In the latter case, the magnesium is lost from the upper, not the lower, GI tract. Magnesium deficiencies are also commonly seen after bowel resection surgery. In acute pancreatitis, magnesium forms soaps with fatty acids. This process takes some of the magnesium out of circulation, causing serum levels to drop.

Urinary problems caused by greater excretion of magnesium in urine can also lead to a low serum magnesium level. Conditions that boost such excretion include:

- ✦ primary aldosteronism (overproduction of aldosterone, an adrenal hormone)
- ✦ hyperparathyroidism (hyperfunction of the parathyroid glands) or hypoparathyroidism (hypofunction of the parathyroid glands)
- ✦ diabetic ketoacidosis
- ✦ use of amphotericin B (Fungizone), cisplatin (Platinol-AQ), cyclosporine (Sandimmune), pentamidine isethionate (NebuPent), or aminoglycoside antibiotics, such as tobramycin (Nebcin) or gentamicin (Garamycin)
- ✦ prolonged administration of loop or thiazide diuretics (see *Drugs associated with hypomagnesemia*)

Drugs associated with hypomagnesemia

Because certain drugs can cause or contribute to hypomagnesemia, you should monitor your patient's serum magnesium levels if he's receiving:

- an aminoglycoside antibiotic, such as amikacin (Amikin), gentamicin (Garamycin), streptomycin, or tobramycin (Nebcin)
- amphotericin B (Fungizone)
- cisplatin (Platinol-AQ)
- cyclosporine (Sandimmune)
- insulin
- a laxative
- loop (such as bumetanide [Bumex], furosemide [Lasix], or torsemide [Demadex]) or thiazide diuretics (such as chlorothiazide [Diuril] or hydrochlorothiazide [HydroDIURIL])
- pentamidine isethionate (NebuPent).

- impaired renal absorption of magnesium resulting from such diseases as glomerulonephritis, pyelonephritis, and renal tubular acidosis.

Magnesium levels may also drop dramatically in patients who are pregnant (second and third trimester); patients who are receiving magnesium-free, sodium-rich I.V. fluids to induce extracellular fluid expansion; and patients who have:

- excessive loss of body fluids (for example, from sweating, breast-feeding, diuretic abuse, or chronic diarrhea)
- hemodialysis
- hypercalcemia or excessive intake of calcium
- hypothermia
- syndrome of inappropriate antidiuretic hormone
- sepsis
- serious burns
- wounds requiring debridement
- any condition that predisposes them to excessive calcium or sodium in the urine.

Assessment findings

Signs and symptoms of hypomagnesemia can range from mild to life-threatening and can involve the central nervous system (CNS), neuromuscular system, cardiovascular system, and GI system.

Identifying hypomagnesemia

When assessing your patient for hypomagnesemia, use this list of signs and symptoms as a guide.

- ✦ Central nervous system: altered level of consciousness, confusion, hallucinations
- ✦ Neuromuscular: muscle weakness, leg and foot cramps, hyperactive deep tendon reflexes, tetany, Chvostek's and Trousseau's signs
- ✦ Cardiovascular: tachycardia, hypertension, characteristic electrocardiogram changes
- ✦ GI: dysphagia, anorexia, nausea, vomiting

Assessment findings

- ✦ May resemble potassium or calcium imbalance

CNS findings

- ✦ Ataxia
- ✦ Depression
- ✦ Vertigo

Neuromuscular findings

- ✦ Weak skeletal muscles
- ✦ Hyperirritable nerves and muscles
- ✦ Hyperactive DTRs
- ✦ Laryngeal stridor
- ✦ Foot or leg cramps
- ✦ Paresthesia
- ✦ Chvostek's and Trousseau's signs (possible hypocalcemia)

In general, your patient's signs and symptoms may resemble those of a potassium or calcium imbalance. However, you can't always count on detecting hypomagnesemia from clinical findings alone. Occasionally, a patient remains symptom-free even though his serum magnesium level measures less than 1.5 mEq/L. (See *Identifying hypomagnesemia.*)

A low serum magnesium level irritates the CNS. Such irritation can lead to an altered level of consciousness, ataxia, confusion, delusions, depression, emotional lability, hallucinations, insomnia, psychosis, seizures, and vertigo.

The body compensates for a low serum magnesium level by moving magnesium out of the cells. Such movement can take an especially high toll on the neuromuscular system. As cells become magnesium starved, skeletal muscles grow weak and nerves and muscles become hyperirritable.

Watch your patient for neuromuscular signs of hypomagnesemia, such as tremors, twitching, tetany, and hyperactive DTRs. (See *Grading DTRs.*)

Respiratory muscles may be affected, too, resulting in breathing difficulties. Your patient may also experience laryngeal stridor, foot or leg cramps, and paresthesia. If you suspect hypomagnesemia, test your patient for hypocalcemia by checking for these signs:

- ✦ Chvostek's sign — facial twitching when the facial nerve is tapped
- ✦ Trousseau's sign — carpal spasm when the upper arm is compressed.

Cardiovascular problems can occur mainly due to the fact that magnesium promotes cardiovascular function. A drop in the magnesium level can irritate the myocardium — with potentially disastrous consequences. Myocardial irritability can lead to cardiac arrhythmias, which can cause a drop in cardiac output. Arrhythmias are especially likely to develop in a

Grading DTRs

If you suspect your patient has hypomagnesemia, you'll want to test his deep tendon reflexes (DTRs) to determine whether his neuromuscular system is irritable—an indication that his magnesium level is too low. When grading your patient's DTRs, use the following scale:

0	Absent
++	Normal
+++	Increased but not necessarily abnormal
++++	Hyperactive, clonic

To record the patient's reflex activity, draw a stick figure and mark the strength of the response at the proper locations. This figure indicates normal DTR activity.

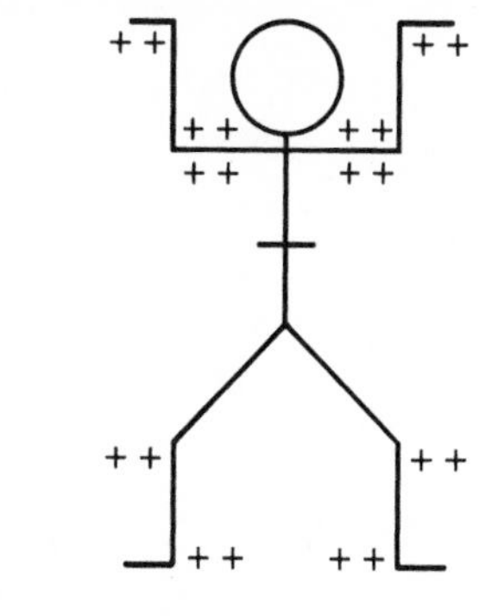

patient with coexisting potassium and calcium imbalances. Arrhythmias triggered by a low serum magnesium level include atrial fibrillation, heart block, paroxysmal atrial tachycardia, premature ventricular contractions, supraventricular tachycardia, torsades de pointes, ventricular fibrillation, and ventricular tachycardia.

Because of the risk of arrhythmia, the patient with severe hypomagnesemia (serum levels below 1 mEq/L) should undergo continuous cardiac monitoring. Sometimes, a patient who has had myocardial infarction or cardiac surgery is given oral magnesium supplements to prevent arrhythmias.

General electrocardiogram (ECG) changes that can occur with a low serum magnesium level include:

Assessment findings *(continued)*

Cardiovascular findings

- Atrial fibrillation
- Heart block
- Paroxysmal atrial tachycardia
- Premature ventricular contractions
- Supraventricular tachycardia
- Torsades de pointes
- Ventricular fibrillation
- Ventricular tachycardia

Assessment findings *(continued)*

ECG findings
- Prolonged PR interval
- Widened QRS complex
- Prolonged QT intervai
- Depressed ST segment
- Broad, flattened T wave
- Prominent U wave

GI findings
- Anorexia
- Dysphagia
- Nausea
- Vomiting

- prolonged PR interval
- widened QRS complex
- prolonged QT interval
- depressed ST segment
- broad, flattened T wave
- prominent U wave.

If your patient with hypomagnesemia is receiving digoxin (Lanoxin), watch him closely for signs and symptoms of digoxin toxicity — another condition that can trigger arrhythmias. A low magnesium level may increase the body's retention of digoxin. Suspect digoxin toxicity if your patient has anorexia, arrhythmias, nausea, vomiting, or yellow-tinged vision.

GI problems may occur in a patient who doesn't have a sufficient amount of magnesium in his bloodstream. He may suffer from such GI problems as anorexia, dysphagia, and nausea and vomiting. These conditions can lead to poor dietary magnesium intake or loss of magnesium through the GI tract, which in turn worsen the patient's condition.

Diagnostic test results

- Serum magnesium level < 1.8 mEq/L
- Other electrolyte abnormalities (below-normal serum potassium or calcium level)
- Characteristic ECG changes

Diagnostic test results

Typical laboratory findings for a patient with hypomagnesemia include:
- a serum magnesium level below 1.8 mEq/L (possibly with a below-normal serum albumin level)
- other electrolyte abnormalities, such as a below-normal serum potassium or calcium level
- characteristic ECG changes
- elevated serum levels of digoxin in a patient receiving the drug.

Treatment

Mild hypomagnesemia
- Dietary change
- Oral magnesium supplementation (magnesium chloride)

Severe hypomagnesemia
- I.V. or deep I.M. injections of magnesium sulfate (if renal function impaired, monitor closely)

TREATMENT

Treatment for hypomagnesemia depends on the underlying cause and the patient's clinical findings. For a patient with a mild magnesium shortage, a change in diet and teaching alone may correct the imbalance. Some physicians also prescribe an oral supplement, such as magnesium chloride, which is preferable to magnesium oxide because the latter is poorly absorbed and can cause alkalosis. Because it may take a few days to replenish magnesium stores inside the cell, magnesium replacement may be necessary for several days after the serum magnesium level returns to normal.

A patient with more severe hypomagnesemia may need I.V. or deep I.M. injections of magnesium sulfate. Before magnesium administration, renal function should be assessed. If renal function is impaired, magnesium levels should be closely monitored.

Nursing interventions

Prevention is the best treatment for hypomagnesemia, so closely watch a patient with risk factors for this imbalance, such as the inability to tolerate oral intake. For a patient previously diagnosed with hypomagnesemia, take these actions:

✦ Assess the patient's mental status and report changes.

✦ Evaluate the patient's neuromuscular status regularly by checking for hyperactive DTRs, tremors, and tetany. Check for Chvostek's and Trousseau's signs if hypocalcemia is also suspected.

✦ Check the patient for dysphagia before giving food, oral fluids, or oral medications. Hypomagnesemia may impair his ability to swallow.

✦ Monitor and record the patient's vital signs. Report findings that indicate hemodynamic instability.

✦ Monitor the patient's respiratory status. A magnesium deficiency can cause laryngeal stridor and compromise the airway.

✦ Connect the patient to a cardiac monitor if his magnesium level is below 1 mEq/L. Watch the rhythm strip closely for arrhythmias.

✦ Monitor the patient if he has lost an excessive amount of fluid, which may occur due to fistula drainage or prolonged diarrhea. A patient who has experienced excessive fluid loss is at risk for magnesium deficiency.

✦ Monitor the patient's urine output at least every 4 hours. Magnesium generally isn't administered if urine output is less than 10 ml in 4 hours.

✦ Assess the patient's vital signs every 15 minutes. If he's experiencing respiratory distress, assess him for a sharp decrease in blood pressure.

✦ If the patient is receiving digoxin, monitor him closely for signs and symptoms of digoxin toxicity, such as nausea, vomiting, and bradycardia. Magnesium deficiency enhances the pharmacologic action of digoxin.

✦ If the patient is receiving a medication — such as an aminoglycoside, amphotericin B (Fungizone), cisplatin (Platinol-AQ), cyclosporine (Sandimmune), gentamicin (Garamycin), insulin, a laxative, a loop or thiazide diuretic, pentamidine isethionate (NebuPent), or torsemide (Demadex) — monitor his serum magnesium levels closely. Certain medications can contribute to low serum magnesium levels.

✦ Monitor the patient's serum electrolyte levels, and notify the physician if the serum potassium level or calcium level is low. Both hypocalcemia and hypokalemia can cause hypomagnesemia.

Key nursing interventions

- Assess mental status
- Evaluate neuromuscular status regularly
- Check for dysphagia before giving food, oral fluids, or oral medications
- Monitor and record patient's vital signs
- Monitor respiratory status
- Connect patient to cardiac monitor
- If patient receiving digoxin, monitor for digoxin toxicity
- Monitor serum electrolyte levels
- Institute seizure precautions
- Establish I.V. access and maintain patent I.V. line
- Check I.V. magnesium orders (proper order states grams or milliliters to administer, volume of desired solution for dilution, and length of time for infusion)
- Keep emergency equipment nearby for airway protection

Checking the label

When you prepare a magnesium sulfate injection, keep in mind that the drug comes in various concentrations, such as 10%, 12.5%, and 50%. Check the label, such as the one shown here, to make sure you're using the correct concentration. The label shows other dosage information as well.

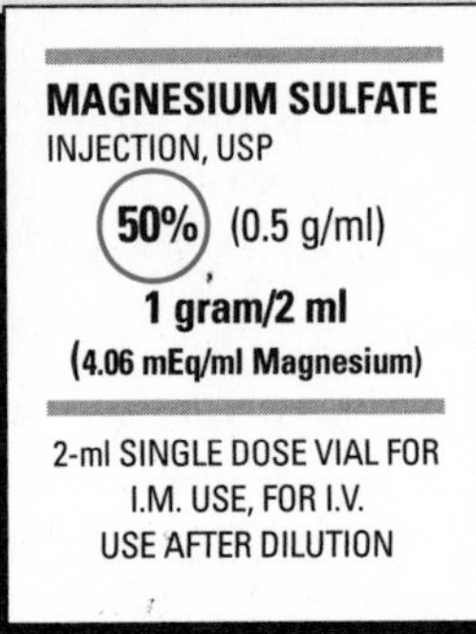

MAGNESIUM SULFATE
INJECTION, USP
50% (0.5 g/ml)
1 gram/2 ml
(4.06 mEq/ml Magnesium)
2-ml SINGLE DOSE VIAL FOR
I.M. USE, FOR I.V.
USE AFTER DILUTION

- Monitor the patient if he has been receiving nothing by mouth and if he has been receiving I.V. fluids without magnesium salts. Prolonged administration of magnesium-free fluids can result in low serum magnesium levels.
- Institute seizure precautions.
- If a seizure occurs, report the type of seizure, its length, and the patient's behavior during the seizure. Reorient him as needed.
- Keep emergency equipment nearby for airway protection.
- Ensure the patient's safety at all times.
- Reorient the patient as needed.
- To ease your patient's anxiety, tell him what to expect before each procedure.
- Establish I.V. access and maintain a patent I.V. line in case your patient needs I.V. magnesium replacement or I.V. fluids.
- When preparing an infusion of magnesium sulfate, keep in mind that I.V. magnesium sulfate comes in various concentrations (such as 10%, 12.5%, and 50%). (See *Checking the label.*) Clarify a physician's order that specifies only the number of ampules or vials to give. A proper order states how many grams or milliliters of a particular concentration to administer, the volume of desired solution for dilution, and the length of time for infusion. (See *Infusing magnesium sulfate.*)

Infusing magnesium sulfate

If the physician prescribes magnesium sulfate to raise your patient's serum magnesium level, you'll need to take some special precautions, such as these listed here:

- ✦ Using an infusion pump, administer magnesium sulfate slowly—no faster than 150 mg/minute. Injecting a bolus dose too rapidly can trigger cardiac arrest.
- ✦ Monitor your patient's vital signs and deep tendon reflexes during magnesium sulfate therapy. Every 15 minutes, check for signs and symptoms of magnesium excess, such as hypotension and respiratory distress.
- ✦ Check the patient's serum magnesium level after each bolus dose or at least every 6 hours if he has a continuous I.V. drip.
- ✦ Stay especially alert for an above-normal serum magnesium level if your patient's renal function is impaired.
- ✦ Place the patient on continuous cardiac monitoring. Observe him closely, especially if he's also receiving digoxin.
- ✦ Monitor urine output before, during, and after magnesium sulfate infusion. Notify the physician if output measures less than 100 ml over 4 hours.
- ✦ Keep calcium gluconate on hand to counteract adverse reactions. Have resuscitation equipment nearby and be prepared to use it if the patient goes into cardiac or respiratory arrest.

Infusing magnesium sulfate

- ✦ Inject magnesium slowly (< 150 mg/minute) using infusion pump
- ✦ Monitor vital signs and DTRs during therapy
- ✦ Stay alert for above-normal magnesium level
- ✦ Place patient on continuous cardiac monitoring
- ✦ Monitor urine output before, during, and after infusion
- ✦ Keep calcium gluconate ready to counteract adverse reactions

✦ When administering magnesium I.M., inject the dose into the deep gluteal muscle. I.M. injections of magnesium are painful. If giving more than one injection, alternate injection sites.

✦ Administer magnesium supplements as needed and ordered. (See *Preventing medication errors.*)

✦ During magnesium replacement, check the cardiac monitor frequently and assess the patient closely for signs of magnesium excess, such as hypotension and respiratory distress. Keep calcium gluconate at the bedside in case such signs occur.

Key nursing interventions *(continued)*

- ✦ When administering magnesium I.M., inject into deep gluteal muscle; if giving more than one injection, alternate injection sites to minimize discomfort
- ✦ Check cardiac monitor frequently during magnesium replacement
- ✦ Monitor and record intake and output

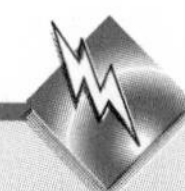

DANGER

Preventing medication errors

When documenting magnesium administration, always write out the word "magnesium" to prevent serious medication errors. The abbreviation for magnesium, $MgSO_4$ is easily confused with that for morphine, MSO_4.

CHARTING CHECKLIST

Documenting hypomagnesemia

If your patient has hypomagnesemia, make sure you document:

- ❑ vital signs
- ❑ heart rhythm
- ❑ neurologic, neuromuscular, and cardiac assessment findings
- ❑ magnesium sulfate or other drugs administered
- ❑ fluid intake and output
- ❑ seizures and safety measures used
- ❑ your interventions and the patient's response
- ❑ pertinent laboratory values, including serum electrolyte, albumin and, if appropriate, digoxin (Lanoxin) levels
- ❑ notification of the physician
- ❑ patient teaching.

✦ Maintain an accurate record of your patient's fluid intake and output. Report any decrease in urine output. (See *Documenting hypomagnesemia.*)

Patient teaching

- ✦ Description of disorder
- ✦ Medications
- ✦ Diet
- ✦ Warning signs and symptoms
- ✦ Referrals

Patient teaching

Be sure to cover these topics and then evaluate your patient's learning:

✦ explanations about hypomagnesemia, its risk factors, and its treatment
✦ prescribed medications
✦ avoidance of drugs that deplete magnesium in the body, such as diuretics and laxatives
✦ consumption of a high-magnesium diet
✦ warning signs and symptoms and when to report them
✦ referral to appropriate support groups such as Alcoholics Anonymous, if necessary.

Hypermagnesemia

- ✦ Indicated by serum magnesium level > 2.5 mEq/L

HYPERMAGNESEMIA

An excess of magnesium in the blood can be as dangerous as having too little. Hypermagnesemia occurs when the body's serum magnesium level rises above 2.5 mEq/L. However, hypermagnesemia is uncommon; typi-

Drugs associated with hypermagnesemia

Closely monitor your patient's serum magnesium level if he's receiving:
- ✦ an antacid (Gaviscon, Maalox)
- ✦ a laxative (Milk of Magnesia, Haley's M-O, magnesium citrate)
- ✦ a magnesium supplement (magnesium oxide, magnesium sulfate).

cally, the kidneys can rapidly reduce the amount of excess magnesium in the body.

Causes and pathophysiology

Hypermagnesemia results from the conditions opposite those that bring on a magnesium shortage. Its main causes are impaired magnesium excretion (for example, from renal dysfunction) and excessive magnesium intake.

Impaired magnesium excretion

Renal dysfunction is the most common cause of hypermagnesemia. Just as some renal conditions boost magnesium excretion to cause hypomagnesemia, others can make the body retain too much magnesium, causing hypermagnesemia. Causes of poor renal excretion of magnesium include advancing age, which tends to reduce renal function; renal failure; Addison's disease; adrenocortical insufficiency; and untreated diabetic ketoacidosis (DKA).

Excessive magnesium intake

Magnesium buildup is common in patients with renal failure who use magnesium-containing antacids or laxatives. (See *Drugs associated with hypermagnesemia.*)

Other causes of excessive magnesium intake include:
- ✦ hemodialysis with a magnesium-rich dialysate
- ✦ total parenteral nutrition solutions that contain too much magnesium
- ✦ continuous infusion of magnesium sulfate to treat such conditions as seizures, pregnancy-induced hypertension (PIH), or preterm labor. (The fetus of a woman receiving magnesium sulfate may develop a higher serum magnesium level, too.)

Causes

- ✦ Main causes: impaired magnesium excretion and excessive magnesium intake

Impaired magnesium excretion
- ✦ Renal dysfunction causing body to retain magnesium (advancing age and renal failure)

Excessive magnesium intake
- ✦ Use of magnesium-containing antacids or laxatives
- ✦ Hemodialysis with magnesium-rich dialysate
- ✦ Total parenteral nutrition solutions that contain too much magnesium
- ✦ Continuous infusion of magnesium sulfate

Assessment findings

Neuromuscular findings
- ✦ Decreased muscle and nerve activity
- ✦ Hypoactive DTRs
- ✦ Facial paresthesia
- ✦ Generalized weakness

CNS findings
- ✦ Drowsiness
- ✦ Lethargy
- ✦ Slow, shallow, depressed respirations

Cardiac findings
- ✦ Weak pulse
- ✦ Bradycardia
- ✦ Heart block
- ✦ Cardiac arrest
- ✦ Vasodilation
- ✦ Warm, flushed feeling

Diagnostic test results
- ✦ Serum magnesium level > 2.5 mEq/L

ASSESSMENT FINDINGS

Just as an abnormally low serum magnesium level overstimulates the neuromuscular system, an abnormally high one depresses it. Specifically, hypermagnesemia blocks neuromuscular transmission, so expect neuromuscular signs and symptoms opposite those of hypomagnesemia, such as:

✦ decreased muscle and nerve activity
✦ hypoactive deep tendon reflexes (DTRs)
✦ facial paresthesia (usually at moderately elevated serum levels)
✦ generalized weakness (for instance, a patient who has a weak hand grasp or difficulty repositioning himself in bed); in severe cases, weakness progresses to flaccid paralysis
✦ occasional nausea and vomiting. (See *Signs and symptoms of hypermagnesemia.*)

Because excess magnesium depresses the central nervous system (CNS), the patient may appear drowsy and lethargic. His level of consciousness (LOC) may even diminish to the point of coma. Hypermagnesemia can pose a danger to the respiratory system — and to life itself — if it weakens the respiratory muscles. Typically, slow, shallow, depressed respirations are indicators of such muscle weakness. Eventually, the patient may suffer respiratory arrest and require mechanical ventilation.

A high serum magnesium level may also trigger serious heart problems — among them a weak pulse, bradycardia, heart block, and cardiac arrest. Arrhythmias may lead to diminished cardiac output. A high serum magnesium level also causes vasodilation, which lowers the blood pressure and may make your patient feel flushed and warm all over.

Diagnostic test results

Typical laboratory findings for a patient with hypermagnesemia include:
✦ a serum magnesium level above 2.5 mEq/L
✦ electrocardiogram (ECG) changes, including a prolonged PR interval, widened QRS complex, and tall T wave. (For more information on how electrolyte imbalances affect ECGs, see the color pages between pages 54 and 55.)

TREATMENT

After hypermagnesemia is confirmed, the physician works to correct both the magnesium imbalance and its underlying cause.

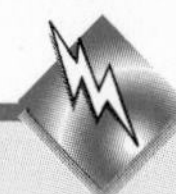

DANGER

Signs and symptoms of hypermagnesemia

Use this chart to compare total serum magnesium levels with the typical signs and symptoms that may appear.

TOTAL SERUM MAGNESIUM LEVEL	SIGNS AND SYMPTOMS
3 mEq/L	✦ Feelings of warmth ✦ Flushed appearance ✦ Mild hypotension ✦ Nausea and vomiting
4 mEq/L	✦ Diminished deep tendon reflexes ✦ Facial paresthesia ✦ Muscle weakness
5 mEq/L	✦ Bradycardia ✦ Drowsiness ✦ Electrocardiogram changes ✦ Worsening hypotension
7 mEq/L	✦ Loss of deep tendon reflexes
8 mEq/L	✦ Respiratory compromise
12 mEq/L	✦ Coma ✦ Heart block
15 mEq/L	✦ Respiratory arrest
20 mEq/L	✦ Cardiac arrest

If the patient has normal renal function, expect the physician to order oral or I.V. fluids. Increased fluid intake raises the patient's urine output, ridding his body of excess magnesium. If the patient doesn't respond to increased fluid intake, the physician may order a loop diuretic to promote magnesium excretion.

In an emergency, expect to give 10% calcium gluconate, a magnesium antagonist. A patient with toxic levels of magnesium in the blood may also need mechanical ventilation to relieve respiratory depression.

A patient with severe renal dysfunction may need hemodialysis with magnesium-free dialysate to lower the serum magnesium level.

Treatment

- ✦ Oral or I.V. fluids (to eliminate excess magnesium by increasing urine output)
- ✦ Loop diuretic (to promote magnesium excretion)
- ✦ 10% calcium gluconate (magnesium antagonist) in emergency
- ✦ Mechanical ventilation (to relieve respiratory depression)
- ✦ Hemodialysis with magnesium-free dialysate (for patient with severe renal dysfunction)

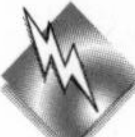

DANGER *If your patient's laboratory test results continue to show that his serum magnesium level is above normal, your first step is to notify the physician. Also, expect to prepare the patient for peritoneal dialysis or hemodialysis using magnesium-free dialysate. The patient needs to get rid of the excess magnesium fast — especially if his renal function is failing.*

Key nursing interventions

- ✦ Monitor patients with hypermagnesemia and those at risk for developing it (pregnant women in preterm labor or with PIH)
- ✦ Monitor vital signs frequently
- ✦ Check for flushed skin and diaphoresis
- ✦ Assess neuromuscular system, including DTRs and muscle strength
- ✦ Monitor serum electrolyte levels
- ✦ Monitor for hypocalcemia (may accompany hypermagnesemia)
- ✦ Monitor urine output
- ✦ Evaluate for changes in mental status

Nursing interventions

✦ Whenever possible, take steps to prevent hypermagnesemia by identifying high-risk patients. People at risk include:

- elderly people
- those with renal insufficiency or failure
- pregnant women in preterm labor or with PIH
- neonates whose mothers received magnesium sulfate during labor
- those receiving magnesium sulfate to control seizures
- those with a high intake of magnesium or magnesium-containing products, such as antacids or laxatives
- those with adrenal insufficiency
- those with severe DKA
- those who are dehydrated
- those with hypothyroidism.

If your patient already has hypermagnesemia, you may need to take these nursing actions:

✦ Monitor your patient's vital signs frequently. Stay especially alert for hypotension and respiratory depression, which are indicators of hypermagnesemia. Notify the physician immediately if the patient's respiratory status deteriorates.

✦ Check for flushed skin and diaphoresis.

✦ Assess the patient's neuromuscular system, including DTRs and muscle strength. (See *Testing the patellar reflex.*)

✦ Monitor laboratory tests and report abnormal results. Monitor serum electrolyte levels and other laboratory test results that reflect renal function, such as blood urea nitrogen and creatinine levels. Monitor the patient for hypocalcemia, which may accompany hypermagnesemia, because a low serum calcium level suppresses parathyroid hormone secretion.

✦ Monitor urine output. The kidneys excrete most of the body's magnesium.

✦ Evaluate the patient for changes in mental status. If his LOC decreases, institute safety measures. Reorient him if he's confused.

Testing the patellar reflex

To gauge your patient's magnesium status, test the patellar reflex, one of the deep tendon reflexes that serum magnesium levels affect. To test this reflex, strike the patellar tendon just below the patella with the patient sitting or lying in a supine position, as shown. Look for leg extension or contraction of the quadriceps muscle in the front of the thigh.

If the patellar reflex is absent, notify the physician immediately. This finding may mean your patient's serum magnesium level is 7 mEq/L or higher.

SITTING POSITION
Have the patient sit on the side of the bed with her legs dangling freely, as shown. Then test the reflex.

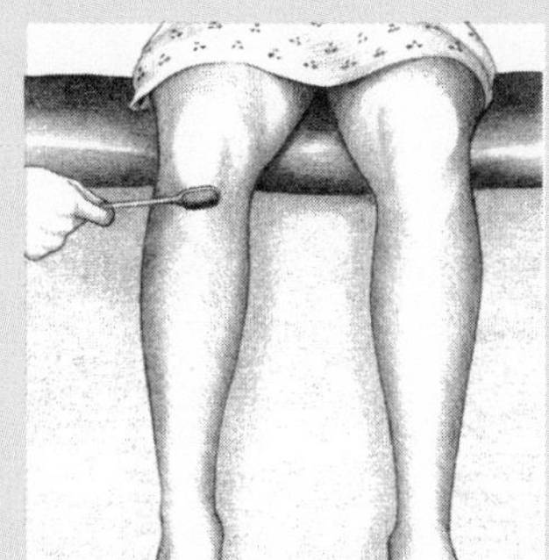

SUPINE POSITION
With the patient in the supine position, flex the knee at a 45-degree angle, and place your nondominant hand behind it for support. Then test the reflex.

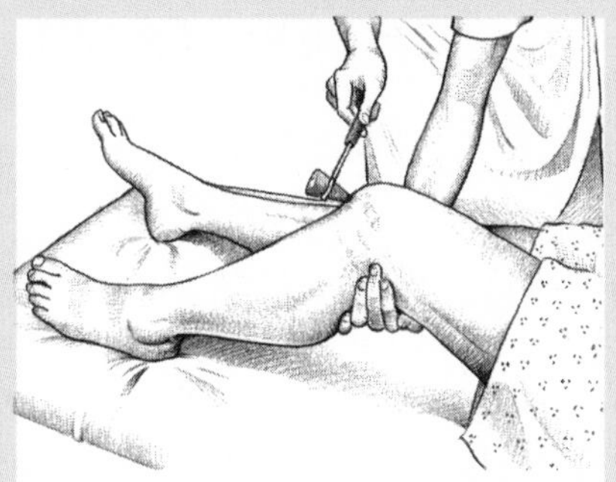

✦ Prepare the patient for continuous cardiac monitoring. Assess ECG tracings for pertinent changes.

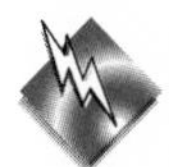

DANGER *If your patient has hypermagnesemia, always be prepared to:*
✦ *administer resuscitation drugs, maintain a patent airway, and provide calcium gluconate, as ordered, in case of a hypermagnesemia emergency*
✦ *get him ready for dialysis as ordered, if the patient's magnesium level becomes dangerously high*
✦ *provide mechanical ventilation, which may be needed if the patient has compromised respiratory function*
✦ *provide a temporary pacemaker, which may be inserted for the patient with bradyarrhythmias.*

✦ Establish I.V. access and maintain a patent I.V. line.
✦ Provide adequate fluids, both I.V. and oral, if prescribed, to help your patient's kidneys excrete excess magnesium. When giving large volumes of fluids, remember to keep accurate intake and output records and to

Key nursing interventions ***(continued)***
✦ Prepare for cardiac monitoring
✦ Assess ECG changes for pertinent changes
✦ Establish I.V. access and maintain patent I.V. line
✦ Provide adequate fluids (I.V. and oral)
✦ Restrict dietary magnesium intake

CHARTING CHECKLIST

Documenting hypermagnesemia

If your patient has hypermagnesemia, make sure you document:

- ❑ vital signs
- ❑ electrocardiogram changes
- ❑ signs and symptoms of hemodynamic instability
- ❑ deep tendon reflex assessment
- ❑ I.V. fluid therapy
- ❑ drugs administered
- ❑ safety measures
- ❑ your interventions and the patient's responses
- ❑ pertinent laboratory values, including serum electrolyte and albumin levels
- ❑ intake and output
- ❑ notification of the physician
- ❑ patient teaching.

watch closely for signs of fluid overload and kidney failure. Both conditions can arise quickly. (See *Documenting hypermagnesemia.*)

✦ Avoid giving your patient medications that contain magnesium. To make sure no other staff members give them, flag the patient's chart and medication administration record with a note that says, "No magnesium products."

✦ Restrict the patient's dietary magnesium intake as needed.

Patient teaching

✦ Description of disorder
✦ Diet
✦ Medications
✦ Warning signs and symptoms
✦ Dialysis

Patient teaching

Be sure you cover these topics and then evaluate your patient's learning:

✦ explanation of hypermagnesemia and its risk factors
✦ hydration requirements
✦ dietary modification if needed
✦ prescribed medications
✦ need to avoid medications that contain magnesium
✦ warning signs and symptoms and when to report them
✦ dialysis if needed.

Calcium imbalances

CALCIUM

Calcium is a positively charged ion, or *cation,* found in both the extracellular fluid and the intracellular fluid. About 99% of the body's calcium is found in the bones and the teeth. Only 1% is found in serum and soft tissue. However, that 1% is what matters when measuring calcium levels in the blood.

Calcium is involved in numerous body functions. Together with phosphorus, it's responsible for the formation and structure of bones and teeth. It helps maintain cell structure and function and plays a role in cell membrane permeability and impulse transmission.

In addition to affecting the contraction of cardiac muscle, smooth muscle, and skeletal muscle, calcium also participates in the blood-clotting process and in the release of certain hormones.

Measuring calcium levels

Calcium can be measured in two ways. The most commonly ordered test is a total serum calcium level, which measures the total amount of calcium in the blood. The normal range for the total serum calcium level is 8.5 to 10.5 mg/dl.

Calcium

- ✦ Positively charged ion (cation) in extracellular and intracellular fluid
- ✦ 99% in bones and teeth; 1% in serum and soft tissue

Functions of calcium

- ✦ Responsible for formation and structure of bones and teeth
- ✦ Helps maintain cell structure and function
- ✦ Helps promote cell membrane permeability and impulse transmission

Calcium levels

- ✦ Normal serum calcium level: 8.5 to 10.5 mg/dl

Calculating calcium and albumin levels

In a noncritically ill patient, for every 1 g/dl that his serum albumin level drops, his total calcium level decreases by 0.8 mg/dl. Use the following calculation to determine what your patient's calcium level would be if his serum albumin level were normal — and to help determine if treatment is necessary.

CORRECTING A LEVEL

The normal albumin level is 4 g/dl. The formula for correcting a patient's calcium level is:

Total serum calcium level + 0.8 (4 – albumin level) =
corrected calcium level

CALCULATING THE ANSWER

For example, if a patient's serum calcium level is 8.2 mg/dl and his albumin level is 3 g/dl, what would his corrected calcium be?

8.2 + 0.8 (4 – 3) = 9 mg/dl

The corrected calcium level is within normal range and probably wouldn't be treated.

AGE ALERT *Children have higher serum calcium levels than adults. In fact, serum levels can rise as high as 7 mg/dl during periods of increased bone growth. Conversely, in elderly patients the normal ranges for calcium levels are narrower. For elderly males, the range is 2.3 to 3.7 mg/dl; for elderly females, the range is 2.8 to 4.1 mg/dl.*

Calcium levels *(continued)*

- Normal ionized calcium level in adults: 4.5 to 5.1 mg/dl; in children, 4.4 to 6 mg/dl

The second test, an ionized calcium level, measures the various forms of calcium in extracellular fluid. About 41% of all extracellular calcium is bound to protein; 9% is bound to citrate or other organic ions. About half is ionized (or free) calcium, the only active form of calcium. Ionized calcium carries out most of the ion's physiologic functions. In adults, the normal range for ionized calcium is 4.5 to 5.1 mg/dl; in children, it's 4.4 to 6 mg/dl.

Because nearly half of all calcium is bound to the protein albumin, serum protein abnormalities can influence total serum calcium levels. For example, in hypoalbuminemia, the total serum calcium level decreases. However, ionized calcium levels — the more important of the two levels — remain unchanged. When considering total serum calcium levels, you should also consider serum albumin levels. (See *Calculating calcium and albumin levels.*)

Dietary sources of calcium

The most common dietary sources of calcium include:
- ✦ bonemeal
- ✦ dairy products, such as milk, cheese, and yogurt
- ✦ green leafy vegetables
- ✦ legumes
- ✦ molasses
- ✦ nuts
- ✦ whole grains.

Regulating calcium

Both intake of dietary calcium and existing stores of calcium affect calcium levels in the body. For adults, the range for the recommended daily requirement of calcium is 800 to 1,200 mg/day. Requirements vary for children, patients who are pregnant, and patients being treated for osteoporosis.

Dairy products are the most common calcium-rich foods, but calcium can also be found in large quantities in green, leafy vegetables. (See *Dietary sources of calcium.*) Calcium is absorbed in the small intestine and is excreted in the urine and stool. Several factors influence calcium levels in the body.

Parathyroid hormone

When serum calcium levels are low, the parathyroid glands release parathyroid hormone (PTH), which draws calcium from the bones and promotes the transfer of calcium (along with phosphorus) into the plasma. That transfer increases serum calcium levels.

PTH also promotes kidney reabsorption of calcium and stimulates the intestines to absorb the mineral. Phosphorus is excreted at the same time. In hypercalcemia, where too much calcium exists in the blood, the body suppresses the release of PTH.

Calcitonin

Calcitonin, produced in the thyroid gland, also helps to regulate calcium levels by acting as an antagonist to PTH. When calcium levels are too high, the thyroid releases calcitonin. High levels of this hormone inhibit bone resorption, which causes a decrease in the amount of calcium available from bone. This causes a decrease in the serum calcium level.

Regulating calcium

- ✦ Recommended daily requirement: 800 to 1,200 mg/day

PTH
- ✦ Promotes transfer of calcium and phosphorus into plasma, increasing serum calcium levels

Calcitonin
- ✦ Antagonist to PTH
- ✦ High levels inhibit bone resorption, decreasing amount of calcium available from bone and decreasing serum calcium level

Calcium in balance

Extracellular calcium levels are normally kept constant by several interrelated processes that move calcium ions into and out of extracellular fluid. Calcium enters the extracellular space through resorption of calcium ions from bone, through the absorption of dietary calcium in the GI tract, and through reabsorption of calcium from the kidneys. Calcium leaves extracellular fluid as it's excreted in stool and urine and deposited in bone tissues. This illustration shows how calcium moves throughout the body.

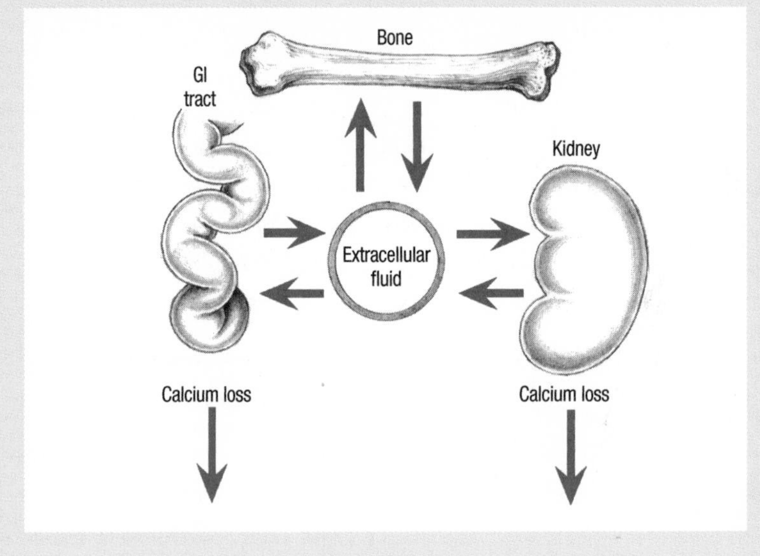

Calcitonin also decreases absorption of calcium and enhances its excretion by the kidneys.

Regulating calcium *(continued)*

Vitamin D

- Active form promotes intestinal calcium absorption and calcium resorption from bone and kidneys, raising serum calcium level

Vitamin D

Another factor that influences calcium levels is vitamin D. Vitamin D is ingested with foods, particularly dairy products. Also, when the skin is exposed to ultraviolet light, it synthesizes vitamin D.

The active form of vitamin D promotes calcium absorption through the intestines, calcium resorption from bone, and kidney reabsorption of calcium, all of which raise the serum calcium level. (See *Calcium in balance.*)

Phosphorus

Phosphorus has the opposite effect of vitamin D: It inhibits calcium absorption in the intestines. When calcium levels are low and the kidneys retain calcium, phosphorus is excreted.

An inverse relationship between calcium and phosphorus exists in the body. When calcium levels rise, phosphorus levels drop. When calcium levels drop, phosphorus levels rise.

Serum pH

The serum pH also has an inverse relationship with the ionized calcium level. If the serum pH level rises and the blood becomes alkaline, more calcium binds with protein and the ionized calcium level drops. Thus, a patient with alkalosis will typically have hypocalcemia.

Conversely, in acidosis, when the pH level drops, less calcium binds to protein and the ionized calcium level rises. When all those regulatory efforts fail to control the level of calcium in the body, one of two conditions may result: hypercalcemia or hypocalcemia.

Regulating calcium *(continued)*

Phosphorus

- Inhibits intestinal calcium absorption
- Inverse relationship with calcium (when calcium levels rise, phosphorus levels drop; when calcium levels drop, phosphorus levels rise)

Serum pH

- Inverse relationship with ionized calcium level
- In alkalosis, more calcium binds to protein, decreasing ionized calcium level
- In acidosis, less calcium binds to protein, increasing ionized calcium level

HYPERCALCEMIA

Hypercalcemia is a common metabolic emergency. It occurs when the serum calcium level rises above 10.5 mg/dl, the ionized serum calcium level rises above 5.1 mg/dl, or the rate of calcium entry into extracellular fluid exceeds the rate of calcium excretion by the kidneys.

Hypercalcemia

- Serum calcium level > 10.5 mg/dl
- Ionized serum calcium level > 5.1 mg/dl
- Rate of calcium entry into extravascular fluid exceeds rate of calcium excretion by kidneys

Causes and pathophysiology

Any situation that causes an increase in the total serum or ionized calcium level can lead to hypercalcemia. The condition is usually caused by an increase in the resorption of calcium from bone. Hyperparathyroidism and cancer are the two major causes of hypercalcemia.

Causes

- Two major causes: hyperparathyroidism and cancer

Hyperparathyroidism

With primary hyperparathyroidism, the most common cause of hypercalcemia, the body excretes more parathyroid (PTH) than normal, which greatly strengthens the effects of the hormone. Calcium resorption from bone and reabsorption from the kidneys are also increased, as is calcium absorption from the intestines.

Cancer

Cancer, the second most common cause of hypercalcemia, causes bone destruction as malignant cells invade the bones and may cause the release of a substance similar to PTH that causes an increase in serum calcium levels.

When serum calcium levels increase, the kidneys can become overwhelmed and unable to excrete the excess calcium, which in turn keeps calcium levels elevated. A patient who has squamous cell carcinoma of the lung is especially prone to hypercalcemia, as well as a patient with myeloma, Hodgkin's lymphoma, renal cell carcinoma, or breast cancer.

Prognosis of hypercalcemia associated with cancer is poor; the 1-year survival rate is only 10% to 30%.

Causes
(continued)

Other causes

- ✦ Increased calcium absorption in GI tract
- ✦ Decreased excretion of calcium by kidneys
- ✦ Multiple fractures
- ✦ Prolonged immobilization
- ✦ Hypophosphatemia and acidosis
- ✦ Certain medications
- ✦ Vitamin A overdose

Other causes

Hypercalcemia can also be caused by an increase in the absorption of calcium in the GI tract or by a decrease in the excretion of calcium by the kidneys. These mechanisms may occur alone or in combination.

Hyperthyroidism can cause an increase in calcium release as more calcium is resorbed from bone. Multiple fractures or prolonged immobilization can also cause an increase in calcium release from bone.

Hypophosphatemia and acidosis, which increase calcium ionization, are linked with hypercalcemia. Certain medications are also associated with the condition. For instance, abusing antacids that contain calcium, receiving an overdose of calcium such as from calcium medications given during cardiopulmonary resuscitation, or ingesting excessive amounts of vitamin D can prompt an increase in serum calcium levels.

Vitamin A overdose can lead to increased bone resorption of calcium. Use of lithium (Lithobid) or thiazide diuretics can decrease calcium excretion by the kidneys. Milk-alkali syndrome, a condition in which calcium and alkali are combined, also raises calcium levels.

Assessment findings

- ✦ Fatigue
- ✦ Confusion
- ✦ Anorexia, nausea, or vomiting
- ✦ Constipation
- ✦ Polyuria
- ✦ Dehydration

Assessment findings

Signs and symptoms of hypercalcemia are intensified if the condition develops acutely. Symptoms are also more severe if calcium levels are greater than 14 mg/dl. Many symptoms stem from the effects of excess calcium in the cells, which causes a decrease in cell membrane excitability, especially in the tissues of the skeletal muscle, the heart muscle, and the nervous system.

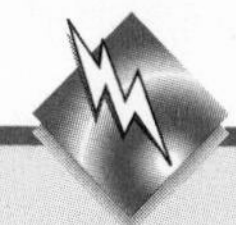

DANGER

Danger signs of hypercalcemia

Watch for these danger signs of hypercalcemia:
- ✦ arrhythmias such as bradycardia
- ✦ cardiac arrest
- ✦ coma
- ✦ paralytic ileus
- ✦ stupor.

The patient with hypercalcemia may complain of fatigue or exhibit confusion, altered mental status, depression, or personality changes. Lethargy can progress to coma in severe cases.

As calcium levels rise, the patient develops muscle weakness, hyporeflexia, and decreased muscle tone. Hypercalcemia may lead to hypertension.

Because heart muscle and the cardiac conduction system are affected by hypercalcemia, arrhythmias, such as bradycardia, can lead to cardiac arrest. Electrocardiography (ECG) may reveal a shortened QT interval and a shortened ST segment. Also observe for digoxin toxicity if the patient is receiving digoxin (Lanoxin).

Hypercalcemia can also lead to GI symptoms, which are commonly the first indicators the patient notices. The patient may experience anorexia, nausea, or vomiting. Bowel sounds are decreased. Constipation can occur because of calcium's effect on smooth muscle and subsequent decrease in GI motility. Abdominal or flank pain and paralytic ileus may result.

Renal problems may also develop, as the kidneys work to remove excess calcium. The patient may experience polyuria and subsequent dehydration. Hypercalcemia can also cause kidney stones and other calcifications. Renal failure may be the end result. Also, the patient may develop pathologic fractures and bone pain. (See *Danger signs of hypercalcemia.*)

Diagnostic test results

Typical laboratory findings for a patient with hypercalcemia include:
- ✦ serum calcium level above 10.5 mg/dl
- ✦ ionized calcium level above 5.1 mg/dl
- ✦ digoxin toxicity (if your patient is taking digoxin)
- ✦ X-rays revealing pathologic fractures

Diagnostic test results

- ✦ Characteristic ECG changes (shortened QT interval, prolonged PT interval, flattened T waves, heart block)

✦ characteristic ECG changes (shortened QT interval, prolonged PT interval, flattened T waves, and heart block).

Treatment
✦ Increase calcium excretion
✦ Inhibit bone resorption

Increasing calcium excretion
✦ Loop diuretics
✦ Hemodialysis

Inhibiting bone resorption
✦ Corticosteroids
✦ Biphosphonates
✦ Etidronate disodium
✦ Pamidronate disodium
✦ Calcitonin

TREATMENT

If hypercalcemia produces no symptoms, treatment may consist only of managing the underlying cause. Dietary intake of calcium may be reduced and medications or infusions containing calcium stopped. Treatment for symptomatic hypercalcemia includes measures to increase the excretion of calcium and to decrease bone resorption.

Increasing calcium excretion

You can help increase excretion of calcium by hydrating the patient, which encourages diuresis. Normal saline solution is typically used for hydration in these cases. The sodium in the solution inhibits renal tubular reabsorption of calcium.

Loop diuretics, such as furosemide (Lasix) and ethacrynic acid (Edecrin), also promote calcium excretion. Thiazide diuretics aren't used for hypercalcemia because they inhibit calcium excretion.

For patients with life-threatening hypercalcemia and those with renal failure, measures to increase calcium excretion may include hemodialysis or peritoneal dialysis with a solution that contains little or no calcium.

Inhibiting bone resorption

Measures to inhibit bone resorption of calcium may also be used to help reduce calcium levels in extracellular fluids. Corticosteroids administered I.V. and then orally can block bone resorption and decrease calcium absorption from the GI tract.

Biphosphonates are used to treat hypercalcemia caused by malignancy. Zoledronate (Zometa) inhibits bone resorption by acting on osteoclasts.

Etidronate disodium (Didronel), commonly used to treat hypercalcemia, also inhibits the action of osteoclasts. This medication takes full effect in 2 to 3 days. Pamidronate disodium (Aredia), which is similar to etidronate disodium, can also be used to inhibit bone resorption.

Calcitonin, a naturally occurring hormone, inhibits bone resorption of calcium, but its effects are short-lived. (See *Decreasing calcium levels.*)

NURSING INTERVENTIONS

Make sure you monitor patients at risk for hypercalcemia, such as those who have cancer or parathyroid disorders, are immobile, or are receiving

Decreasing calcium levels

If your patient doesn't seem to be responding to treatment for hypercalcemia, make sure he isn't still taking vitamin D supplements.

Keep in mind that calcitonin may be given to decrease calcium levels rapidly, but the effects are only temporary. If hypercalcemia is severe, you may give one or two doses with fluids and furosemide to provide rapid reduction of calcium levels.

a calcium supplement. For a patient who develops hypercalcemia, you'll want to take these actions:

✦ Monitor vital signs and assess the patient frequently.

✦ Watch the patient for arrhythmias. Assess neurologic and neuromuscular function and report changes.

✦ Monitor the patient's fluid intake and output.

✦ Monitor serum electrolyte levels, especially calcium, to determine the effectiveness of treatment and to detect new imbalances that might result from therapy.

✦ Make sure that treatment for the underlying disease is addressed.

✦ Insert and maintain I.V. access. Normal saline solution is usually administered at a rate of 200 to 500 ml/hour. Monitor the patient for signs of pulmonary edema, such as crackles and dyspnea.

✦ If administering a diuretic, make sure the patient is properly hydrated first so he doesn't experience volume depletion.

✦ Encourage the patient to drink 3 to 4 qt (3 to 4 L) of fluid daily, unless contraindicated, to stimulate calcium excretion from the kidneys and to decrease the risk of calculi formation.

✦ Strain the urine for calculi. Also check for flank pain, which can indicate the presence of renal calculi.

✦ If the patient is receiving digoxin, watch for signs and symptoms of a toxic reaction, such as anorexia, nausea, vomiting, or an irregular heart rate.

✦ Ambulate the patient as soon as possible to prevent bones from releasing calcium.

✦ Handle a patient who has chronic hypercalcemia gently to prevent pathologic fractures. Reposition bedridden patients frequently. Perform active or passive range-of-motion exercises to prevent complications from immobility.

Key nursing interventions

✦ Watch for arrhythmias
✦ Monitor serum calcium levels
✦ Make sure patient is hydrated
✦ Strain urine for calculi
✦ Watch for digoxin toxicity, if appropriate
✦ Ambulate patient as soon as possible

CHARTING CHECKLIST

Documenting hypercalcemia

If your patient has hypercalcemia, make sure you document:

- ❑ assessments, including neurologic examination and level of consciousness
- ❑ vital signs, including cardiac rhythm
- ❑ intake and output
- ❑ interventions, including I.V. therapy, and the patient's response
- ❑ signs and symptoms
- ❑ safety measures taken
- ❑ time that you notified the physician
- ❑ pertinent laboratory results, including calcium levels
- ❑ patient teaching provided and the patient's response.

✦ Provide a safe environment. Keep side rails raised as needed, the bed in its lowest position, and the wheels locked. Make sure the patient's belongings and call button are within reach. If the patient is confused, reorient him.

✦ Offer emotional support to the patient and his family throughout treatment. Overt signs of hypercalcemia can be emotionally distressing for all involved.

✦ Chart all care given and the patient's response to it. (See *Documenting hypercalcemia.*)

Patient teaching

- ✦ Description of disorder
- ✦ Risk factors
- ✦ Fluid intake
- ✦ Diet
- ✦ Medications
- ✦ Warning signs and symptoms

Patient teaching

Be sure to cover these topics and then evaluate your patient's learning:

- ✦ description of hypercalcemia, its causes, and treatment
- ✦ risk factors
- ✦ importance of increased fluid intake
- ✦ dietary guidelines for a low-calcium diet
- ✦ prescribed medications, including possible adverse effects
- ✦ warning signs and symptoms and when to report them
- ✦ avoidance of supplements and antacids that contain calcium.

Hypocalcemia

- ✦ Serum calcium level < 8.5 mg/dl
- ✦ Ionized calcium level < 4.5 mg/dl

HYPOCALCEMIA

Hypocalcemia occurs when calcium levels fall below the normal range—that is, when total serum calcium levels fall below 8.5 mg/dl or ionized calcium levels fall below 4.5 mg/dl.

Causes and pathophysiology

Hypocalcemia can occur when a person doesn't take in enough calcium, when the body doesn't absorb the mineral properly, or when excessive amounts of calcium are lost from the body. A decreased level of ionized calcium can also cause hypocalcemia.

Inadequate calcium intake

Inadequate intake of calcium can put a patient at risk for hypocalcemia. Alcoholics — with their typically poor nutritional intake, poor calcium absorption, and low magnesium level (magnesium affects parathyroid hormone [PTH] secretion) — are especially at risk. A breast-fed infant can have low calcium and vitamin D levels if his mother's intake of those nutrients is inadequate. Also, anyone who doesn't receive sufficient exposure to sunlight may suffer from vitamin D deficiency and subsequently lower calcium levels.

Impaired calcium absorption

Hypocalcemia can result when calcium isn't absorbed properly from the GI tract, a condition commonly caused by malabsorption. Malabsorption can result from increased intestinal motility from severe diarrhea, laxative abuse, or chronic malabsorption syndrome. Absorption is also affected by a lack of vitamin D in the diet. Anticonvulsants, such as phenobarbital (Luminal) and phenytoin (Dilantin), can interfere with vitamin D metabolism and calcium absorption. A high phosphorus level in the intestines can also interfere with absorption, as can a reduction in gastric acidity, which decreases the solubility of calcium salts.

Excessive calcium loss

Pancreatic insufficiency can cause malabsorption of calcium and a subsequent loss of calcium in stool. Acute pancreatitis can cause hypocalcemia as well, although the causative mechanism isn't well understood. PTH or possibly the combining of free fatty acids and calcium in pancreatic tissue may be involved.

Hypocalcemia can also occur when PTH secretion is reduced or eliminated. Thyroid surgery, surgical removal of the parathyroid gland, removal of a parathyroid tumor, or injury or disease of the parathyroid gland (such as hypoparathyroidism) can all reduce or prevent PTH secretion.

Hypocalcemia can also result from medications that decrease calcium resorption from bone, such as calcitonin and mithramycin. The kidneys

Causes

- Inadequate calcium intake
- Impaired calcium absorption
- Excessive calcium loss

Inadequate calcium intake

- At risk: alcoholics, breast-fed infants, people without sufficient exposure to sunlight

Impaired calcium absorption

- Malabsorption
- Lack of dietary vitamin D
- Anticonvulsants
- High intestinal phosphorus level
- Reduced gastric acidity

Excessive calcium loss

- Acute pancreatitis
- Reduced or eliminated PTH secretion
- Certain medications

may excrete excess calcium and cause hypocalcemia. Diuretics, especially loop diuretics such as furosemide (Lasix) and ethacrynic acid (Edecrin), increase renal excretion of calcium as well as water and other electrolytes. Renal failure may also harm the kidneys' ability to activate vitamin D, which affects calcium absorption. Edetate disodium (disodium EDTA), which is used to treat lead poisoning, can combine with calcium and carry it out of the body when excreted.

Causes *(continued)*

Additional causes
- Hypomagnesemia
- Hypoalbuminemia
- Hyperphosphatemia
- Alkalosis
- Citrate
- Severe burns or infections

Additional causes

Hypomagnesemia, a low magnesium level, can affect the function of the parathyroid gland and cause a decrease in calcium reabsorption in the GI tract and the kidneys. Drugs that lower serum magnesium levels, such as cisplatin (Platinol) and gentamicin (Garamycin), may decrease calcium absorption from bone.

Hypoalbuminemia, low serum albumin, is the most common cause of hypocalcemia. It may result from cirrhosis, nephrosis, malnutrition, burns, chronic illness, and sepsis.

Hyperphosphatemia, a high level of phosphorus in the blood, can cause calcium levels to fall as phosphorus levels rise. Excess phosphorus combines with calcium to form salts, which are then deposited in tissues.

When phosphates are administered orally, I.V., or rectally, the phosphorus binds with calcium and serum calcium levels drop. Infants receiving cow's milk are predisposed to hypocalcemic tetany because of its high levels of phosphorus.

Alkalosis can cause calcium to bind to albumin, thereby decreasing ionized calcium levels. Citrate, added to stored blood to prevent clotting, binds with calcium and renders it unavailable for use. Therefore, patients receiving massive blood transfusions are at risk for hypocalcemia. That risk also applies to pediatric patients.

Age alert
- Factors contributing to hypocalcemia in elderly patients: inadequate dietary intake of calcium, poor calcium absorption, reduced activity or inactivity

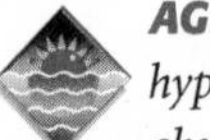

AGE ALERT *In elderly patients there are several factors that contribute to hypocalcemia, including inadequate dietary intake of calcium, poor calcium absorption (especially in postmenopausal women lacking estrogen), and reduced activity or inactivity. Inactivity causes a loss of calcium from the bone and osteoporosis, in which serum levels may be normal but bone stores of the mineral are depleted.*

Severe burns and infections are other causes of hypocalcemia. Burned or diseased tissues trap calcium ions from extracellular fluid, thereby reducing serum calcium levels.

Checking for Trousseau's and Chvostek's signs

Testing for Trousseau's and Chvostek's signs can aid in the diagnosis of tetany and hypocalcemia. Use the guidelines below to check for these important signs.

TROUSSEAU'S SIGN

To check for Trousseau's sign, apply a blood pressure cuff to the patient's upper arm and inflate it to a pressure 20 mm Hg above the systolic pressure. Trousseau's sign may appear after 1 to 4 minutes. The patient will experience an adducted thumb, flexed wrist and metacarpophalangeal joints, and extended interphalangeal joints (with fingers together)—carpopedal spasm—indicating tetany, a major sign of hypocalcemia.

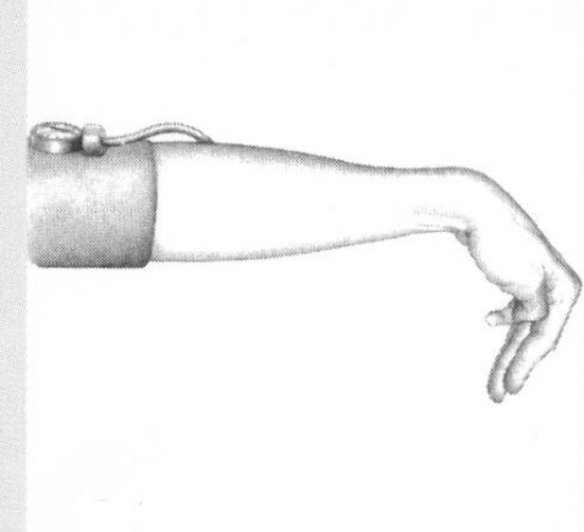

CHVOSTEK'S SIGN

You can induce Chvostek's sign by tapping the patient's facial nerve adjacent to the ear. A brief contraction of the upper lip, nose, or side of the face indicates Chvostek's sign.

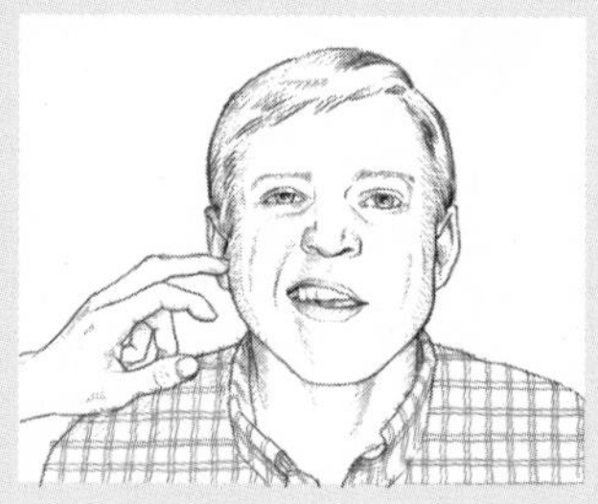

Assessment findings

Signs and symptoms of hypocalcemia reflect calcium's effects on nerve transmission and muscle and heart function; therefore, neuromuscular and cardiovascular findings are most common. The neurologic effects of a low calcium level include anxiety, confusion, and irritability, which can progress to seizures.

Neuromuscular symptoms may develop. The patient may experience paresthesia of the toes, fingers, or face, especially around the mouth. He may also experience twitching, muscle cramps, or tremors. Laryngeal and abdominal muscles are particularly prone to spasm, leading to laryngospasm and bronchospasm. An increase in nerve excitability can lead to the classic manifestation of tetany, which may be evidenced by positive Trousseau's or Chvostek's signs. (See *Checking for Trousseau's and Chvostek's signs.*)

Assessment findings

Neuromuscular findings

- Paresthesia of toes, fingers, or face
- Twitching, muscle cramps, or tremors
- Tetany

Cardiovascular findings

- Diminished response to digoxin
- Decreased cardiac output
- Prolonged ST segment
- Lengthened QT interval

Administering I.V. calcium

- Clarify if physician ordered calcium gluconate or calcium chloride
- Dilute prescribed I.V. calcium preparation in dextrose 5% in water
- Administer preparation slowly
- Watch for signs and symptoms of hypercalcemia
- Institute cardiac monitoring
- Observe I.V. site for signs of infiltration

Administering I.V. calcium safely

Be prepared to administer parenteral calcium to a patient who has symptomatic hypocalcemia. Always clarify whether the physician orders calcium gluconate or calcium chloride. Doses vary according to the specific drug. Note the type and dosage of each calcium preparation carefully, and follow these steps when administering it.

PREPARING

Dilute the prescribed I.V. calcium preparation in dextrose 5% in water. Never dilute calcium in solutions containing bicarbonate because precipitation will occur. Avoid giving the patient calcium diluted in normal saline solution because the sodium chloride will increase renal calcium loss.

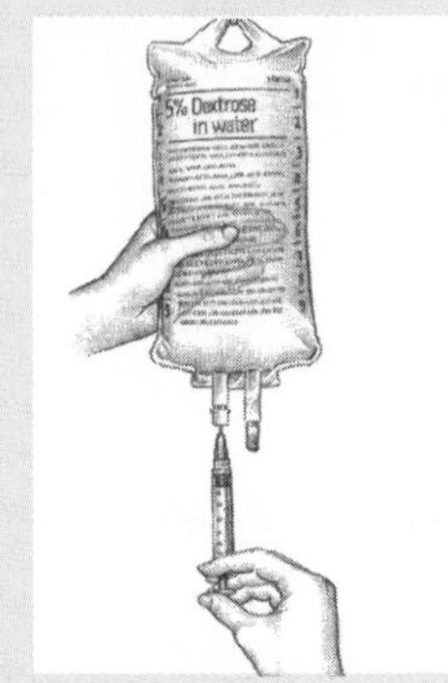

ADMINISTERING

Always administer I.V. calcium slowly, according to the physician's order or established protocol. Never give it rapidly because it may result in syncope, hypotension, or cardiac arrhythmias. Initially, calcium may be given as a slow I.V. bolus. If hypocalcemia persists, the initial bolus may be followed by a slow I.V. drip using an infusion pump.

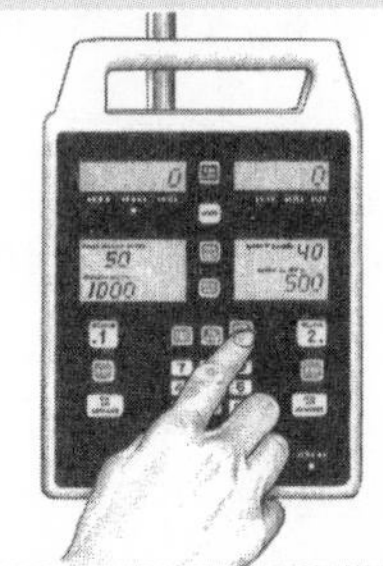

MONITORING

Overcorrection may lead to hypercalcemia. Watch for signs and symptoms of hypercalcemia, including anorexia, nausea, vomiting, lethargy, and confusion. Institute cardiac monitoring, and observe the patient for cardiac arrhythmias, especially if the patient is receiving digoxin. Observe the I.V. site for signs of infiltration; calcium can cause tissue sloughing and necrosis. Closely monitor serum calcium levels.

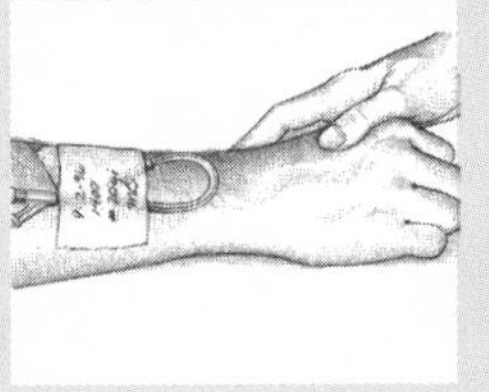

Fractures may occur more easily in a patient with hypocalcemia for an extended period. He may also have brittle nails or dry skin and hair. Other signs of hypocalcemia include diarrhea; hyperactive deep tendon reflexes; diminished response to digoxin; decreased cardiac output and subsequent arrhythmias; prolonged ST segment on the electrocardiogram (ECG); lengthened QT interval on the ECG; which puts the patient at risk for *torsades de pointes* (a form of ventricular tachycardia); or decreased myocardial contractility, leading to angina, bradycardia, hypotension, and heart failure.

Treating hypocalcemia

If treatment for hypocalcemia doesn't seem to be working:
- ✦ check the magnesium level. A low magnesium level must be corrected before I.V. calcium will increase serum calcium levels.
- ✦ check the phosphate level. If the phosphate level is too high, calcium won't be absorbed. Reduce the phosphate level first.
- ✦ mix I.V. calcium in dextrose solutions only. Normal saline may cause calcium to be excreted.

Diagnostic test results

Typical laboratory findings for a patient with hypocalcemia include:
- ✦ total serum calcium level less than 8.5 mg/dl
- ✦ ionized calcium level below 4.5 mg/dl (ionized calcium measurement is the definitive method to diagnose hypocalcemia)
- ✦ low albumin level
- ✦ characteristic ECG changes.

Note that falsely decreased levels may be seen with hyperbilirubinemia or administration of heparin, oxalate, or citrate.

Diagnostic test results
- ✦ Total serum calcium level < 8.5 mg/dl
- ✦ Ionized calcium level < 4.5 mg/dl
- ✦ Low albumin level
- ✦ ECG changes

Treatment

Treatment for hypocalcemia focuses on correcting the imbalance as quickly and as safely as possible. The underlying cause should be addressed to prevent recurrence.

Acute hypocalcemia requires immediate correction by administering either I.V. calcium gluconate or I.V. calcium chloride. Although calcium chloride contains three times as much available calcium as calcium gluconate, the latter is more commonly used. Calcium chloride is advised for patients in cardiac arrest, while calcium gluconate is preferred in patients who aren't in cardiac arrest. Magnesium replacement may also be needed because hypocalcemia doesn't respond to calcium therapy alone. (See *Administering I.V. calcium safely.*)

Chronic hypocalcemia requires vitamin D supplements to facilitate GI absorption of calcium. Oral calcium supplements also help increase calcium levels.

In addition, the patient's diet should also be adjusted to allow for an adequate intake of calcium, vitamin D, and protein. In cases where the patient also has a high phosphorus level, aluminum hydroxide antacids may be given to bind with excess phosphorus. (See *Treating hypocalcemia.*)

Treatment
- ✦ For acute hypocalcemia: I.V. calcium gluconate or I.V. calcium chloride
- ✦ For chronic hypocalcemia: vitamin D supplements and oral calcium supplements

Key nursing interventions

- ✦ Monitor respiratory status
- ✦ Place patient on cardiac monitor
- ✦ Check for Chvostek's and Trousseau's signs
- ✦ Monitor patient receiving I.V. calcium for arrhythmias
- ✦ Administer I.V. calcium replacement therapy carefully
- ✦ Monitor pertinent laboratory test results

NURSING INTERVENTIONS

If your patient is at increased risk for hypocalcemia, assess him carefully, especially if he has had parathyroid or thyroid surgery or has received massive blood transfusions. If your patient is breast-feeding, assess her for adequate vitamin D intake and exposure to sunlight.

When assessing a patient you suspect has hypocalcemia, obtain a complete medical history. Note if the patient has ever had neck surgery. Hypoparathyroidism may develop immediately or several years after neck surgery. Ask a patient who has chronic hypocalcemia if he has a history of fractures. Obtain a list of medications the patient is taking; the list may help you determine the underlying cause of hypocalcemia. Make sure you also assess the effects of symptoms on the patient's ability to perform activities of daily living.

If your patient is recovering from parathyroid or thyroid surgery, keep calcium gluconate at the bedside, which ensures a quick response to signs of a sudden drop in calcium levels. If the patient develops hypocalcemia, take these nursing actions:

✦ Monitor vital signs, and assess the patient frequently.

✦ Monitor respiratory status, including rate, depth, and rhythm.

✦ Watch for stridor, dyspnea, and crowing.

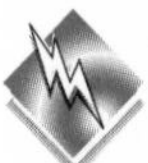

DANGER *If the patient shows overt signs of hypocalcemia, keep a tracheotomy tray and a handheld resuscitation bag at the bedside in case laryngospasm occurs.*

✦ Place your patient on a cardiac monitor, and evaluate him for changes in heart rate and rhythm. Notify the physician if the patient develops arrhythmias, such as ventricular tachycardia or heart block.

✦ Check the patient for Chvostek's sign or Trousseau's sign.

✦ Monitor a patient receiving I.V. calcium for arrhythmias, especially if he's also taking digoxin. Calcium and digoxin have similar effects on the heart.

✦ Insert and maintain a patent I.V. line for calcium therapy.

✦ Administer I.V. calcium replacement therapy carefully. Ensure the patency of the I.V. line because infiltration can cause tissue necrosis and sloughing.

✦ Administer oral replacements as ordered. Give calcium supplements 1 to 1½ hours after meals. If GI upset occurs, give the supplement with milk.

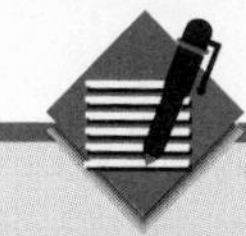

CHARTING CHECKLIST

Documenting hypocalcemia

If your patient has hypocalcemia, make sure you document:
- ❑ vital signs, including cardiac rhythm
- ❑ intake and output
- ❑ seizure activity
- ❑ safety measures
- ❑ assessments, interventions, and the patient's response
- ❑ patency and appearance of the I.V. site, before and after calcium infusion
- ❑ pertinent laboratory results, including calcium levels
- ❑ time that you notified the physician
- ❑ patient teaching provided and the patient's response.

✦ Monitor pertinent laboratory test results, including not only calcium levels but also albumin levels and those of other electrolytes such as magnesium. Remember to check the ionized calcium level after every 4 units of blood transfused.
✦ Encourage the older patient to take a calcium supplement as ordered and to exercise as much as he can tolerate to prevent calcium loss from bones.
✦ Take precautions for seizures such as padding bed side rails.
✦ Reorient a confused patient. Provide a calm, quiet environment.
✦ Document all care given to the patient and all observations made. (See *Documenting hypocalcemia.*)

Patient teaching

Be sure to cover these topics and then evaluate your patient's learning:
✦ description of hypocalcemia, its causes, and treatment
✦ importance of a high-calcium diet
✦ sources of dietary calcium
✦ avoidance of long-term laxative use
✦ prescribed medications
✦ importance of exercise
✦ warning signs and symptoms and when to report them
✦ need to report pain during I.V. infusion of calcium
✦ possible use of female hormones in patients with osteoporosis.

Patient teaching
✦ Description of disorder
✦ Diet
✦ Medications
✦ Exercise
✦ Warning signs and symptoms
✦ Pain during I.V. infusion
✦ Female hormones for patients with osteoporosis

Phosphorus imbalances

Phosphorus

- Primary anion (negatively charged ion) in intracellular fluid
- 85% in bones and teeth; 14% in soft tissue; < 1% in extracellular fluid

Major functions of phosphorus

- Helps metabolize carbohydrates, fat, and protein
- Promotes energy transfer to cells through formation of energy-storing substances (adenosine triphosphate)
- Essential for healthy bones and teeth

PHOSPHORUS

Phosphorus is the primary anion, or *negatively charged ion,* found in the intracellular fluid. It's contained in the body as phosphate. About 85% of phosphorus exists in bone and teeth, combined in a 1:2 ratio with calcium. About 14% is in soft tissue, and less than 1% is in extracellular fluid.

An essential element of all body tissues, phosphorus is vital to various body functions. It plays a crucial role in cell membrane integrity (phospholipids make up the cell membranes), muscle function, neurologic function, and the metabolism of carbohydrates, fat, and protein. Phosphorus is a primary ingredient in 2,3-diphosphoglycerate (2,3-DPG), a compound in red blood cells (RBCs) that facilitates oxygen delivery from RBCs to the tissues.

Phosphorus is also involved in the buffering of acids and bases. It promotes energy transfer to cells through the formation of energy-storing substances such as adenosine triphosphate. It's also important for white blood cell phagocytosis and for platelet function. Lastly, along with calcium, phosphorus is essential for healthy bones and teeth.

Dietary sources of phosphorus

Major dietary sources of phosphorus include:
- cheese
- dried beans
- eggs
- fish
- milk products
- nuts and seeds
- organ meats (such as brain and liver)
- poultry
- whole grains.

Normal serum levels

Normal serum phosphorus levels in adults range from 2.5 to 4.5 mg/dl (or 1.8 to 2.6 mEq/L). In comparison, the normal phosphorus level in the cells is 100 mEq/L. Because phosphorus is located primarily within the cells, serum levels may not always reflect the total amount of phosphorus in the body. For example, it's important to distinguish between a decrease in the level of serum phosphate, which causes hypophosphatemia, and a decrease in total body storage of phosphate, which causes a phosphate deficiency.

Normal serum levels
- Normal serum phosphorus levels in adults: 2.5 to 4.5 mg/dl
- Normal phosphorus level in cells: 100 mEq/L

Regulating phosphorus

The total amount of phosphorus in the body is related to dietary intake, hormonal regulation, kidney excretion, and transcellular shifts. For adults, the range for the recommended daily requirement of phosphorus is 800 to 1,200 mg. Phosphorus is readily absorbed through the GI tract; the amount absorbed is proportional to the amount ingested. (See *Dietary sources of phosphorus.*)

Most ingested phosphorus is absorbed through the jejunum. The kidneys excrete about 90% of phosphorus as they regulate serum levels and the GI tract excretes the rest. If dietary intake of phosphorus increases, the kidneys increase excretion to maintain normal levels of phosphorus. A low-phosphorus diet causes the kidneys to reabsorb more phosphorus in the proximal tubules in order to conserve it.

Regulating phosphorus
- Total amount of phosphorus in body related to dietary intake, hormonal regulation, kidney excretion, and transcellular shifts
- Kidneys excrete about 90% of phosphorus
- If dietary intake of phosphorus increases, kidneys increase excretion
- If dietary intake of phosphorus decreases, kidneys reabsorb more phosphorus in proximal tubules

How PTH affects phosphorus levels

- Increases phosphorus release from bone
- Increases phosphorus absorption from intestines
- Decreases phosphorus reabsorption in renal tubules

Regulating phosphorus *(continued)*

Calcium and PTH

- Changes in calcium levels — not changes in phosphorus levels — affect release of PTH
- Calcium and phosphorus have inverse relationship

Phosphorus shifts

- Caused by insulin and alkalosis

How PTH affects phosphorus levels

This illustration shows how parathyroid hormone (PTH) affects serum phosphorus (P) levels. PTH increases phosphorus release from bone, increases phosphorus absorption from the intestines, and decreases phosphorus reabsorption in the renal tubules.

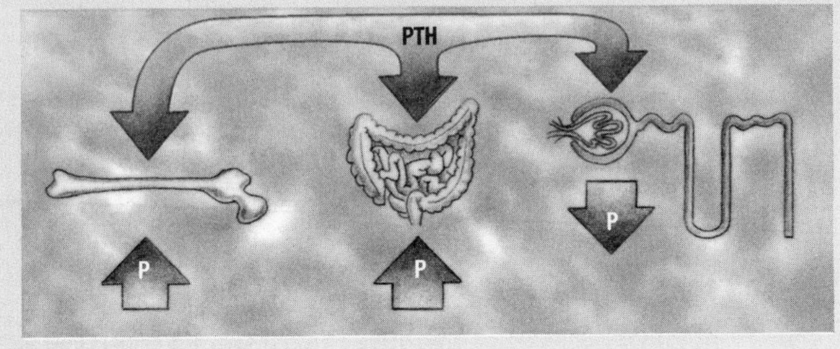

Calcium and PTH

The parathyroid gland controls hormonal regulation of phosphorus levels by affecting the activity of parathyroid hormone (PTH). (See *How PTH affects phosphorus levels.*) Changes in calcium levels, rather than changes in phosphorus levels, affect the release of PTH. You may recall that phosphorus balance is closely related to that of calcium.

Normally, calcium and phosphorus have an inverse relationship. For instance, when serum calcium level is low, phosphorus level is high. PTH is released, causing an increase in calcium and phosphorus resorption from bone and raising both calcium and phosphorus levels. Phosphorus absorption from the intestines is also increased. Activated vitamin D — calcitriol — also enhances its absorption in the intestines.

PTH then acts on the kidneys to increase excretion of phosphorus. The renal effect of PTH outweighs its other effects on serum phosphorus levels, particularly the action of returning phosphorus levels to normal. Reduced PTH levels allow for phosphorus reabsorption by the kidneys and as a result, serum levels rise.

Phosphorus shifts

Certain conditions cause phosphorus to move, or shift, in and out of cells. Insulin moves not only glucose but also phosphorus into the cell. Alkalosis results in the same kind of phosphorus shift that affects serum phosphorus levels.

AGE ALERT *Elderly patients are at risk for altered electrolyte levels due to their lower ratio of lean body weight to total body weight, which places them at risk for water deficit. In addition, their thirst response is diminished and renal function is decreased, which makes maintaining electrolyte balance more difficult. Other age-related renal changes include alteration in renal blood flow and glomerular filtration rate. Medication can also alter electrolyte levels by affecting the absorption of phosphate. Therefore, ask your elderly patients if they use over-the-counter medications, such as antacids, laxatives, herbs, and teas.*

Age alert
- Elderly patients at risk for altered electrolyte levels (lower ratio of lean to total body weight, diminished thirst response, decreased renal function, medication)
- Other age-related renal changes: altered renal blood flow and glomerular filtration rate

HYPERPHOSPHATEMIA

Hyperphosphatemia occurs when the serum phosphorus level exceeds 4.5 mg/dl (or 2.6 mEq/L). It usually reflects the kidneys' inability to excrete excess phosphorus and commonly occurs along with an increased release of phosphorus from damaged cells. Severe hyperphosphatemia occurs when the serum phosphorus levels reach 6 mg/dl or higher.

Hyperphosphatemia
- Serum phosphorus level > 4.5 mg/dl
- Reflects kidneys' inability to excrete phosphorus
- Commonly occurs with increased release of phosphorus from damaged cells

CAUSES AND PATHOPHYSIOLOGY

Hyperphosphatemia results from a number of underlying mechanisms, including impaired renal excretion of phosphorus, hypoparathyroidism, a shift of phosphorus from the intracellular fluid to the extracellular fluid, and an increase in dietary intake of phosphorus.

Impaired renal excretion

Normally, renal excretion of phosphorus equals that which the GI tract absorbs daily. Hyperphosphatemia most commonly results from renal failure due to the kidneys' inability to excrete excess phosphorus. When the glomerular filtration rate begins to drop below 30 ml/minute, the kidneys can't filter excess phosphorus adequately. Because the kidneys are responsible for most of the excretion of phosphorus, their inability to filter phosphorus leads to an elevated serum phosphorus level.

Hypoparathyroidism

A risk after thyroid or parathyroid surgery, hypoparathyroidism impairs synthesis of parathyroid hormone. When less parathyroid hormone is synthesized, less phosphorus is excreted from the kidneys resulting in elevated serum phosphorus levels.

Causes

Impaired renal excretion
- Most common cause

Hypoparathyroidism
- Risk of thyroid or parathyroid surgery
- Impairs synthesis of parathyroid hormone

Causes
(continued)

Shifting phosphorus
- Acid-base imbalances
- Conditions that cause cellular destruction
- Chemotherapy
- Muscle necrosis
- Rhabdomyolysis

Increased phosphorus intake
- Overadministration of phosphorus supplements or of laxatives or enemas that contain phosphorus
- Excessive intake of vitamin D

Shifting phosphorous

Several conditions can cause phosphorus to shift from the intracellular fluid to the extracellular fluid. Acid-base imbalances, such as respiratory acidosis and diabetic ketoacidosis (DKA), are common examples. Any condition that causes cellular destruction can also result in a transcellular shift of phosphorus.

Destruction of cells can trigger the release of intracellular phosphorus into the extracellular fluid, causing serum phosphorus levels to rise. Chemotherapy, for example, causes significant cell destruction, as do muscle necrosis and rhabdomyolysis, conditions that can stem from infection, heatstroke, and trauma.

Increased phosphorus intake

Excessive intake of phosphorus can result from overadministration of phosphorus supplements or of laxatives or enemas that contain phosphorus such as Fleet enemas.

Excessive intake of vitamin D can result in increased absorption of phosphorus and lead to an elevated serum phosphorus level.

AGE ALERT *Infants have naturally higher phosphorus levels. When fed cow's milk, which contains more phosphorus than breast milk, they're more at risk for hyperphosphatemia. Children and postmenopausal women also have naturally higher phosphorus levels, predisposing them to hyperphosphatemia.*

Assessment findings
- Hypocalcemia (signs and symptoms of acute hyperphosphatemia usually caused by hypocalcemia)
- Paresthesia in fingertips and around mouth
- Muscle spasm, cramps, pain, and weakness
- Hyperreflexia
- Positive Chvostek's and Trousseau's signs
- Tetany

ASSESSMENT FINDINGS

Hyperphosphatemia causes few clinical problems by itself. However, because phosphorus and calcium levels have an inverse relationship, hyperphosphatemia may lead to hypocalcemia, which can be life-threatening. Signs and symptoms of acute hyperphosphatemia are usually caused by the effects of hypocalcemia.

The patient may develop paresthesia in the fingertips and around the mouth, which may increase in severity and spread proximally along the limbs and to the face. Muscle spasm, cramps, pain, and weakness may also occur and may be severe enough to prevent the patient from performing normal activities. The patient may also exhibit hyperreflexia and positive Chvostek's and Trousseau's signs that are due to low calcium levels and may progress to tetany and neurologic disorders.

Neurologic signs and symptoms include decreased mental status, delirium, and seizures. Electrocardiogram (ECG) changes include a prolonged QT interval and ST segment. The patient may also experience hypotension, heart failure, anorexia, nausea, and vomiting. Bone development may also be affected.

When phosphorus levels rise, phosphorus binds with calcium, forming an insoluble compound called *calcium phosphate.* Organ dysfunction can result when calcium phosphate precipitates, or is deposited, in the heart, lungs, kidneys, corneas, or other soft tissues. This process, called *calcification,* usually occurs as a result of chronically elevated phosphorus levels. With calcification, the patient may experience arrhythmias, an irregular heart rate, and decreased urine output. Corneal haziness, conjunctivitis, cataracts, and impaired vision may occur, and papular eruptions may develop on the skin.

Diagnostic test results

Typical laboratory findings for a patient with hyperphosphatemia include:

- ✦ serum phosphorus level above 4.5 mg/dl (or 2.6 mEq/L)
- ✦ serum calcium level below 8.5 mg/dl
- ✦ X-ray studies that may reveal skeletal changes due to osteodystrophy (defective bone development) in chronic hyperphosphatemia
- ✦ increased blood urea nitrogen (BUN) and creatinine levels, which reflect worsening renal function
- ✦ ECG changes characteristic of hypocalcemia (prolonged QT interval).

Treatment

An elevated serum phosphorus level may be treated with drugs and other therapeutic measures. The treatment is aimed at correcting the underlying disorder, if one exists, and correcting hypocalcemia.

If a patient's elevated serum phosphorus level is due to excessive phosphorus intake, the condition may be easily remedied by reducing phosphorus intake. Therapeutic measures include reducing dietary intake of phosphorus and eliminating the use of phosphorus-based laxatives and enemas. (See *Lowering phosphorus levels,* page 144.)

Drug therapy may help decrease absorption of phosphorus in the GI system. Drug therapy may include aluminum, magnesium, or calcium gel or phosphate-binding antacids. Calcium salts, such as calcium carbonate (Cal-Plus) and calcium acetate (PhosLo), are widely used but may cause hypercalcemia, so careful dosing is needed. Polymeric phosphate binders such as sevelamer hydrochloride (Renagel) may also be given. For pa-

Assessment findings *(continued)*

- ✦ Calcification accompanied by arrhythmias, irregular heart rate, decreased urine output, corneal haziness, conjunctivitis, cataracts, impaired vision, papular eruptions

Diagnostic test results

- ✦ Serum phosphorus level > 4.5 mg/dl
- ✦ Serum calcium level < 8.5 mg/dl
- ✦ ECG changes characteristic of hypocalcemia

Treatment

- ✦ Therapeutic measures, including reducing dietary intake of phosphorus
- ✦ Polymeric phosphate binders such as sevelamer hydrochloride

Lowering phosphorus levels

If your patient is following a low-phosphorus diet that hasn't lowered his serum phosphorus levels, you should investigate these factors:

- ✦ medication compliance (especially of phosphorus-binding antacids)
- ✦ continued use of phosphate-containing laxatives or enemas
- ✦ kidney function
- ✦ correction of underlying causes.

Treatment
(continued)

- ✦ For severe hypophosphatemia: I.V. saline solution, proximal diuretics, hemodialysis or peritoneal dialysis

tients with underlying renal insufficiency or renal failure, use of magnesium antacids may result in hypermagnesemia and should be avoided.

Keep in mind that a mildly elevated phosphorus level may benefit a patient with renal failure. High phosphorus levels allow more oxygen to move from the red blood cells to tissues, which can help prevent hypoxemia and limit the effects of chronic anemia on oxygen delivery.

Treatment for the underlying cause of respiratory acidosis or DKA can lower serum phosphorus levels. In a patient with diabetes, the administration of insulin causes phosphorus to shift back into the cell, which can result in a decrease in serum phosphorus levels.

For patients with severe hyperphosphatemia, I.V. saline solution may be given to promote renal excretion of phosphorus. However, this treatment requires that the patient have functional kidneys and can tolerate the increased load of sodium and fluid. Proximal diuretics such as acetazolamide (Diamox) may also be given to increase renal excretion of phosphorus.

As a final therapeutic intervention, hemodialysis or peritoneal dialysis may be initiated if the patient has chronic renal failure or an extreme case of acute hyperphosphatemia with symptomatic hypocalcemia.

Nursing interventions

Identify patients at risk for hyperphosphatemia, and carefully monitor them. Use caution when administering phosphorus in I.V. infusions, enemas, and laxatives because the extra phosphorus may cause hyperphosphatemia. If your patient has already developed hyperphosphatemia, your nursing care should focus on careful monitoring, safety measures, and interventions to restore normal serum phosphorus levels. Follow these steps to provide care for the patient:

CHARTING CHECKLIST

Documenting hyperphosphatemia

If your patient has hyperphosphatemia, make sure you document:

- ❑ assessment findings
- ❑ intake and output
- ❑ I.V. therapy and medications given
- ❑ muscle spasms, cramps, pain, strength
- ❑ paresthesia in the fingertips and around the mouth
- ❑ visual disturbances
- ❑ safety measures to protect the patient
- ❑ time that you notified the physician
- ❑ your interventions, including patient teaching and the patient's response.

✦ Monitor vital signs, keeping in mind the signs and symptoms of hypocalcemia. If you note any signs or symptoms of worsening hypocalcemia, such as paresthesia in the fingers or around the mouth, hyperactive reflexes, or muscle cramps, promptly notify the physician. Also notify the physician if you detect signs or symptoms of calcification, including oliguria, visual impairment, conjunctivitis, irregular heart rate or palpitations, and papular eruptions.

✦ Monitor fluid intake and output. If urine output falls below 30 ml/hour, immediately notify the physician. Decreased urine output can seriously affect renal clearance of excess serum phosphorus.

✦ Carefully monitor serum electrolyte levels, especially calcium and phosphorus. Report changes immediately. Also monitor BUN and serum creatinine levels, because hyperphosphatemia can impair renal tubules when calcification occurs.

✦ Keep a flow sheet of daily laboratory test results for a patient at risk. Include BUN and serum phosphorus, calcium, and creatinine levels as well as fluid intake and output. Keep the flow sheet on a clipboard so changes can be detected immediately. (See *Documenting hyperphosphatemia.*)

✦ Administer prescribed medications, monitor their effectiveness, and assess the patient for possible adverse reactions. Give antacids with meals to increase their effectiveness in binding phosphorus.

✦ Prepare the patient for possible dialysis if hyperphosphatemia is severe.

✦ If a patient's condition results from chronic renal failure or if his treatment includes a low-phosphorus diet, consult a dietitian to assist the pa-

Key nursing interventions

- ✦ Monitor vital signs
- ✦ Watch for hypocalcemia
- ✦ Notify physician if signs or symptoms of calcification develop
- ✦ Monitor fluid intake and output
- ✦ Monitor serum electrolyte levels (especially calcium and phosphorus)
- ✦ Monitor BUN and serum creatinine levels
- ✦ Administer prescribed medications

tient in complying with dietary restrictions. Dietary phosphorus should be restricted to 0.6 to 0.9 g/day.

Patient teaching
- Description of disorder
- Medications
- Diet
- Warning signs and symptoms
- Referrals

Patient teaching

Be sure to cover these topics and then evaluate your patient's learning:
- description of hypercalcemia, its causes, and treatment
- prescribed medications
- avoidance of preparations that contain phosphorus (laxatives, enemas, supplements)
- avoidance of high-phosphorus foods (dairy products, meat, fish, poultry, eggs, and peanuts)
- warning signs and symptoms and when to report them
- referrals to dietitian and social services, if indicated.

Hypophosphatemia
- Serum phosphorus level < 2.5 mg/dl (can be severe if < 1 mg/dl)
- Can occur when total body phosphorus stores are normal

HYPOPHOSPHATEMIA

Hypophosphatemia occurs when the serum phosphorus level falls below 2.5 mg/dl (or 1.8 mEq/L). Although this condition generally indicates a deficiency of phosphorus, it can occur under various circumstances when total body phosphorus stores are normal. Severe hypophosphatemia occurs when serum phosphorus levels are less than 1 mg/dl and the body can't support its energy needs, leading to possible organ failure.

Causes
- Three underlying mechanisms: shifting of phosphorus from extracellular to intracellular fluid, decreased intestinal absorption of phosphorus, and increased kidney excretion of phosphorus

Hyperventilation
- Can result from heatstroke, sepsis, pain, anxiety, and DKA
- Can result in respiratory alkalosis, which shifts phosphorus from serum to cells

CAUSES AND PATHOPHYSIOLOGY

Three underlying mechanisms can lead to hypophosphatemia: a shift of phosphorus from extracellular fluid to intracellular fluid, a decrease in intestinal absorption of phosphorus, and an increased loss of phosphorus through the kidneys. Some causes of hypophosphatemia may involve more than one mechanism. Hyperventilation, insulin, absorption problems, and kidney excretion are some of the factors that may cause phosphorus to shift from extracellular fluid into the cell.

Hyperventilation

Respiratory alkalosis, one of the most common causes of hypophosphatemia, can stem from a number of conditions that produce hyperventilation, including sepsis, alcohol withdrawal, heatstroke, pain, anxiety, diabetic ketoacidosis (DKA), hepatic encephalopathy, and acute salicylate poisoning. Although the mechanism that prompts respiratory alkalosis to induce hypophosphatemia is unknown, the response is a shift of phosphorus into the cells and a resulting decrease in serum phosphorus levels.

Insulin

Hyperglycemia, an elevated serum glucose level, causes the release of insulin, which transports glucose and phosphorus into the cells. The same effect may occur in a patient with diabetes who's receiving insulin or in a significantly malnourished patient; at particular risk for malnourishment are patients who are elderly, debilitated, or alcoholic and those with anorexia nervosa.

Phosphorus also shifts into cells after initiation of enteral or parenteral feeding and when phosphorus supplementation is insufficient. This shift is called *refeeding syndrome* and usually occurs 3 or more days after feedings begin. Patients recovering from hypothermia can also develop hypophosphatemia as phosphorus moves into the cells.

Absorption problems

Malabsorption syndromes, starvation, and prolonged or excessive use of phosphorus-binding antacids or sucralfate are among the many causes of impaired intestinal absorption of phosphorus. Because vitamin D contributes to intestinal absorption of phosphorus, inadequate vitamin D intake or synthesis can inhibit phosphorus absorption. Chronic diarrhea or laxative abuse can also result in increased GI loss of phosphorus. Decreased dietary intake rarely causes hypophosphatemia because phosphate is found in most foods.

Kidney excretion

Diuretic use is the most common cause of phosphorus loss through the kidneys. Thiazides, loop diuretics, and acetazolamide are the diuretics that most commonly cause hypophosphatemia. The second most common cause is DKA in diabetic patients who have poorly controlled blood glucose levels. In DKA, an osmotic diuresis is induced from high glucose levels. This results in a significant loss of phosphorus from the kidneys. Ethanol affects phosphorus reabsorption in the kidney so that more phosphorus is excreted in the urine.

A buildup of parathyroid hormone (PTH), which occurs with hyperparathyroidism and hypocalcemia, also leads to hypophosphatemia because PTH stimulates the kidneys to excrete phosphate. Finally, hypophosphatemia occurs in patients who have extensive burns. Although the causative mechanism is unclear, the condition is suspected to occur in re-

Causes *(continued)*

Insulin
- Transports glucose and phosphorus into cells
- Release caused by hyperglycemia
- Effects mimicked by initiation of enteral or parenteral feeding, insufficient phosphorus supplementation, and hypothermia

Absorption problems
- Malabsorption syndromes
- Starvation
- Prolonged or excessive use of phosphorus-binding antacids or sucralfate
- Inadequate vitamin D intake or synthesis
- Chronic diarrhea or laxative abuse

Kidney excretion
- Diuretics (most common cause of phosphorus loss through kidneys)
- DKA in diabetic patients (second most common cause of phosphorus loss through kidneys)
- Buildup of PTH
- Extensive burns

sponse to the extensive diuresis of salt and water that typically occurs during the first 2 to 4 days after a burn injury. Respiratory alkalosis and carbohydrate administration may also play a role.

Assessment findings

Most common
- Muscle weakness
- Diplopia
- Malaise
- Anorexia
- Shallow, ineffective respirations

Neurologic
- Paresthesia
- Irritability
- Apprehension
- Memory loss
- Confusion

Cardiovascular
- Hypotension
- Low cardiac output
- Cardiomyopathy
- Decreased oxygen delivery to tissues

Hematologic
- Hemolytic anemia
- Susceptibility to infection
- Bruising and bleeding, particularly mild GI bleeding

ASSESSMENT FINDINGS

Mild to moderate hypophosphatemia is typically asymptomatic. Noticeable effects of hypophosphatemia typically occur only in severe cases. The characteristics of severe hypophosphatemia are apparent in many organ systems. Signs and symptoms may develop acutely due to rapid decreases in phosphorus or gradually as the result of slow, chronic decreases in phosphorus. Hypophosphatemia affects the musculoskeletal, central nervous, cardiac, and hematologic systems. Because phosphorus is required to make high-energy adenosine triphosphate (ATP), many of the signs and symptoms of hypophosphatemia are related to low energy stores.

With hypophosphatemia, muscle weakness is the most common symptom. Other symptoms may include diplopia, malaise, and anorexia. The patient may experience a weakened hand grasp, slurred speech, or dysphagia, and also may develop myalgia.

Respiratory failure may result from weakened respiratory muscles and poor contractility of the diaphragm. Respirations may appear shallow and ineffective. In later stages, the patient may be cyanotic. Keep in mind that it may be difficult to wean a mechanically ventilated patient with hypophosphatemia from the ventilator.

With severe hypophosphatemia, rhabdomyolysis, which causes skeletal muscle destruction, can occur with altered muscle cell activity. Muscle enzymes such as creatine kinase are released from the cells into the extracellular fluid. Loss of bone density, osteomalacia, and bone pain may also occur with prolonged hypophosphatemia. In addition, fractures can result.

Without adequate phosphorus, the body can't make enough ATP, a cornerstone of energy metabolism. As a result, central nervous system cells can malfunction, causing paresthesia, irritability, apprehension, memory loss, and confusion. The neurologic effects of hypophosphatemia may progress to seizures or coma.

The cardiovascular effects of hypophosphatemia result in the heart's decreased contractility due to low energy stores of ATP. As a result, the patient may develop hypotension and a low cardiac output. Severe hypophosphatemia may lead to cardiomyopathy, which can be reversed with treatment. A drop in production of 2,3-DPG causes a decrease in oxygen delivery to tissues. Because hemoglobin has a stronger affinity for oxygen than for other gases, oxygen is less likely to be given up to the tissues as it circulates through the body. Consequently, less oxygen is delivered to the myocardium, which can cause chest pain.

Hypophosphatemia may also cause hemolytic anemia because of changes in the structure and function of red blood cells. Patients with hypophosphatemia are more susceptible to infection because of the effect of low levels of ATP in white blood cells. Lack of ATP results in a decreased functioning of leukocytes. Chronic hypophosphatemia also affects platelet function, resulting in bruising and bleeding, particularly mild GI bleeding.

Diagnostic test results

Typical laboratory findings for a patient with hypophosphatemia include:

- serum phosphorus level of less than 2.5 mg/dl (or 1.8 mEq/L); severe hypophosphatemia is less than 1 mg/dl
- elevated creatine kinase level with rhabdomyolysis
- X-ray studies revealing the skeletal changes typical of osteomalacia or bone fractures
- abnormal electrolytes (decreased magnesium levels and increased calcium levels).

Treatment

Treatment varies with the severity and cause of the hypophosphatemia. It includes treating the underlying cause and correcting the imbalance with phosphorus replacement and a high-phosphorus diet. The route of replacement therapy depends on the severity of the imbalance.

Treatment for mild to moderate hypophosphatemia includes a diet high in phosphorus-rich foods, such as eggs, nuts, whole grains, meat, fish, poultry, and milk products. However, if calcium is contraindicated or the patient can't tolerate milk, oral phosphorus supplements should be used. Oral supplements include Neutra-Phos and Neutra-Phos-K and can be used for moderate hypophosphatemia. Dosage limitations are related to the adverse effects, most notably nausea and diarrhea. (See *Raising phosphorus levels*, page 150.)

For patients with severe hypophosphatemia or a nonfunctioning GI tract, I.V. phosphorus replacement is the recommended choice. Dosages of I.V. potassium phosphate and I.V. sodium phosphate are guided by the patient's response to treatment and serum phosphorus levels. Potassi-

Diagnostic test results

- Serum phosphorus level < 2.5 mg/dl (severe hypophosphatemia, < 1 mg/dl)
- X-ray studies revealing skeletal changes typical of osteomalacia or bone fractures
- Decreased magnesium levels
- Increased calcium levels

Treatment

- Diet high in phosphorous-rich foods (oral phosphorus supplements if calcium is contraindicated or patient can't tolerate milk) for mild to moderate hypophosphatemia
- I.V. phosphorus replacement for severe hypophosphatemia or patients with nonfunctioning GI tract
- Assess for evidence of decreasing muscle strength
- Administer prescribed phosphorus supplements
- During infusions, watch for signs of hypocalcemia, hyperphosphatemia, and I.V. infiltration
- Monitor serum electrolyte levels, especially calcium and phosphorus levels

Raising phosphorus levels

If your patient is following a phosphorus-rich diet that hasn't raised his serum phosphorus levels, you should investigate these factors:
- ✦ GI problems, which make phosphorus digestion difficult
- ✦ phosphate-binding antacid use
- ✦ alcohol abuse
- ✦ thiazide diuretic use
- ✦ treatment regimen compliance for diabetes.

um phosphate should be administered slowly (no more than 10 mEq/hour). Adverse effects of I.V. replacement for hypophosphatemia include hyperphosphatemia and hypocalcemia.

Key nursing interventions

- ✦ Monitor vital signs
- ✦ Assess LOC and neurologic status
- ✦ Ensure patient safety
- ✦ Restore normal serum phosphorus levels
- ✦ Monitor for signs of heart failure (crackles, shortness of breath, decreased blood pressure, elevated heart rate)

Nursing interventions

If your patient is beginning total parenteral nutrition or is otherwise at risk for developing hypophosphatemia, monitor him for signs and symptoms of this imbalance. If the patient has already developed hypophosphatemia, your nursing care should focus on careful monitoring, safety measures, and interventions to restore normal serum phosphorus levels. Immediately notify the physician to any changes in the patient's condition and take these other actions:

✦ Monitor vital signs. Remember, hypophosphatemia can lead to respiratory failure, low cardiac output, confusion, seizures, or coma.

✦ Assess the patient's level of consciousness (LOC) and neurologic status each time you check his vital signs. Document your observations and the patient's neurologic status on a flow sheet so changes can be noted immediately, even on other shifts. (See *Documenting hypophosphatemia.*)

DANGER *If the patient has severe hypophosphatemia, monitor the rate and depth of respirations. Report signs and symptoms of hypoxia, such as confusion, restlessness, increased respiratory rate and, in later stages, cyanosis. If possible, take steps to prevent hyperventilation, because it worsens respiratory alkalosis and can lower phosphorus levels. Follow arterial blood gas results and pulse oximetry levels to monitor the effectiveness of ventilation. Wean patients from the ventilator slowly.*

✦ Monitor the patient for evidence of heart failure related to reduced myocardial functioning. Such evidence includes crackles, shortness of breath, decreased blood pressure, and elevated heart rate.

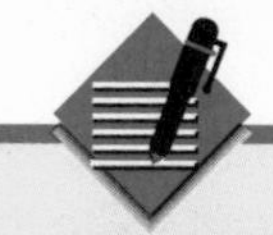

CHARTING CHECKLIST

Documenting hypophosphatemia

If your patient has hypophosphatemia, make sure you document:
- ❑ vital signs
- ❑ neurologic status, including level of consciousness, restlessness, apprehension
- ❑ muscle strength
- ❑ respiratory assessment
- ❑ serum electrolyte levels and other pertinent laboratory data
- ❑ time that you notified the physician
- ❑ I.V. therapy, including condition of the I.V. site, medication, dose, and the patient's response
- ❑ seizures, if any
- ❑ your interventions and the patient's response
- ❑ safety measures to protect the patient
- ❑ patient teaching provide and the patient's response.

✦ Monitor the patient's temperature at least every 4 hours. Check WBC counts. Follow strict sterile technique in changing dressings and report signs of infection.

✦ Assess the patient frequently for evidence of decreasing muscle strength, such as weak hand grasps or slurred speech, and document your findings regularly.

✦ Administer prescribed phosphorus supplements. Keep in mind that oral supplements may cause diarrhea. To improve their taste, mix them with juice. Vitamin D may also be ordered with the oral phosphate supplements to increase absorption.

✦ Insert an I.V. line, as ordered, and keep it patent. Infuse phosphorus solutions slowly, using an infusion device to control the rate. During infusions, watch for signs of hypocalcemia, hyperphosphatemia, and I.V. infiltration. Potassium phosphate can cause tissue sloughing and necrosis. Monitor serum phosphate levels every 6 hours.

✦ Administer an analgesic, if ordered.

✦ Make sure the patient maintains bed rest, if ordered, for his own safety. Keep the bed in its lowest position, with wheels locked and side rails raised. If the patient is at risk for seizures, pad the side rails and keep an artificial airway at the patient's bedside.

✦ Orient the patient as needed. Keep clocks, calendars, and familiar personal objects within his sight.

Key nursing interventions *(continued)*

- ✦ Monitor temperature every 4 hours
- ✦ Assess for decreased muscle strength
- ✦ Monitor serum phosphate levels every 6 hours during phosphorus infusions

✦ Inform the patient and his family that confusion caused by a low phosphorus level is only temporary and will most likely decrease with therapy.
✦ Record the patient's fluid intake and output.
✦ Carefully monitor serum electrolyte levels, especially calcium and phosphorus levels as well as other pertinent laboratory test results and make sure to report abnormalities.
✦ Assist the patient with ambulation and activities of daily living, if needed, and keep essential objects near him.

Patient teaching
✦ Description of disorder
✦ Medications
✦ Diet
✦ Warning signs and symptoms
✦ Follow-up appointments

Patient teaching

If your patient has hypophosphatemia, cover these topics with the patient and then evaluate his learning:
✦ description of hypophosphatemia and its risk factors, prevention, and treatment
✦ medications ordered
✦ need to consult with a dietitian
✦ need for a high-phosphorus diet
✦ avoidance of antacids that contain phosphorus
✦ warning signs and symptoms and when to report them
✦ need to maintain follow-up appointments.

Chloride imbalances

CHLORIDE

Chloride is the most abundant anion, or negatively charged ion, in extracellular fluid. It moves in and out of the cells with sodium and potassium and combines with major cations, or positively charged ions, to form sodium chloride, hydrochloric acid, potassium chloride, calcium chloride, and other important compounds. High levels of chloride are found in cerebrospinal fluid (CSF), but it can also be found in bile and in gastric and pancreatic juices.

Because of its negative charge, chloride travels with positively charged sodium and helps maintain serum osmolality and water balance. Chloride and sodium also work together to form CSF. The choroid plexus, a tangled mass of tiny blood vessels inside the ventricles of the brain, depends on these two electrolytes to attract water and to form the fluid component of CSF.

In the stomach, chloride is secreted by the gastric mucosa as hydrochloric acid, providing the acid medium conducive to digestion and enzyme activation. Chloride helps maintain acid-base balance and assists in carbon dioxide transport in the red blood cells.

Chloride

- ✦ Most abundant anion (negatively charged ion) in extracellular fluid
- ✦ Combines with major cations (positively charged ions) to form important compounds
- ✦ High levels found in CSF; also found in bile and in gastric and pancreatic juices

Functions of chloride

- ✦ Helps maintain serum osmolality and water balance
- ✦ Works with sodium to form CSF
- ✦ Helps maintain acid-base balance
- ✦ Assists in carbon dioxide transport in red blood cells

NORMAL CHLORIDE LEVELS

Serum chloride levels normally range between 96 and 106 mEq/L. By comparison, the chloride level inside a cell is 4 mEq/L. Chloride levels re-

Normal chloride levels

- ✦ Normal serum chloride level: 96 to 106 mEq/L
- ✦ Changes in direct proportion with sodium level

Dietary sources of chloride

Common dietary sources of chloride include:
- canned vegetables
- fruits
- processed meats
- raw vegetables, such as lettuce and celery
- salty foods
- table salt.

main relatively stable with age. Because chloride balance is closely associated with sodium balance, the levels of both electrolytes usually change in direct proportion to one another.

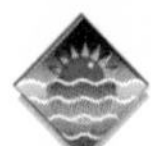

AGE ALERT *Patients between ages 60 and 90 have chloride levels between 98 and 107 mEq/L; patients age 90 and older, between 98 and 111 mEq/L.*

Regulating chloride
- Depends on intake and excretion of chloride and reabsorption of chloride ions in kidney

Sodium and chloride
- Closely linked; change in one electrolyte level causes comparable change in other

Acids and bases
- Chloride reabsorbed and excreted in direct opposition to bicarbonate

REGULATING CHLORIDE

Chloride regulation depends on intake and excretion of chloride and reabsorption of chloride ions in the kidneys. The normal daily chloride requirement for adults is 750 mg. Most diets provide sufficient chloride in the form of salt, usually as sodium chloride, in the same foods that contain sodium. (See *Dietary sources of chloride.*)

Most chloride is absorbed in the intestines with only a small portion lost in stool. It's produced mainly in the stomach as hydrochloric acid, so chloride levels can be influenced by GI disorders.

Sodium and chloride

Because chloride and sodium are closely linked, a change in one electrolyte level causes a comparable change in the other. For example, chloride levels can be indirectly affected by aldosterone secretion, which causes the renal tubules to reabsorb sodium. As positively charged sodium ions are reabsorbed, negatively charged chloride ions are passively reabsorbed because of their electrical attraction to sodium.

Acids and bases

Regulation of chloride levels also involves acid-base balance. Chloride is reabsorbed and excreted in direct opposition to bicarbonate. When chloride levels change, the body attempts to keep its positive-negative balance by making corresponding changes in the levels of bicarbonate, another negatively charged ion—which is alkaline—in the kidneys.

Chloride and bicarbonate have an inverse relationship. When chloride levels decrease, the kidneys retain bicarbonate and bicarbonate levels increase. When chloride levels increase, the kidneys excrete bicarbonate and bicarbonate levels decrease. Therefore, changes in chloride and bicarbonate levels can lead to acidosis or alkalosis.

HYPERCHLOREMIA

Hyperchloremia, an excess of chloride in extracellular fluid, occurs when serum chloride levels exceed 108 mEq/L. This condition is associated with other acid-base imbalances, such as metabolic acidosis, and rarely occurs alone.

Causes and pathophysiology

Because chloride regulation and sodium regulation are closely related, hyperchloremia may also be associated with hypernatremia. Chloride and bicarbonate have an inverse relationship, so an excess of chloride ions may be linked to a decrease in bicarbonate. Excess serum chloride results from increased chloride intake or absorption, from acidosis, or from chloride retention by the kidneys.

Increased intake and absorption

Increased intake of chloride as sodium chloride can cause hyperchloremia, especially if water is lost from the body at the same time. That water loss raises the chloride level even more. Increased chloride absorption by the bowel can occur in patients who have had anastomoses joining the ureter and intestines.

Conditions that alter electrolyte and acid-base balance and cause metabolic acidosis include dehydration, renal tubular acidosis, renal failure, respiratory alkalosis, salicylate toxicity, hyperparathyroidism, hyperaldosteronism, and hypernatremia.

Drug-related retention

Several medications can also contribute to hyperchloremia. Direct ingestion of ammonium chloride or other drugs that contain chloride or cause chloride retention can lead to hyperchloremia. Ion exchange resins that contain sodium, such as Kayexalate, can cause chloride to be exchanged

Hyperchloremia

- ✦ Serum chloride level > 108 mEq/L
- ✦ Excess of chloride in extracellular fluid
- ✦ Rarely occurs alone; associated with other acid-base imbalances

Causes

- ✦ Can result from increased chloride intake or absorption, acidosis, or chloride retention by kidneys

Increased intake and absorption

- ✦ Increased intake as sodium chloride
- ✦ Increased chloride absorption by the bowel
- ✦ Metabolic acidosis

Drug-related retention

- ✦ Ammonium chloride
- ✦ Ion exchange resins containing sodium (Kayexalate)
- ✦ Carbonic anhydrase inhibitors (acetazolamide)

Anion gap and metabolic acidosis

Hyperchloremia increases the likelihood that a patient will develop hyperchloremic metabolic acidosis. The illustration below shows the relationship between chloride and bicarbonate in the development of hyperchloremic metabolic acidosis.

A normal anion gap in a patient with metabolic acidosis indicates that the acidosis is most likely caused by a loss of bicarbonate ions by the kidneys or the GI tract. In such cases, a corresponding increase in chloride ions also occurs.

Acidosis can also result from an accumulation of chloride ions in the form of acidifying salts. A corresponding decrease in bicarbonate ions occurs at the same time. In this illustration, the chloride level is high (> 106 mEq/L) and the bicarbonate level is low (< 22 mEq/L).

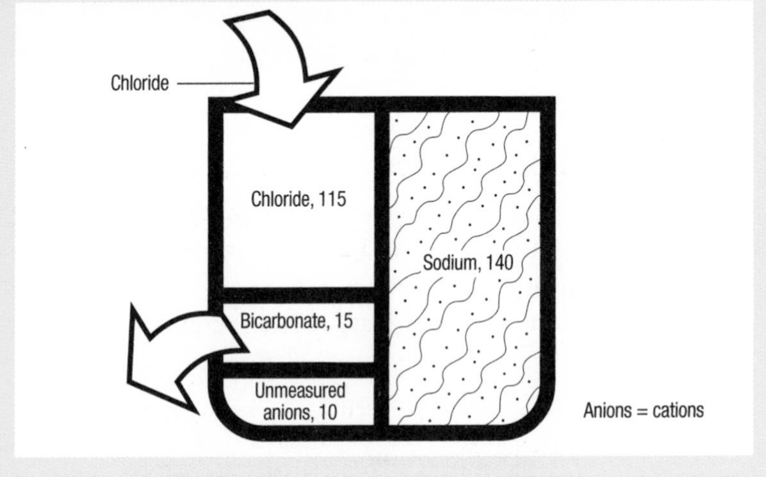

for potassium in the bowel. When chloride follows sodium into the bloodstream, serum chloride levels rise. Carbonic anhydrase inhibitors, such as acetazolamide, also promote chloride retention in the body by increasing bicarbonate ion loss.

Assessment findings
- Tachypnea
- Lethargy
- Weakness
- Diminished cognitive ability
- Deep, rapid respirations (Kussmaul's respirations)
- If untreated, arrhythmias, decreased cardiac output, decreased LOC, and coma

Assessment findings

Hyperchloremia rarely produces signs and symptoms on its own. Instead, the major signs and symptoms are essentially those of metabolic acidosis, including tachypnea, lethargy, weakness, diminished cognitive ability, and deep, rapid respirations such as Kussmaul's respirations.

Left untreated, acidosis can lead to arrhythmias, decreased cardiac output, a further decrease in the patient's level of consciousness (LOC), and even coma. Metabolic acidosis related to a high chloride level is called *hyperchloremic metabolic acidosis.* (See *Anion gap and metabolic acidosis.*)

Treatment with diuretics

If your patient with hyperchloremia doesn't respond to therapy, the physician may order diuretics to eliminate chloride. Although other electrolytes will be lost, the patient's chloride level should decrease.

If a patient has an increased serum chloride level, his serum sodium level is probably high as well, which can lead to fluid retention. He also may be agitated and have dyspnea, tachycardia, hypertension, or pitting edema — signs of hypernatremia and hypervolemia.

Diagnostic test results

Typical laboratory findings for a patient with hyperchloremia include:

✦ serum chloride level greater than 106 mEq/L

✦ serum sodium level greater than 145 mEq/L

✦ serum pH level less than 7.35, a serum bicarbonate level less than 22 mEq/L, and a normal anion gap (8 to 14 mEq/L), suggesting metabolic acidosis.

Diagnostic test results

✦ Serum chloride level > 106 mEq/L

✦ Serum sodium level > 145 mEq/L

✦ Serum pH < 7.35, serum bicarbonate level < 22 mEq/L, and normal anion gap (8 to 14 mEq/L), suggesting metabolic acidosis

Treatment

Treatment for hyperchloremia includes correcting the underlying cause as well as restoring fluid, electrolyte, and acid-base balance. (See *Treatment with diuretics.*) Dehydrated patients may receive fluids to dilute the chloride and speed renal excretion of chloride ions. Sodium and chloride intake also may be restricted.

If the patient's liver function is adequate, he may receive an infusion of lactated Ringer's solution to convert lactate to bicarbonate in the liver and to increase the base bicarbonate level and correct acidosis. In severe hyperchloremia, I.V. sodium bicarbonate may be administered to raise serum bicarbonate levels. Because bicarbonate and chloride compete for sodium, I.V. sodium bicarbonate therapy can lead to renal excretion of chloride ions and correction of acidosis.

Treatment

✦ Fluids and sodium and chloride restrictions for dehydrated patients

✦ Infusion of lactated Ringer's solution if patient's liver function is adequate

✦ I.V. sodium bicarbonate for severe hyperchloremia

Nursing interventions

Try to prevent hyperchloremia by monitoring high-risk patients. If your patient develops a chloride imbalance follow these interventions:

✦ Monitor vital signs, including cardiac rhythm.

CHARTING CHECKLIST

Documenting hyperchloremia

If your patient has hyperchloremia, make sure you document:
- ❑ vital signs, including cardiac rhythm
- ❑ level of consciousness, muscle strength, and activity level
- ❑ serum electrolyte and arterial blood gas levels
- ❑ fluid intake and output
- ❑ safety precautions taken
- ❑ assessment and interventions and the patient's responses
- ❑ patient teaching provided and the patient's response.

Key nursing interventions
- ✦ Monitor vital signs, including cardiac rhythm
- ✦ Reorient confused patient
- ✦ Continually assess patient, paying particular attention to neurologic, cardiac, and respiratory examinations
- ✦ Insert I.V. line, and maintain its patency
- ✦ Restrict fluids, sodium, and chloride, if ordered

✦ If the patient is confused, reorient him as needed, and provide a safe, quiet environment to prevent injury. Teach the patient's family to do the same.
✦ Continually assess the patient, paying particular attention to the neurologic, cardiac, and respiratory examinations. Immediately report changes to the physician.
✦ Look for changes in the respiratory pattern that may indicate a worsening of the acid-base imbalance.
✦ Insert an I.V. line and maintain its patency. Administer I.V. fluids and medications as ordered. Watch for signs of fluid overload.
✦ Evaluate muscle strength, and adjust activity level accordingly.
✦ If the patient is receiving high doses of sodium bicarbonate, watch for signs and symptoms of overcompensation, such as metabolic alkalosis, which may cause central and peripheral nervous system overstimulation. Also watch for signs of hypokalemia as potassium is forced into the cells.
✦ Restrict fluids, sodium, and chloride, if ordered.
✦ Monitor and record serum electrolyte levels and arterial blood gas results.
✦ Monitor and record fluid intake and output. (See *Documenting hyperchloremia.*)

Patient teaching
- ✦ Description of disorder
- ✦ Warning signs and symptoms
- ✦ Diet
- ✦ Medications

Patient teaching

Be sure to cover these topics and then evaluate your patient's learning:
✦ description of hyperchloremia and its risk factors, prevention, and treatment
✦ warning signs and symptoms and when to report them
✦ dietary restrictions if ordered

✦ medications if prescribed
✦ importance of replenishing lost fluids during hot weather.

HYPOCHLOREMIA

Hypochloremia is a deficiency of chloride in extracellular fluid. It occurs when serum chloride levels fall below 96 mEq/L. When serum chloride levels drop, levels of sodium, potassium, calcium, and other electrolytes may be affected. If much more chloride than sodium is lost, hypochloremic alkalosis may occur.

Causes and pathophysiology

Serum chloride levels drop when chloride intake or absorption decreases or when chloride losses increase. Losses may occur through the skin (in sweat), the GI tract, or the kidneys. Changes in sodium levels or acid-base balance also alter chloride levels.

Decreased chloride intake

Reduced chloride intake may occur in infants being fed chloride-deficient formula and in people on salt-restricted diets. Patients dependent on I.V. fluids are also at risk if the fluids lack chloride such as a dextrose solution without electrolytes.

AGE ALERT *In infants, hypochloremic alkalosis isn't uncommon. In the past, some infants were fed a chloride-deficient formula, which caused hypochloremic alkalosis to develop, resulting in cognitive delays, language disorders, and impaired visual motor skills. In 1980, the U.S. Congress passed a law regulating chloride content in infant formula so that it contains a minimum of 55 to 65 mg/100 kcal and a maximum of 150 mg/100 kcal of chloride. Human milk contains about 420 mg/L and undiluted cow's milk contains 900 to 1,020 mg/L. Infant formula contains 10.6 to13.5 mEq/L; formula for older infants (follow-up formula), 14 to 19.2 mEq/L. Recommended daily chloride intake is 2 to 4 mEq/L/kg for infants and children and 60 to150 mEq/L for adolescents.*

Hypochloremic alkalosis is also commonly seen in children and neonates. Poor dietary intake of chloride, diuretic therapy in chronic lung disease, or nasogastric (NG) suctioning can all cause this condition. It may also be seen in infants with chloride-wasting syndromes resulting from renal causes such as Bartter syndrome, intestinal causes such as congenital chloride-losing diarrhea, or chloride loss from cystic fibrosis.

Excessive chloride losses

Excessive chloride losses can occur with prolonged vomiting, diarrhea, severe diaphoresis, gastric surgery, NG suctioning, and other GI tube

Hypochloremia
✦ Deficiency of chloride in extracellular fluid
✦ Serum chloride levels < 96 mEq/L

Causes
✦ Serum chloride levels decrease when chloride intake or absorption decreases or chloride losses increase
✦ Losses occur through skin (sweat), GI tract, or kidneys

Decreased chloride intake
✦ Infants being fed chloride-deficient formula
✦ People on salt-restricted diets
✦ Patients dependent on I.V. fluids

Age alert
✦ Recommended daily chloride intake for infants and children: 2 to 4 mEq/L; for adolescents, 60 to 150 mEq/L

Hypochloremic alkalosis
✦ Commonly seen in children and neonates
✦ Caused by poor dietary intake of chloride, diuretic therapy in chronic lung disease, NG suctioning, and chloride-wasting syndromes

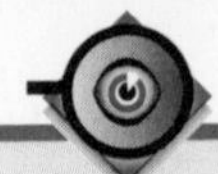

CLOSER LOOK

How hypochloremic metabolic alkalosis develops

A dangerous development, hypochloremia can lead to hypochloremic metabolic alkalosis. Below is an illustration of how this happens.

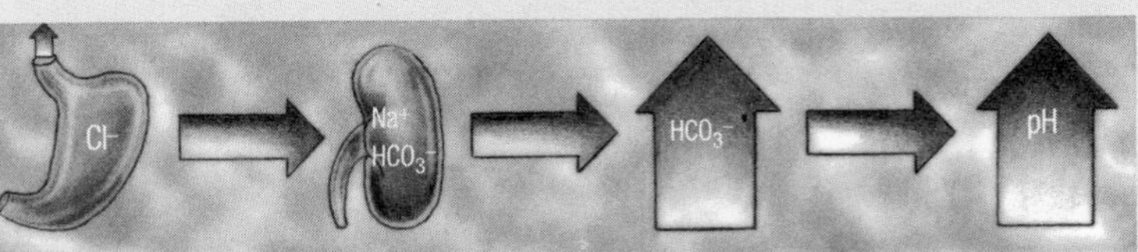

Nasogastric suctioning can deplete chloride ions (Cl^-).	Kidneys retain sodium ions (Na^+) and bicarbonate ions (HCO_3^-) to balance chloride loss.	HCO_3^- accumulate in extracellular fluid.	Excess HCO_3^- raises pH level and leads to hypochloremic metabolic alkalosis.

Excessive chloride losses

- Can occur with prolonged vomiting, diarrhea, severe diaphoresis, gastric surgery, NG suctioning, and GI tube drainage
- May be caused by bicarbonate, corticosteroids, laxatives, theophylline, and such diuretics as furosemide, ethacrynic acid, and hydrochlorothiazide

drainage. Severe vomiting can cause a loss of hydrochloric acid from the stomach, an acid deficit in the body, and subsequent metabolic alkalosis. Patients with cystic fibrosis can also lose more chloride than normal. Any prolonged and untreated hypochloremic state can result in hypochloremic alkalosis. (See *How hypochloremic metabolic alkalosis develops.*)

People at risk for hypochloremia include children with prolonged vomiting from pyloric obstruction and those with draining fistulas and ileostomies that can cause a loss of chloride from the GI tract. Various drugs may decrease chloride, including bicarbonate, corticosteroids, laxatives, and theophylline (Slo-Phyllin). Diuretics, such as furosemide (Lasix), ethacrynic acid (Edecrin), and hydrochlorothiazide (HydroDIURIL) can also cause an excessive loss of chloride because chloride ions are excreted by the kidneys with cations.

Additional causes

Other causes of hypochloremia include sodium and potassium deficiency or metabolic alkalosis; conditions that affect acid-base or electrolyte balance, such as untreated diabetic ketoacidosis and Addison's disease; and rapid removal of ascitic fluid (which contains sodium) during paracentesis. Also, patients who have heart failure may develop hypochloremia because serum chloride levels are diluted by excess fluid in the body.

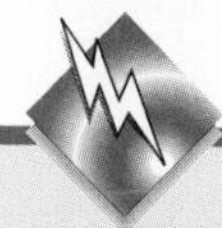

DANGER

Danger signs of hypochloremia

Suspect that your patient with hypochloremia is in extreme danger if he has any of these life-threatening conditions:
✦ arrhythmias
✦ respiratory arrest
✦ seizures and coma.

Assessment findings

Patients who have hypochloremia may have signs and symptoms of acid-base and electrolyte imbalances. You may notice signs of hyponatremia, hypokalemia, or metabolic alkalosis. Alkalosis results in a high pH and, to compensate, respirations become slow and shallow as the body tries to retain carbon dioxide and restore the pH level to normal.

The nerves also become more excitable, so observe for tetany, hyperactive deep tendon reflexes, and muscle hypertonicity. (See *Danger signs of hypochloremia.*) The patient may have muscle cramps, twitching, and weakness and be agitated or irritable. If hypochloremia goes unrecognized, it can become life-threatening. As the chloride imbalance worsens, along with other imbalances, the patient may suffer arrhythmias, seizures, coma, or respiratory arrest.

Assessment findings
✦ Slow, shallow respirations
✦ Tetany
✦ Hyperactive deep tendon reflexes
✦ Muscle hypertonicity
✦ Muscle cramps
✦ Twitching
✦ Weakness
✦ Agitated or irritable disposition

Diagnostic test results

Typical laboratory findings for a patient with hypochloremia include:
✦ serum chloride level below 98 mEq/L
✦ serum sodium level below 135 mEq/L indicating hyponatremia
✦ serum pH greater than 7.45 and serum bicarbonate level greater than 26 mEq/L indicating metabolic alkalosis.

Diagnostic test results
✦ Serum chloride level < 98 mEq/L
✦ Serum sodium level < 135 mEq/L
✦ Serum pH > 7.45 and serum bicarbonate level > 26 mEq/L

Treatment

Treatment for hypochloremia focuses on correcting the underlying cause, such as low dietary chloride intake, prolonged vomiting, or gastric suctioning. Chloride may be replaced through fluid administration or drug therapy. The patient may also require treatment for associated metabolic alkalosis or electrolyte imbalances such as hypokalemia.

Treatment
✦ Correction of underlying cause
✦ Chloride replacement through fluid administration or drug therapy

Treating hypochloremia

If treatment for hypochloremia isn't successful, make sure the patient isn't drinking large amounts of water, which can cause him to excrete large amounts of chloride. In addition, review the causes of hypochloremia to identify new or coexisting conditions that might be causing chloride loss.

Chloride may be given orally; for example, in a salty broth. If the patient can't take oral supplements, he may receive medications or normal saline solution I.V. To avoid hypernatremia, which causes a high sodium level, or to treat hypokalemia, potassium chloride may be administered I.V.

Treatment for associated metabolic alkalosis usually addresses the underlying causes. The underlying cause of diaphoresis, vomiting or other GI losses, or renal losses should be investigated. Rarely, metabolic alkalosis may be treated by administering ammonium chloride, an acidifying agent that's used when alkalosis is caused by chloride loss. Drug dosage depends on the severity of the alkalosis. The effects of ammonium chloride last only 3 days. After that, the kidneys begin to excrete the extra acid. (See *Treating hypochloremia*.)

NURSING INTERVENTIONS

Key nursing interventions

- ✦ Monitor LOC, muscle strength, and movement
- ✦ Monitor vital signs, especially respiratory rate and pattern, and observe for worsening respiratory function
- ✦ Monitor cardiac rhythm
- ✦ Monitor and record serum electrolyte levels, especially chloride, sodium, potassium, and bicarbonate
- ✦ Provide high-chloride foods (tomato juice, salty broth)

Be sure to monitor patients at risk for hypochloremia, such as those receiving diuretic therapy or NG suctioning. When caring for a patient with hypochloremia, you'll also want to take these nursing actions:

✦ Monitor level of consciousness (LOC), muscle strength, and movement.

✦ Notify the physician if the patient's condition worsens.

DANGER *In patients with hypochloremia, monitor vital signs, especially respiratory rate and pattern, and observe for worsening respiratory function. Also monitor cardiac rhythm because hypokalemia may be present with hypochloremia. Have emergency equipment handy in case the patient's condition deteriorates.*

✦ Monitor and record serum electrolyte levels, especially chloride, sodium, potassium, and bicarbonate. Also assess arterial blood gas results for acid-base imbalance.

✦ If the patient is alert and can swallow without difficulty, offer foods high in chloride, such as tomato juice or salty broth. Don't let the patient fill up on plain drinking water.

CHARTING CHECKLIST

Documenting hypochloremia

If your patient has hypochloremia, make sure you document:
- ❑ vital signs, including cardiac rhythm
- ❑ intake and output
- ❑ serum electrolyte levels and arterial blood gas results
- ❑ your assessment, including level of consciousness, seizure activity, and respiratory status
- ❑ time that you notified the physician
- ❑ I.V. therapy, along with other interventions, and the patient's response
- ❑ safety measures implemented
- ❑ patient teaching and the patient's response.

✦ Insert an I.V. line, as ordered, and keep it patent. Administer chloride and potassium replacements as ordered.

✦ If administering ammonium chloride, assess the patient for pain at the infusion site and adjust the rate, if needed. Because ammonium chloride is metabolized by the liver, don't give it to patients with severe hepatic disease.

✦ Use normal saline solution, not tap water, to flush the patient's NG tube.

✦ Accurately measure and record intake and output, including the volume of vomitus and gastric contents from suction and other GI drainage tubes.

✦ Provide a safe environment. Help the patient ambulate, and keep his personal items and call button within reach. Institute seizure precautions, as needed.

✦ Provide a quiet environment, explain interventions, and reorient the patient as needed.

✦ Document all care and the patient's response. (See *Documenting hypochloremia*.)

Key nursing interventions *(continued)*

- ✦ Monitor intake and output
- ✦ Use normal saline solution to flush NG tube
- ✦ Ensure patient safety
- ✦ Reorient patient as needed

Patient teaching

Be sure to cover these topics and then evaluate your patient's learning:

✦ description of hypochloremia and its risk factors, prevention, and treatment

✦ warning signs and symptoms and when to report them

✦ dietary supplements

✦ medications if prescribed.

Patient teaching

- ✦ Description of disorder
- ✦ Warning signs and symptoms
- ✦ Dietary supplements
- ✦ Medications

Acid-base imbalances

Acid-base imbalances

- Cells use nutrients to produce energy to function, forming carbon dioxide and hydrogen (by-products)

ABG analysis

- pH — measures H^+ concentration and indicates blood acidity or alkalinity
- $Paco_2$ — reflects adequacy of lung ventilation
- HCO_3^- level — reflects kidney retention or excretion of bicarbonate

Compensatory mechanisms

- Chemical buffers
- Respiratory reactions
- Kidney reactions

UNDERSTANDING ACID-BASE IMBALANCES

The body constantly works to maintain homeostasis between acids and bases. Without that balance, cells can't function properly. As cells use nutrients to produce the energy they need to function, two by-products are formed — carbon dioxide and hydrogen. Acid-base balance depends on the regulation of free hydrogen ions (H^+). The concentration of H^+ in body fluids determines the extent of acidity or alkalinity, both of which are measured in pH. Remember, pH levels are inversely proportional to H^+ concentration, which means when H^+ concentration increases, pH decreases causing acidosis. Conversely, when H^+ concentration decreases, pH increases causing alkalosis. (For more information about pH, see chapter 3, Acid-base balance.)

Blood gas measurements remain the major diagnostic tool for evaluating acid-base states. An arterial blood gas (ABG) analysis includes these tests: pH, which measures the H^+ concentration and is an indication of the blood's acidity or alkalinity; partial pressure of arterial carbon dioxide ($Paco_2$), which reflects the adequacy of lung ventilation; and bicarbonate level (HCO_3^-), which reflects the activity of the kidneys in retaining or excreting bicarbonate. (See *Analyzing ABG results.*)

Most of the time, the body's compensatory mechanisms restore acid-base balance — or at least prevent the life-threatening consequences of an

Analyzing ABG results

When analyzing your patient's arterial blood gas (ABG), use these three main normal values:

pH	7.35 to 7.45
$Paco_2$	35 to 45 mm Hg
HCO_3^-	22 to 26 mEq/L

imbalance. Those compensatory mechanisms include chemical buffers, certain respiratory reactions, and certain kidney reactions.

For example, the body compensates for a primary respiratory disturbance such as respiratory acidosis by inducing metabolic alkalosis. Unfortunately, not all attempts to compensate are equal. The respiratory system is efficient and can compensate for metabolic disturbances quickly, whereas the metabolic system, working through the kidneys, can take hours or days to compensate for an imbalance. This chapter discusses each of the four major acid-base imbalances.

METABOLIC ACIDOSIS

Metabolic acidosis is caused by an increase in hydrogen ion (H^+) production and is characterized by a pH below 7.35 and a bicarbonate (HCO_3^-) level below 22 mEq/L. This disorder depresses the central nervous system (CNS) and if left untreated, it may lead to ventricular arrhythmias, coma, and cardiac arrest.

CAUSES AND PATHOPHYSIOLOGY

The underlying mechanisms in metabolic acidosis are a loss of HCO_3^- from extracellular fluid, an accumulation of metabolic acids, or a combination of the two. If the patient's anion gap, which is the measurement of the difference between the amount of sodium and the amount of HCO_3^- in the blood, is greater than 14 mEq/L, then the acidosis is due to an accumulation of metabolic acids or unmeasured anions.

If the metabolic acidosis is associated with a normal anion gap (8 to 14 mEq/L), loss of HCO_3^- may be the cause. (See *How metabolic acidosis develops,* pages 166 to 167.)

(Text continues on page 168.)

Metabolic acidosis

- Indicated by pH < 7.35 and HCO_3^- < 22 mEq/L
- Caused by increase in H^+ production
- If untreated, may lead to ventricular arrhythmias, coma, and cardiac arrest

Pathophysiology

- Underlying mechanisms: Loss of HCO_3^- from extracellular fluid, accumulation of metabolic acids, or combination of both
- Characterized by gain in acids or loss of bases from plasma

Metabolic acidosis development

Step 1

- H^+ accumulates in body, binding with chemical buffers in cells and extracellular fluid

Step 2

- Excess H^+ decrease pH and stimulate chemoreceptors in medulla, increasing respiratory rate
- Respiratory compensation occurs within minutes, but insufficient to correct imbalance

Step 3

- Kidneys try compensating for acidosis by secreting excess H^+ into renal tubules
- Secreted H^+ forms weak acid after being excreted into urine

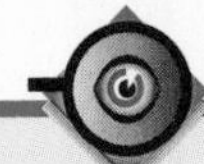

CLOSER LOOK

How metabolic acidosis develops

This series of illustrations shows how metabolic acidosis develops at the cellular level.

STEP 1

As hydrogen ions (H^+) start to accumulate in the body, chemical buffers (plasma bicarbonate and proteins) in the cells and extracellular fluid bind with them. *No signs are detectable at this stage.*

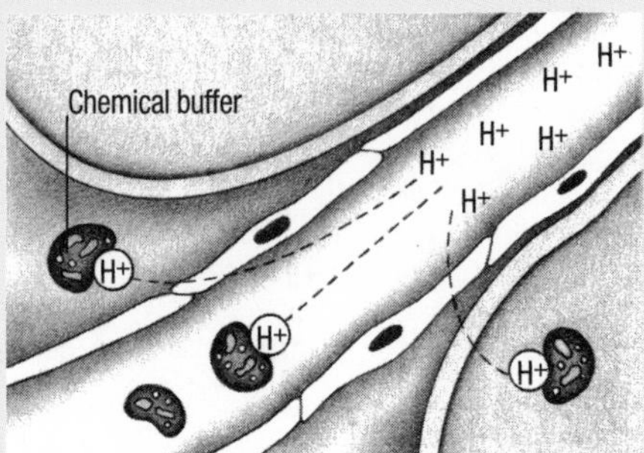

STEP 2

Excess H^+ that the buffers can't bind with decrease pH and stimulate chemoreceptors in the medulla to increase the respiratory rate. The increased respiratory rate lowers partial pressure of arterial carbon dioxide ($Paco_2$), which allows more H^+ to bind with bicarbonate ions (HCO_3^-). Respiratory compensation occurs within minutes but isn't sufficient to correct the imbalance. *Look for a pH level below 7.35, an HCO_3^- level below 22 mEq/L, a decreasing $Paco_2$ level, and rapid, deeper respirations.*

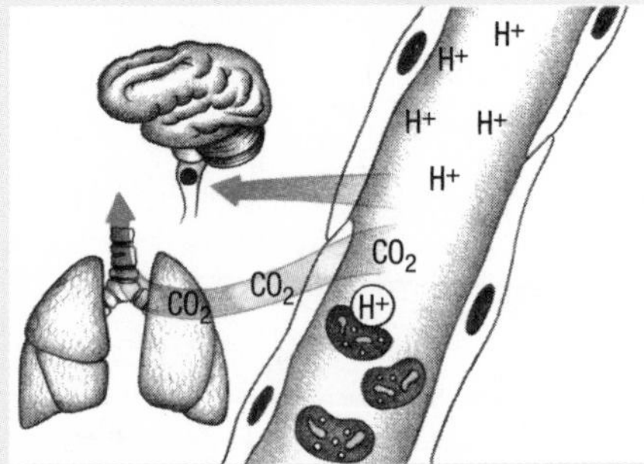

STEP 3

Healthy kidneys try to compensate for acidosis by secreting excess H^+ into the renal tubules. Those ions are buffered by phosphate or ammonia and then are excreted into the urine in the form of a weak acid. *Look for acidic urine.*

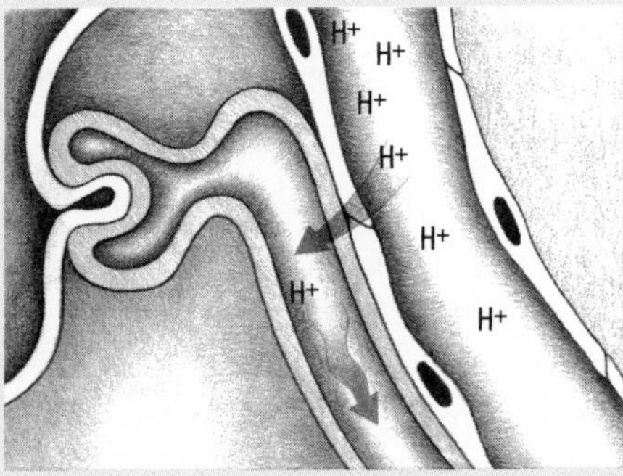

STEP 4

Each time H^+ is secreted into the renal tubules, a sodium ion (Na^+) and HCO_3^- are absorbed from the tubules and returned to the blood. *Look for pH and HCO_3^- levels that return slowly to normal.*

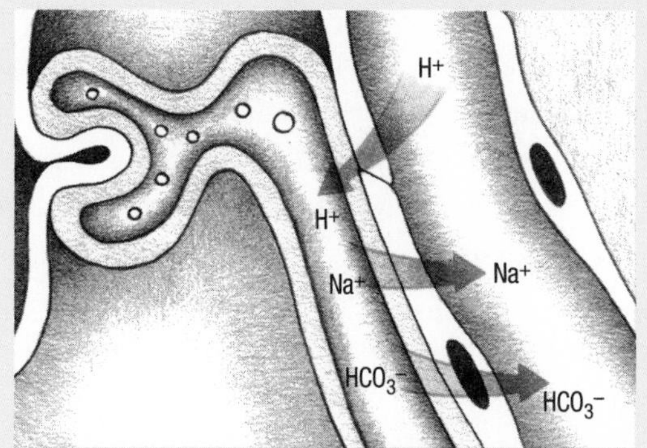

STEP 5

Excess H^+ in the extracellular fluid diffuse into cells. To maintain the balance of the charge across the membrane, the cells release potassium ions (K^+) into the blood. *Look for signs and symptoms of hyperkalemia, including colic and diarrhea, weakness or flaccid paralysis, tingling and numbness in the extremities, bradycardia, a tall T wave, a prolonged PR interval, and a wide QRS complex.*

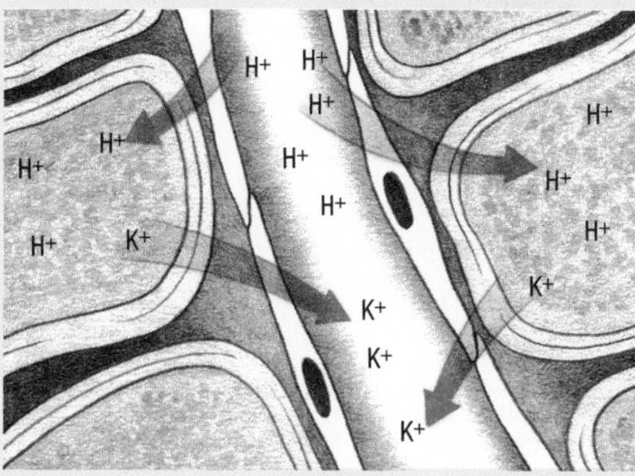

STEP 6

Excess H^+ alters the normal balance of K^+, Na^+, and calcium ions (Ca^{++}), leading to reduced excitability of nerve cells. *Look for signs and symptoms of progressive central nervous system depression, including lethargy, dull headache, confusion, stupor, and coma.*

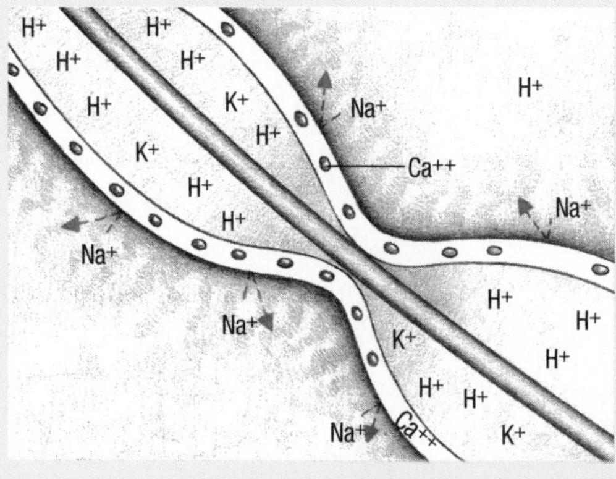

Metabolic acidosis development
(continued)

Step 4

- Each time H^+ secreted into renal tubules, Na^+ and HCO_3^- are absorbed from tubules and returned to blood

Step 5

- Excess H^+ in extracellular fluid diffuse into cells
- Cells release K^+ into blood to maintain charge balance across membrane

Step 6

- Excess H^+ alters normal balance of K^+, Na^+, and Ca^{++}, reducing excitability of nerve cells

Metabolic acidosis is characterized by a gain in acids or a loss of bases from plasma. The condition may be related to an overproduction of ketone bodies. Fatty acids are converted to ketone bodies when glucose supplies have been used and the body draws on fat stores for energy. Conditions that cause an overproduction of ketone bodies include diabetes mellitus, chronic alcoholism, severe malnutrition or starvation, poor dietary intake of carbohydrates, hyperthyroidism, and severe infection with accompanying fever.

Lactic acidosis can cause or worsen metabolic acidosis and can occur secondarily to shock, heart failure, pulmonary disease, hepatic disorders, seizures, or strenuous exercise.

Metabolic acidosis can also stem from a decreased ability of the kidneys to excrete acids, as occurs in renal insufficiency or renal failure with acute tubular necrosis. Metabolic acidosis also occurs with excessive GI losses from diarrhea, intestinal malabsorption, a draining fistula of the pancreas or liver, or a urinary diversion to the ileum. Other causes include hyperaldosteronism and use of a potassium-sparing diuretic such as acetazolamide, which inhibits the secretion of acid.

Risk factors

- ✦ Patient with poisoning
- ✦ Patient with toxic reaction to medication (toluene, salicylates, methanol, ethylene glycol, paraldehyde; hydrochloric acid, ammonium chloride)

At particular risk for metabolic acidosis are patients with poisoning or a toxic reaction to a drug, which can occur following inhalation of toluene or ingestion of a salicylate, such as aspirin or an aspirin-containing medication; methanol; ethylene glycol; paraldehyde; hydrochloric acid; or ammonium chloride.

Assessment findings

Assessment findings

- ✦ Kussmaul's respirations
- ✦ Depressed CNS
- ✦ Decreased blood pressure
- ✦ Weakness
- ✦ Headache
- ✦ Deteriorated LOC, from confusion to stupor and coma
- ✦ Anorexia, nausea, and vomiting

Metabolic acidosis typically produces respiratory, neurologic, and cardiac signs and symptoms. As acid builds up in the bloodstream, the lungs compensate by blowing off carbon dioxide (CO_2).

Hyperventilation, especially increased depth of respirations, is the first clue to metabolic acidosis. Called *Kussmaul's respirations,* the breathing is rapid and deep. A patient with diabetes who experiences Kussmaul's respirations may have a fruity odor to his breath, which stems from catabolism of fats and excretion of acetone through the lungs.

As the pH drops, the CNS is further depressed, as is myocardial function. Cardiac output and blood pressure drop, and arrhythmias may occur if the patient also has hyperkalemia.

Initially, the skin is warm and dry as a result of peripheral vasodilation, but as shock develops, the skin becomes cold and clammy. The patient may complain of weakness and a dull headache as the cerebral ves-

ABG results in metabolic acidosis

This chart shows typical arterial blood gas (ABG) findings in uncompensated and compensated metabolic acidosis.

	UNCOMPENSATED	COMPENSATED
pH	<7.35	Normal
$Paco_2$ (mm Hg)	Normal	< 35
HCO_3^- (mEq/L)	< 22	< 22

sels dilate. The patient's level of consciousness (LOC) may deteriorate from confusion to stupor and coma. A neuromuscular examination may show diminished muscle tone and deep tendon reflexes. Metabolic acidosis also has an effect on the GI system, causing anorexia, nausea, and vomiting.

Diagnostic test results

Typical laboratory findings for a patient with metabolic acidosis include:

✦ arterial blood gas (ABG) analysis is the key diagnostic test for detecting metabolic acidosis. Typically, the pH is below 7.35. $Paco_2$ may be less than 35 mm Hg, indicating compensatory attempts by the lungs to rid the body of excess CO_2. (See *ABG results in metabolic acidosis.*)

✦ Serum potassium levels are usually elevated as H^+ move into the cells and potassium moves out to maintain electroneutrality.

✦ Blood glucose and serum ketone levels rise in patients with diabetic ketoacidosis (DKA).

✦ Plasma lactate levels rise in patients with lactic acidosis. (See *Understanding lactic acidosis,* page 170.)

✦ The anion gap is increased—this measurement is calculated by subtracting the amount of negative ion (chloride plus bicarbonate) from the amount of the positive ion (sodium). Sometimes the amount of potassium ion is added to the amount of positive ion, but the amount of potassium ion is usually so small that the calculation doesn't change. The normal anion gap is 8 to 14 mEq/L.

✦ Electrocardiogram changes associated with hyperkalemia—such as tall T waves, prolonged PR intervals, and wide QRS complexes—may be found.

Diagnostic test results

✦ ABG analysis (key test): pH < 7.35 and $Paco_2 < 35$ mm Hg

✦ Elevated serum potassium level

✦ Increased blood glucose and serum ketone levels with DKA

✦ Increased plasma lactate levels in patients with lactic acidosis

✦ Increased anion gap

✦ ECG showing tall T waves, prolonged PR intervals, and wide QRS complexes

Understanding lactic acidosis

- Lactate — produced as result of carbohydrate metabolism and metabolized by liver; normal level, 0.93 to 1.65 mEq/L
- Lactic acidosis — occurs when lactate accumulates faster than it can be metabolized

Causes

- Septic shock
- Cardiac arrest
- Pulmonary disease
- Seizures
- Strenuous exercise

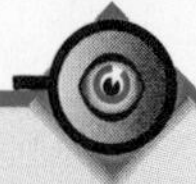

CLOSER LOOK

Understanding lactic acidosis

Lactate, produced as a result of carbohydrate metabolism, is metabolized by the liver. The normal lactate level is 0.93 to 1.65 mEq/L. With tissue hypoxia, however, cells are forced to switch to anaerobic metabolism and more lactate is produced. When lactate accumulates in the body faster than it can be metabolized, lactic acidosis occurs. It can happen any time the demand for oxygen in the body is greater than its availability. Causes of lactic acidosis include septic shock, cardiac arrest, pulmonary disease, seizures, and strenuous exercise. The latter two cause transient lactic acidosis. Hepatic disorders can also cause lactic acidosis because the liver can't metabolize lactate.

TREATMENT

Treatment focuses on eliminating the underlying cause. If the pH is below 7.1, sodium bicarbonate may be given. Use caution when administering sodium bicarbonate, however, because it may cause alkalosis.

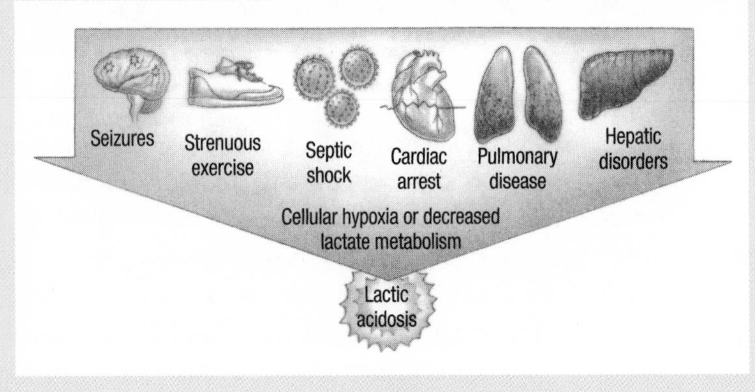

Treatment

- Respiratory compensation (first line of therapy), including mechanical ventilation
- I.V. sodium bicarbonate
- Dialysis

TREATMENT

Treatment aims to correct metabolic acidosis as quickly as possible by addressing both the symptoms and the underlying cause. Respiratory compensation is usually the first line of therapy, including mechanical ventilation, if needed.

For patients with diabetes, expect to administer rapid-acting insulin to reverse DKA and drive potassium back into the cell. For any patient with metabolic acidosis, monitor serum potassium levels. Even though high serum levels exist initially, serum potassium levels will drop as the acidosis is corrected and may result in hypokalemia. Any other electrolyte imbalances are evaluated and corrected.

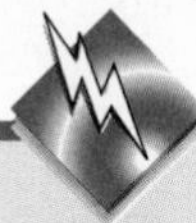

DANGER

Acidosis and dopamine

If you're administering dopamine (Intropin) to a patient and it isn't raising his blood pressure as you expected, investigate your patient's pH. A pH level below 7.1, which can happen in severe metabolic acidosis, causes resistance to vasopressor therapy. Correct the pH level, and the dopamine may prove to be more effective.

Sodium bicarbonate is administered I.V. to neutralize blood acidity in patients with a pH lower than 7.1 and bicarbonate loss. Fluids are replaced parenterally as required. Dialysis may be initiated in patients with renal failure or a toxic reaction to a drug. Such patients may receive an antibiotic to treat sources of infection or an antidiarrheal to treat diarrhea-induced bicarbonate loss.

DANGER *Watch for worsening of CNS status or deteriorating laboratory and ABG test results. Ventilatory support may be needed, so prepare for intubation. Dialysis may be needed for patients with renal failure, especially when complicated by diabetes. Maintain a patent I.V. line to administer emergency drugs, and flush the line with normal saline solution before and after administering sodium bicarbonate because the bicarbonate may inactivate or cause precipitation of many drugs.* *(See* Acidosis and dopamine.*)*

Nursing interventions

If your patient is at risk for metabolic acidosis, careful monitoring can help prevent it from developing. If your patient has metabolic acidosis, nursing care includes immediate emergency interventions and long-term treatment of the condition and its underlying causes. Observe these guidelines:

✦ Monitor vital signs, and assess cardiac rhythm.

✦ Prepare for mechanical ventilation or dialysis as required.

✦ Monitor the patient's neurologic status closely because changes can occur rapidly. Notify the physician of any changes in the patient's condition.

✦ Insert an I.V. line, as ordered, and maintain patent I.V. access. Have a large-bore catheter in place for emergency situations. Administer I.V. fluid, a vasopressor, an antibiotic, and other medications, as prescribed.

Key nursing interventions

✦ Monitor vital signs
✦ Assess cardiac rhythm
✦ Prepare for mechanical ventilation or dialysis, as required
✦ Monitor neurologic status
✦ Insert I.V. line and maintain patent access

CHARTING CHECKLIST

Documenting metabolic acidosis

If your patient has metabolic acidosis, make sure you document:

- ❑ assessment findings, including results of neurologic examination
- ❑ intake and output
- ❑ time you notified the physician
- ❑ prescribed medications and I.V. therapy, and the patient's response
- ❑ safety measures implemented
- ❑ serum electrolyte levels and arterial blood gas results
- ❑ ventilator or dialysis data
- ❑ vital signs and cardiac rhythm
- ❑ patient teaching provided and the patient's response.

Key nursing interventions *(continued)*

- ✦ Administer sodium bicarbonate as ordered
- ✦ Eliminate underlying cause
- ✦ Monitor renal function by recording intake and output
- ✦ Monitor serum electrolyte levels
- ✦ Monitor ABG results

✦ Administer sodium bicarbonate as ordered. Remember to flush the I.V. line with normal saline solution before and after giving bicarbonate because the chemical can inactivate many drugs or cause them to precipitate. Be aware that too much bicarbonate can cause metabolic alkalosis and pulmonary edema.

✦ Position the patient to promote chest expansion and facilitate breathing. If the patient is stuporous, turn him frequently.

✦ Take steps to help eliminate the underlying cause. For example, administer insulin and I.V. fluids as prescribed to reverse DKA.

✦ Watch for any secondary changes, such as declining blood pressure, that hypovolemia may cause.

✦ Monitor the patient's renal function by recording intake and output. (See *Documenting metabolic acidosis.*)

✦ Watch for changes in the serum electrolyte levels, and monitor ABG results throughout treatment to check for overcorrection.

✦ Orient the patient as needed. If he's confused, take steps to ensure his safety, such as keeping his bed in the lowest position.

✦ Investigate reasons for the patient's ingestion of toxic substances.

Physical examination and further diagnostic tests may provide additional information about your patient's metabolic acidosis. As you reevaluate the patient's condition, consider these questions:

✦ Has the patient's LOC returned to normal?

✦ Have his vital signs stabilized?

- Have his ABG results, blood glucose levels, and serum electrolyte levels improved?
- Is his cardiac output normal?
- Has he regained a normal sinus rhythm or his previously stable underlying rhythm?
- Is he ventilating adequately?

Patient teaching

Be sure to cover these topics and then evaluate your patient's learning:

- description of metabolic acidosis and its treatment
- testing of blood glucose levels, if indicated
- need for strict adherence to antidiabetic therapy, if appropriate
- avoidance of alcohol
- warning signs and symptoms and when to report them
- prescribed medications
- avoidance of ingestion of toxic substances.

Patient teaching

- Description of disorder
- Testing of blood glucose levels
- Antidiuretic therapy
- Alcohol avoidance
- Warning signs and symptoms
- Toxic substances

METABOLIC ALKALOSIS

Metabolic alkalosis, caused by a decrease in hydrogen ion (H^+) production, is characterized by a blood pH above 7.45 and is accompanied by a bicarbonate (HCO_3^-) level above 26 mEq/L. In acute metabolic alkalosis, the HCO_3^- level may be as high as 50 mEq/L. With early diagnosis and prompt treatment, the prognosis for effective treatment is good. Left untreated, metabolic alkalosis can result in coma, arrhythmias, and death.

Metabolic alkalosis

- Indicated by blood pH > 7.45 and bicarbonate level > 26 mEq/L
- Caused by decrease in H^+ production
- If untreated, may lead to coma, arrhythmias, and death

Causes and pathophysiology

In metabolic alkalosis, the underlying mechanisms include a loss of H^+ (acid), a gain in HCO_3^-, or both. Partial pressure of arterial carbon dioxide ($Paco_2$) greater than 45 mm Hg (possibly as high as 60 mm Hg) indicates that the lungs are compensating for the alkalosis. Renal compensation is more effective but slower as well. Metabolic alkalosis is commonly associated with hypokalemia, particularly from the use of thiazides, furosemide (Lasix), ethacrynic acid (Edecrin), and other diuretics that deplete potassium stores. In hypokalemia, the kidneys conserve potassium. At the same time, the kidneys also increase the excretion of hydrogen ions, which prompts alkalosis from the loss of acid. Metabolic alkalosis may also occur with hypochloremia and hypocalcemia. (See *How metabolic alkalosis develops*, pages 174 and 175.)

(Text continues on page 176.)

Pathophysiology

- Underlying mechanisms include loss of H^+, gain in HCO_3^-, or both
- Commonly associated with hypokalemia, but may also occur with hypochloremia and hypocalcemia

Metabolic alkalosis development

Step 1

- Chemical buffers in extracellular fluid and cells bind with HCO_3^- as it accumulates

Step 2

- Excess HCO_3^- elevates pH levels, causing decreased respiratory rate and, in turn, increased $Paco_2$

Step 3

- When HCO_3^- exceeds 28 mEq/L, renal glomeruli can't reabsorb excess HCO_3^- and it's excreted into urine (H^+ retained)

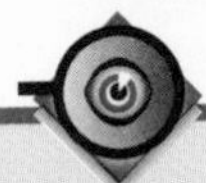

CLOSER LOOK

How metabolic alkalosis develops

This series of illustrations shows how metabolic alkalosis develops at the cellular level.

STEP 1

As bicarbonate ions (HCO_3^-) start to accumulate in the body, chemical buffers in extracellular fluid and cells bind with the ions. *No signs are detectable at this stage.*

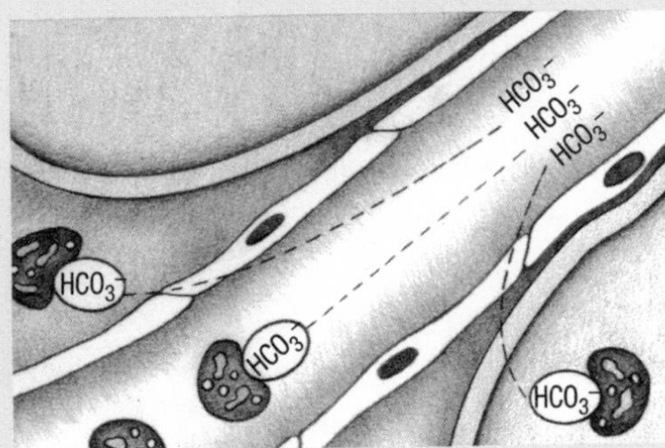

STEP 2

Excess HCO_3^- ions that don't bind with chemical buffers elevate serum pH levels, which in turn depresses chemoreceptors in the medulla. Depression of those chemoreceptors causes a decrease in respiratory rate, which increases the partial pressure of arterial carbon dioxide ($Paco_2$). The additional carbon dioxide (CO_2) combines with water (H_2O) to form carbonic acid (H_2CO_3). *Note:* Lowered oxygen levels limit respiratory compensation. *Look for a serum pH level above 7.45, an HCO_3^- level above 26 mEq/L, a rising $Paco_2$, and slow, shallow respirations.*

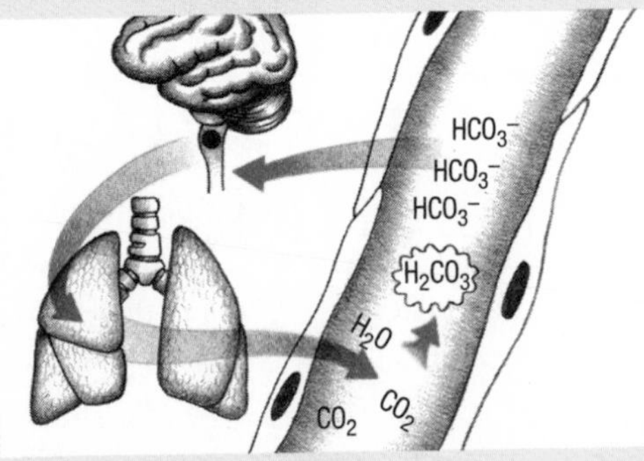

STEP 3

When the HCO_3^- level exceeds 28 mEq/L, the renal glomeruli can no longer reabsorb excess HCO_3^-. That excess HCO_3^- is excreted in the urine; hydrogen ions (H^+) are retained. *Look for alkaline urine and pH and HCO_3^- levels that return slowly to normal.*

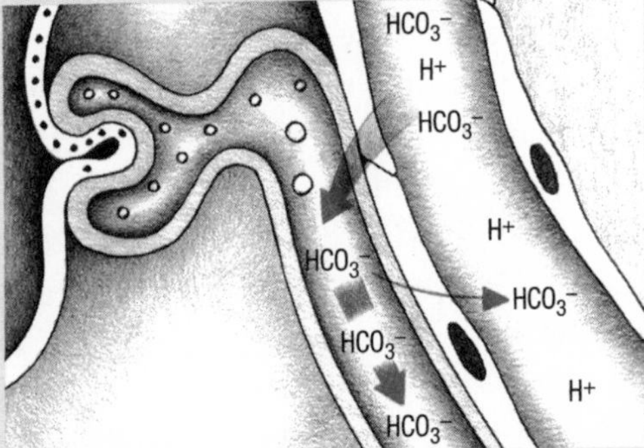

STEP 4

To maintain electrochemical balance, the kidneys excrete excess sodium ions (Na^+), H_2O, and HCO_3^-. *Look for polyuria initially, then signs and symptoms of hypovolemia, including thirst and dry mucous membranes.*

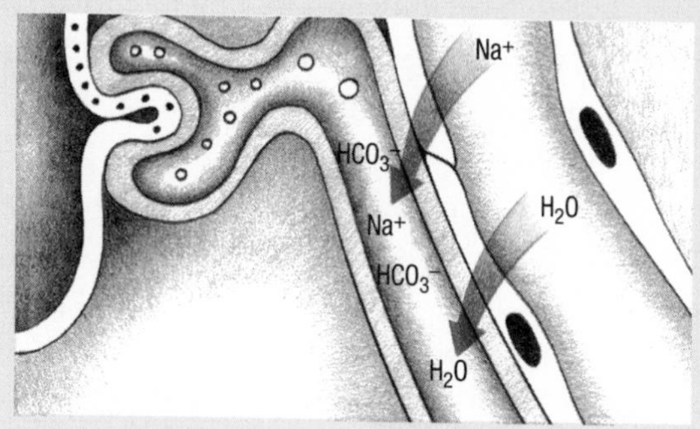

STEP 5

Lowered H^+ levels in the extracellular fluid cause the ions to diffuse out of the cells. To maintain the balance of charge across the cell membrane, extracellular potassium ions (K^+) move into the cells. *Look for signs and symptoms of hypokalemia, including anorexia, muscle weakness, loss of reflexes, and others.*

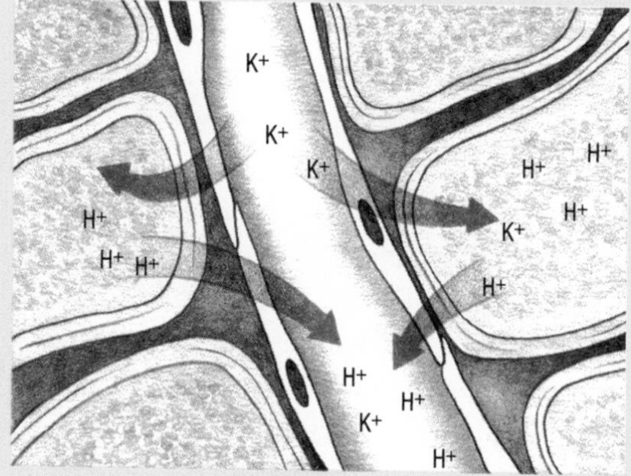

STEP 6

As H^+ levels decline, calcium ionization (Ca^{++}) decreases. That decrease in ionization makes nerve cells more permeable to Na^+. Na^+ moving into nerve cells stimulate neural impulses and produce overexcitability of the peripheral and central nervous systems. *Look for tetany, belligerence, irritability, disorientation, and seizures.*

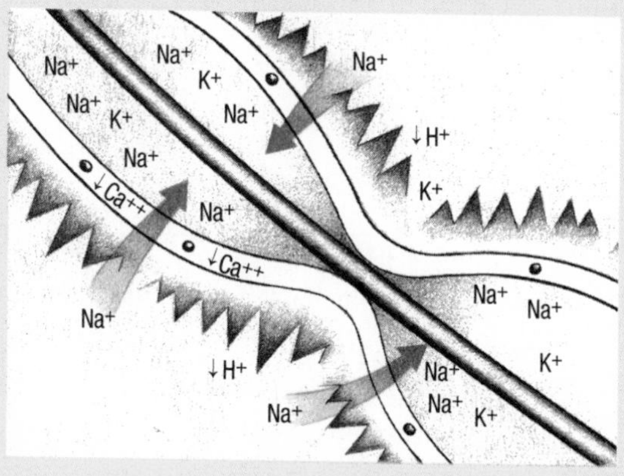

Metabolic alkalosis development *(continued)*

Step 4

- Kidneys excrete excess Na^+, H_2O, and HCO_3^- to maintain electro-chemical balance

Step 5

- Lowered H^+ levels in extracellular fluid cause ions to diffuse out of cells and extracellular K^+ to move into cells

Step 6

- Ca^{++} ionization decreases as H^+ levels decline, making cells more permeable to Na^+
- Na^+ moving into nerve cells stimulate neural impulses, producing overexcitability of peripheral and central nervous systems

Causes

- ✦ Excessive acid loss from GI tract (most common)
- ✦ Vomiting
- ✦ Pyloric stenosis
- ✦ Prolonged NG suctioning
- ✦ Diuretic therapy

Metabolic alkalosis can result from many causes, the most common of which is excessive acid loss from the GI tract. Vomiting causes loss of hydrochloric acid from the stomach. Children who have pyloric stenosis can develop this disorder. Alkalosis also results from prolonged nasogastric (NG) suctioning, presenting a risk for surgical patients and patients with GI disorders.

Diuretic therapy presents another risk of metabolic alkalosis. Thiazide and loop diuretics can lead to a loss of hydrogen, potassium, and chloride ions from the kidneys. Hypokalemia causes H^+ excretion from the kidneys as they try to conserve potassium. Potassium moves out of the cell as hydrogen moves in, resulting in alkalosis.

With the fluid loss of diuresis, the kidneys attempt to conserve sodium and water. For sodium to be reabsorbed, H^+ must be excreted. In a process known as contraction alkalosis, bicarbonate is reabsorbed and metabolic alkalosis results.

Other causes of metabolic alkalosis include Cushing's disease, which causes retention of sodium and chloride and urinary loss of potassium and hydrogen. Rebound alkalosis following correction of organic acidosis, such as after cardiac arrest and administration of sodium bicarbonate, can also cause metabolic alkalosis. Posthypercapnic alkalosis occurs when chronic carbon dioxide retention is corrected by mechanical ventilation and the kidneys haven't yet corrected the chronically high HCO_3^- levels.

Metabolic alkalosis can also result from kidney disease, such as renal artery stenosis, or from multiple transfusions. Certain drugs, such as corticosteroids and antacids that contain sodium bicarbonate, can also lead to metabolic alkalosis.

Assessment findings

Initial

- ✦ Slow, shallow respirations (hypoventilation)

Neuromuscular

- ✦ Muscle twitching
- ✦ Weakness
- ✦ Tetany
- ✦ Hyperactive reflexes
- ✦ Numbness and tingling of fingers, toes, and mouth

Assessment findings

Initially, your patient may have slow, shallow respirations as hypoventilation, a compensatory mechanism, occurs. However, this mechanism is limited because hypoxemia soon develops, which stimulates ventilation. The signs and symptoms of metabolic alkalosis are commonly associated with an underlying condition. The resulting hypokalemic or hypocalcemic electrocardiogram (ECG) changes may be seen, as well as hypotension.

Metabolic alkalosis results in neuromuscular excitability, which causes muscle twitching, weakness, tetany, and hyperactive reflexes. The patient may experience numbness and tingling of the fingers, toes, and mouth

ABG results in metabolic alkalosis

This chart shows typical arterial blood gas (ABG) findings in uncompensated and compensated metabolic alkalosis.

	UNCOMPENSATED	COMPENSATED
pH	> 7.45	Normal
$Paco_2$ (mm Hg)	Normal	> 45
HCO_3^- (mEq/L)	> 26	> 26

area. Neurologic symptoms include apathy and confusion. Seizures, stupor, and coma may result.

If hypokalemia affects the GI tract, the patient will probably experience anorexia, nausea, and vomiting. If it affects the genitourinary (GU) tract—that is, if the kidneys are affected—polyuria may result. If left untreated, metabolic alkalosis can result in arrhythmias and death.

Diagnostic test results

Typical laboratory findings for a patient with metabolic alkalosis include:

✦ arterial blood gas (ABG) analysis may reveal a blood pH above 7.45 and an HCO_3^- level above 26 mEq/L. If the underlying cause is excessive acid loss, the HCO_3^- level may be normal. $Paco_2$ level may be above 45 mm Hg, indicating respiratory compensation. (See *ABG results in metabolic alkalosis.*)

✦ Serum electrolyte levels usually indicate low potassium, calcium, and chloride levels. HCO_3^- levels are elevated.

✦ ECG changes may occur, such as a low T wave that merges with the P wave.

Treatment

Treatment aims to correct the acid-base imbalance by providing the patient's body sufficient time to rid itself of excess HCO_3^- and increase its H^+ concentration.

✦ I.V. administration of ammonium chloride is rarely done but may be necessary in severe cases.

✦ Thiazide diuretics and NG suctioning are discontinued. An antiemetic may be administered to treat underlying nausea and vomiting.

Assessment findings *(continued)*

Neurologic
- ✦ Apathy
- ✦ Confusion
- ✦ Seizures
- ✦ Stupor
- ✦ Coma

GI
- ✦ Anorexia
- ✦ Nausea
- ✦ Vomiting

GU
- ✦ Polyuria

Diagnostic test results

- ✦ ABG analysis: blood pH > 7.45, HCO_3^- level > 26 mEq/L, and $Paco_2$ level > 45 mm Hg
- ✦ ECG may show low T wave that merges with the P wave

Treatment

- ✦ Discontinuation of thiazide diuretics and NG suctioning
- ✦ Antiemetics
- ✦ Acetazolamide

CHARTING CHECKLIST

Documenting metabolic alkalosis

If your patient has metabolic alkalosis, make sure you document:

❑ vital signs, including cardiac rhythm
❑ level of consciousness, muscle strength, and activity level
❑ serum electrolyte and arterial blood gas levels
❑ fluid intake and output
❑ safety precautions taken
❑ assessment and interventions and the patient's responses
❑ patient teaching provided and the patient's response.

✦ Acetazolamide (Diamox) may be added to increase renal excretion of HCO_3^-.

Key nursing interventions

- Monitor vital signs, including cardiac rhythm and respiratory pattern
- Assess LOC
- Administer oxygen as ordered
- Maintain patent I.V. access as ordered
- Monitor intake and output
- Irrigate NG tube with normal saline solution instead of tap water
- Assess laboratory test results
- Watch for signs of muscle weakness, tetany, or decreased activity

NURSING INTERVENTIONS

If your patient is at risk for metabolic alkalosis, careful monitoring can help prevent its development. If your patient has metabolic alkalosis, follow these guidelines:

✦ Monitor vital signs, including cardiac rhythm and respiratory pattern.

✦ Assess the patient's level of consciousness (LOC) when taking his health history or by talking with him while you're performing the physical examination. For instance, apathy and confusion may be evident in a patient's conversation.

✦ Administer oxygen, as ordered, to treat hypoxemia.

✦ Institute seizure precautions when needed, and explain them to the patient and his family.

✦ Maintain patent I.V. access as ordered.

✦ Administer diluted potassium solutions with an infusion device.

✦ Monitor intake and output. (See *Documenting metabolic alkalosis.*)

✦ Infuse 0.9% ammonium chloride no faster than 1 L over 4 hours. Faster administration may cause hemolysis of red blood cells. Don't administer the drug to a patient who has hepatic or renal disease.

✦ Irrigate an NG tube with normal saline solution instead of tap water, to prevent loss of gastric electrolytes.

✦ Assess laboratory test results, such as ABG and serum electrolyte levels. Notify the physician of any changes.

✦ Watch closely for signs of muscle weakness, tetany, or decreased activity.

Patient teaching

Be sure to cover these topics and then evaluate your patient's learning:
✦ description of metabolic alkalosis and its treatment
✦ need to avoid overuse of alkaline agents and diuretics
✦ prescribed medications, especially adverse effects of potassium-wasting diuretics or potassium chloride supplements
✦ warning signs and symptoms and when to report them.

Patient teaching
✦ Description of disorder
✦ Medications
✦ Warning signs and symptoms

RESPIRATORY ACIDOSIS

A compromise in any of the three essential parts of breathing — ventilation, perfusion, or diffusion — may result in respiratory acidosis. This acid-base disturbance is characterized by alveolar hypoventilation that occurs when the pulmonary system is unable to rid the body of enough carbon dioxide (CO_2) to maintain a healthy pH balance. This imbalance is due to decreased respiration or inadequate gas exchange.

The lack of efficient CO_2 release leads to hypercapnia, in which the partial pressure of arterial carbon dioxide ($Paco_2$) is greater than 45 mm Hg. The condition can be acute, resulting from sudden failure in ventilation, or chronic, resulting from chronic pulmonary disease.

In acute respiratory acidosis, the pH drops below normal (lower than 7.35). In chronic respiratory acidosis, commonly due to chronic obstructive pulmonary disease (COPD), pH stays within normal limits (7.35 to 7.45) because the kidneys have had time to compensate for the imbalance.

Respiratory acidosis
✦ Can result from compromised essential parts of breathing (ventilation, perfusion, diffusion) resulting in decreased respiration or inadequate gas exchange
✦ Indicated by $Paco_2$ level > 45 mm Hg
✦ In acute form, pH drops below normal (< 7.35)
✦ In chronic form, pH stays within normal range

Causes and pathophysiology

When a patient hypoventilates, CO_2 builds up in the bloodstream and pH drops below normal causing respiratory acidosis. The kidneys try to compensate for a drop in pH by conserving bicarbonate or base ions, or generating them in the kidney, which in turn raises the pH. (See *How respiratory acidosis develops*, pages 180 and 181.)

Respiratory acidosis can result from neuromuscular problems, depression of the respiratory center in the brain, lung disease, or an airway obstruction.

(Text continues on page 182.)

Pathophysiology
✦ Hypoventilation causes increased CO_2 in bloodstream and decreased pH, resulting in respiratory acidosis
✦ Kidneys compensate for drop in pH by conserving bicarbonate or base ions, or generating them in kidney

Respiratory acidosis development

Step 1

- Decreased pulmonary ventilation causes retained CO_2 to combine with H_2O to form increased H_2CO_3
- Excessive H_2CO_3 causes decreased pH

Step 2

- Decreased pH causes 2,3-DPG increase in red blood cells and Hb to release O_2
- Altered Hb, now strongly alkaline, eliminates excess H^+ and CO_2 by picking it up

Step 3

- Increased $Paco_2$ causes increased CO_2 in all tissues and fluids, including cerebrospinal fluid and medulla's respiratory center
- Increased CO_2 and free H^+ stimulate respiratory center to increase respiratory rate
- Increased respiratory rate expels more CO_2, reducing its level in blood and tissues

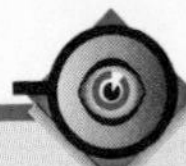

CLOSER LOOK

How respiratory acidosis develops

This series of illustrations shows how respiratory acidosis develops at the cellular level.

STEP 1

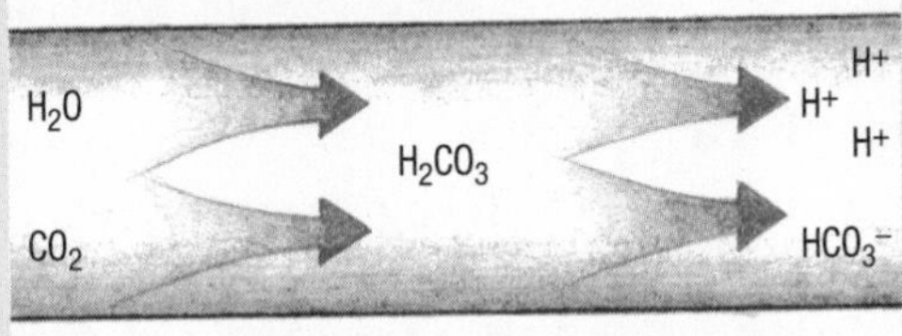

When pulmonary ventilation decreases, retained carbon dioxide (CO_2) combines with water (H_2O) to form carbonic acid (H_2CO_3) in larger-than-normal amounts. The H_2CO_3 dissociates to release free hydrogen ions (H^+) and bicarbonate ions (HCO_3^-). The excessive H_2CO_3 causes a drop in pH. *Look for a $Paco_2$ level above 45 mm Hg and a pH level below 7.35.*

STEP 2

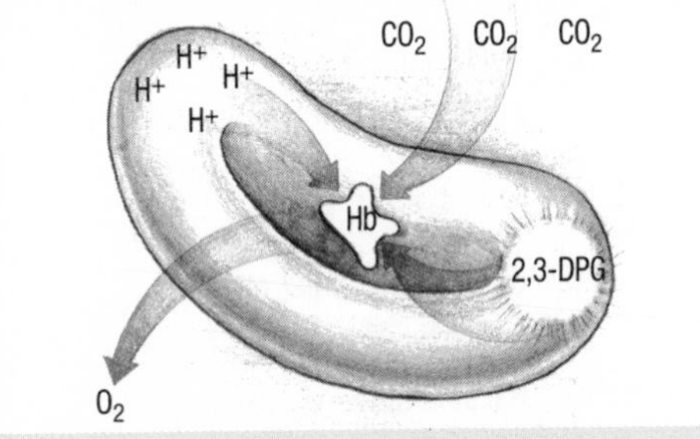

As the pH level falls, 2, 3-diphosphoglycerate (2, 3-DPG) increases in the red blood cells and causes a change in hemoglobin (Hb) that makes the Hb release oxygen (O_2). The altered Hb, now strongly alkaline, picks up H^+ and CO_2, thus eliminating some of the H^+ and excess CO_2. *Look for decreased arterial oxygen saturation.*

STEP 3

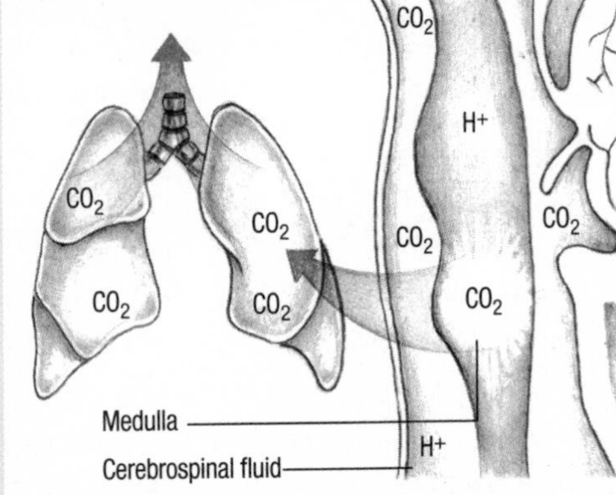

Whenever $Paco_2$ increases, CO_2 builds up in all tissues and fluids, including cerebrospinal fluid and the respiratory center in the medulla. The CO_2 reacts with water to form H_2CO_3, which then breaks into H^+ and HCO_3^-. The increased amount of CO_2 and free H^+ stimulate the respiratory center to increase the respiratory rate. An increased respiratory rate expels more CO_2 and helps to reduce the CO_2 level in the blood and other tissues. *Look for rapid, shallow respirations and a decreasing $Paco_2$.*

STEP 4

Eventually, CO_2 and H^+ cause cerebral blood vessels to dilate, which increases blood flow to the brain. That increased flow can cause cerebral edema and depress central nervous system activity. *Look for headache, confusion, lethargy, nausea, or vomiting.*

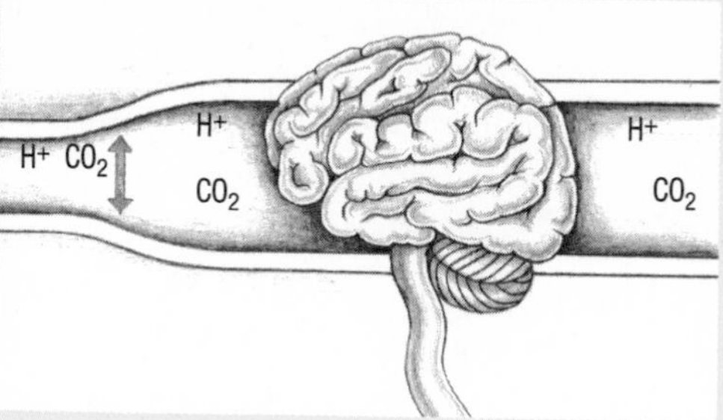

STEP 5

As respiratory mechanisms fail, the increasing $Paco_2$ stimulates the kidneys to conserve bicarbonate and sodium ions and to excrete H^+, some in the form of ammonium (NH_4). The additional HCO_3^- and sodium combine to form extra sodium bicarbonate ($NaHCO_3$), which is then able to buffer more free hydrogen ions. *Look for increased acid content in the urine, increasing serum pH and bicarbonate levels, and shallow, depressed respirations.*

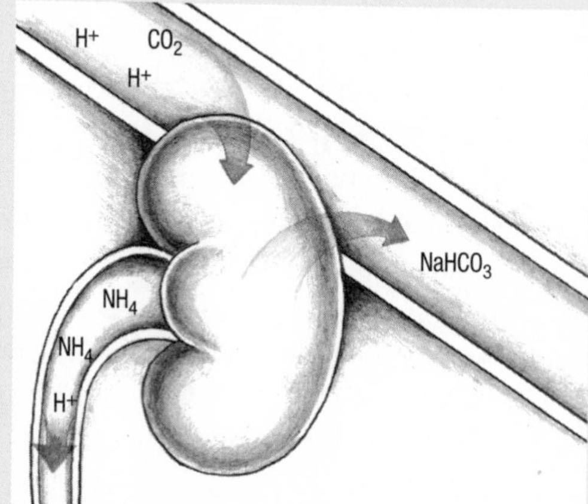

STEP 6

As the concentration of H^+ overwhelms the body's compensatory mechanisms, H^+ move into the cells, and potassium ions (K^+) move out. A concurrent lack of oxygen (O_2) causes an increase in the anaerobic production of lactic acid, which further skews the acid-base balance and critically depresses neurologic and cardiac functions. *Look for hyperkalemia, arrhythmias, increased $Paco_2$, decreased Pao_2, decreased pH, and decreased level of consciousness.*

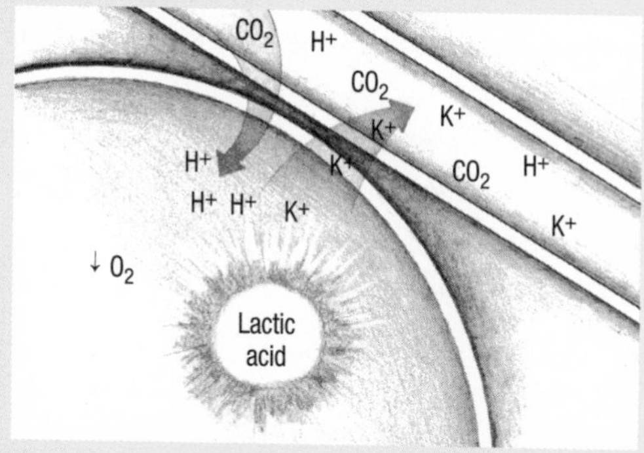

Respiratory acidosis development *(continued)*

Step 4

- CO_2 and H^+ cause cerebral vessels to dilate, increasing blood flow to brain
- Increased blood flow to brain may cause cerebral edema and depressed central nervous system activity

Step 5

- Increased $Paco_2$ stimulates kidneys to conserve bicarbonate and sodium ions and to excrete H+, partially in form of NH_4
- Additional HCO_3^- and sodium combine to form $NaHCO_3$, a compound able to buffer more free hydrogen ions

Step 6

- As concentration of H^+ overwhelms compensatory mechanisms, H^+ move into cells and K^+ move out
- Concurrent lack of O_2 increases anaerobic production of lactic acid, further skewing acid-base balance and critically depressing neurologic and cardiac functions

Causes

- Medications, including anesthetics, hypnotics, opioids, and sedatives (depress brain's respiratory center)
- Lung diseases
- Chest wall trauma that leads to pneumothorax or flail chest
- Airway obstruction
- Treatments

In certain neuromuscular diseases — such as Guillain-Barré syndrome, myasthenia gravis, and poliomyelitis — the respiratory muscles fail to respond properly to the respiratory drive, resulting in respiratory acidosis. Diaphragmatic paralysis, which commonly occurs with spinal cord injury, works the same way to cause respiratory acidosis.

Hypoventilation from central nervous system (CNS) trauma or brain lesions — such as tumors, vascular disorders, or infections — may impair the patient's ventilatory drive. Obesity, as in pickwickian syndrome, or primary hypoventilation, as in Ondine's curse, may contribute to this imbalance as well. Also, certain drugs — including anesthetics, hypnotics, opioids, and sedatives — can depress the respiratory center of the brain, leading to hypercapnia.

Lung diseases that decrease the amount of pulmonary surface area available for gas exchange can prompt respiratory acidosis. Less surface area decreases the amount of gas exchange that can occur, thus impeding CO_2 exchange. Examples of pulmonary problems that can decrease surface area include respiratory infections, COPD, acute asthma attacks, chronic bronchitis, late stages of acute respiratory distress syndrome, pulmonary edema, conditions in which there's increased dead space in the lungs such as hypoventilation, and physiologic or anatomic shunts.

Chest-wall trauma, leading to pneumothorax or flail chest, can also cause respiratory acidosis. The ventilatory drive remains intact, but the chest-wall mechanics of the collapsed lung don't allow for sufficient alveolar ventilation to meet the body's needs. Chest-wall mechanics can also be impeded as a result of the rib cage distortion caused by fibrothorax or kyphoscoliosis.

Respiratory acidosis can also be caused by airway obstruction, which leads to carbon dioxide retention in the lungs. Airway obstruction can occur as a result of retained secretions, tumors, anaphylaxis, laryngeal spasm, or lung diseases that interfere with alveolar ventilation.

AGE ALERT *Keep in mind that children are prone to airway obstruction, as are patients who are elderly and debilitated, who may not be able to effectively clear secretions.*

Treatments can induce respiratory acidosis. For instance, mechanical ventilation that underventilates a patient can cause CO_2 retention. A postoperative patient is at risk for respiratory acidosis if fear of pain prevents him from participating in pulmonary hygiene measures, such as coughing and deep breathing. Also, analgesics or sedatives can depress the medulla, which is responsible for controlling respirations. Depressing the medulla can lead to inadequate ventilation and subsequent respiratory acidosis.

AGE ALERT *Infants commonly have problems with acid-base imbalances, particularly acidosis. Because of their low residual lung volume, any alteration in respiration can rapidly and dramatically change their* $Pa{CO_2}$*, leading to acidosis. Infants also have a high metabolic rate, which yields large amounts of metabolic wastes and acids that must be excreted by the kidneys. This, along with their immature buffer system, leaves infants prone to acidosis.*

Age alert
- ✦ Infants commonly have acid-base imbalances (particularly acidosis) because of low residual lung volume
- ✦ High infantile metabolic rates problematic because kidneys must excrete large amounts of metabolic wastes and acids

Assessment findings

Signs and symptoms of respiratory acidosis depend on the cause of the condition. The patient may complain of a headache because carbon dioxide dilates cerebral blood vessels.

CNS depression may result in an altered level of consciousness (LOC), ranging from restlessness, confusion, and apprehension to somnolence and coma. If the acidosis remains untreated, a fine flapping tremor and depressed reflexes may develop. The patient may also report nausea and vomiting, and the skin may be warm and flushed.

Most patients with respiratory acidosis have rapid, shallow respirations. They will be dyspneic and possibly diaphoretic. Auscultation will reveal diminished or absent breath sounds over the affected area. However, if acidosis stems from CNS trauma or lesions or drug overdose, the respiratory rate will be greatly decreased.

In a patient with acidosis, hyperkalemia, and hypoxemia, you may note tachycardia and ventricular arrhythmias. Cyanosis is a late sign of the condition. Resulting myocardial depression may lead to shock and, ultimately, cardiac arrest.

Assessment findings
- ✦ Headache
- ✦ Altered LOC (restlessness, confusion, apprehension, somnolence, and coma)
- ✦ Nausea
- ✦ Vomiting
- ✦ Warm, flushed skin
- ✦ Rapid, shallow respirations
- ✦ Dyspnea
- ✦ Diaphoresis (possibly)
- ✦ Diminished or absent breath sounds over affected area
- ✦ Cyanosis (late sign)

Diagnostic test results

Typical laboratory findings for a patient with respiratory acidosis include:
- ✦ arterial blood gas (ABG) analysis reveals pH below 7.35 and $Pa{CO_2}$ above 45 mm Hg. HCO_3^- level varies, depending on how long the acidosis has been present. In a patient with acute respiratory acidosis, HCO_3^- level may be normal; in a patient with chronic respiratory acidosis, it may be above 26 mEq/L. (See *ABG results in respiratory acidosis*, page 184.)
- ✦ Chest X-rays can help pinpoint some causes, such as COPD, pneumonia, pneumothorax, and pulmonary edema.

Diagnostic test results
- ✦ ABG analysis: pH < 7.35, $Pa{CO_2}$ > 45 mm Hg , and variable HCO_3^- level
- ✦ Abnormal chest X-rays

ABG results in respiratory acidosis

This chart shows typical arterial blood gas (ABG) findings in uncompensated and compensated respiratory acidosis.

	UNCOMPENSATED	COMPENSATED
pH	< 7.35	Normal
$PaCO_2$ (mm Hg)	> 45	> 45
HCO_3^- (mEq/L)	Normal	> 26

✦ Serum electrolyte levels with potassium greater than 5 mEq/L typically indicate hyperkalemia. In acidosis, potassium leaves the cell, so expect the serum level to be elevated.
✦ Drug screening may confirm a suspected overdose.

Treatment

Nonpulmonary cause
- ✦ Correction of underlying cause

Pulmonary cause
- ✦ Bronchodilator to open constricted airways
- ✦ Supplemental oxygen
- ✦ Drug therapy to treat hyperkalemia
- ✦ Antibiotics for infection
- ✦ Chest physiotherapy to remove secretions from lungs
- ✦ Removal of foreign body from patient's airway, if appropriate

Key nursing interventions

- ✦ Monitor vital signs
- ✦ Assess cardiac rhythm
- ✦ Assess for respiratory patterns, and report changes quickly

TREATMENT

Treatment of respiratory acidosis focuses on improving ventilation and lowering the $PaCO_2$ level. If respiratory acidosis stems from nonpulmonary conditions, such as neuromuscular disorders or a drug overdose, treatment goals involve correcting or improving the underlying cause.

Treatment for respiratory acidosis with a pulmonary cause includes a bronchodilator to open constricted airways, supplemental oxygen as needed, drug therapy to treat hyperkalemia, an antibiotic to treat infection, chest physiotherapy to remove secretions from the lungs, or removal of a foreign body from the patient's airway, if needed. (See *When hypoventilation can't be corrected.*)

NURSING INTERVENTIONS

If your patient develops respiratory acidosis, maintain a patent airway. Help remove any foreign bodies from the airway and establish an artificial airway. Provide adequate humidification to ensure moist secretions. Additional measures include these interventions:

✦ Monitor vital signs, and assess cardiac rhythm. Respiratory acidosis can cause tachycardia, alterations in respiratory rate and rhythm, hypotension, and arrhythmias.
✦ Continue to assess respiratory patterns, and report changes quickly. Prepare for mechanical ventilation, if indicated.

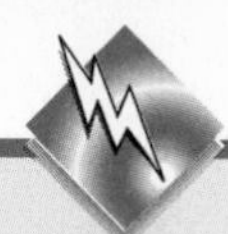

DANGER

When hypoventilation can't be corrected

If hypoventilation can't be corrected, expect your patient to have an artificial airway inserted and to be placed on mechanical ventilation. Be aware that bronchoscopy may be needed to remove retained secretions.

✦ Monitor the patient's neurologic status, and report significant changes. Also monitor the patient's cardiac function, because respiratory acidosis may progress to shock and cardiac arrest.

✦ Report variations in ABG, pulse oximetry, or serum electrolyte levels.

✦ Give medications, such as an antibiotic or a bronchodilator, as prescribed.

✦ Administer oxygen as ordered. Generally, lower concentrations of oxygen are given to patients with COPD. The medulla of a patient with COPD is accustomed to high CO_2 levels. A lack of oxygen, called the *hypoxic drive,* stimulates those patients to breathe. Too much oxygen diminishes that drive and depresses respiratory efforts.

✦ Perform tracheal suctioning, incentive spirometry, postural drainage, and coughing and deep breathing, as indicated.

✦ Make sure the patient takes in enough fluids, both oral and I.V., and maintain accurate intake and output records. (See *Documenting respiratory acidosis,* page 186.)

✦ Provide reassurance to the patient and family.

✦ Keep in mind that any sedatives you give to the patient can decrease his respiratory rate.

✦ Institute safety measures as needed to protect a confused patient.

As you reevaluate your patient's condition, consider these questions:

✦ Have the patient's respiratory rate and LOC returned to normal?

✦ Does auscultation of the patient's chest reveal reduced adventitious breath sounds?

✦ Have all tachycardias or ventricular arrhythmias been stabilized?

✦ Have the patient's cyanosis and dyspnea diminished?

✦ Have the patient's ABG results and serum electrolyte levels returned to normal?

✦ Do chest X-rays show improvement in the condition of the patient's lungs?

Key nursing interventions *(continued)*

✦ Monitor neurologic status

✦ Report variations in ABG, pulse oximetry, or serum electrolyte levels

✦ Give medications as prescribed

✦ Administer oxygen as ordered

✦ Ensure adequate fluid intake, both oral and I.V.

✦ Maintain accurate intake and output records

✦ Institute safety measures

CHARTING CHECKLIST

Documenting respiratory acidosis

If your patient has respiratory acidosis, make sure you document:

- ❑ vital signs and cardiac rhythm
- ❑ intake and output
- ❑ assessment and interventions and the patient's response
- ❑ time you notified the physician
- ❑ medications administered, oxygen therapy, and ventilator settings
- ❑ character of pulmonary secretions
- ❑ serum electrolyte levels and arterial blood gas results
- ❑ patient teaching provided and the patient's response.

Patient teaching

- ✦ Description of disorder
- ✦ ABG analysis
- ✦ Medications
- ✦ Home oxygen therapy
- ✦ Warning signs and symptoms
- ✦ Activity level
- ✦ Diet

Patient teaching

Be sure to cover these topics and then evaluate your patient's learning:

- ✦ description of respiratory acidosis and prevention measures
- ✦ reasons for repeated ABG analyses
- ✦ deep-breathing exercises
- ✦ prescribed medications
- ✦ home oxygen therapy, if indicated
- ✦ warning signs and symptoms and when to report them
- ✦ proper technique for using bronchodilators, if appropriate
- ✦ need for frequent rest
- ✦ need for increased caloric intake, if appropriate.

Respiratory alkalosis

- ✦ Results from alveolar hyperventilation and hypocapnia
- ✦ Indicated by pH > 7.45 and $Paco_2$ < 35 mm Hg

RESPIRATORY ALKALOSIS

Respiratory alkalosis, which is the opposite of respiratory acidosis, results from alveolar hyperventilation and hypocapnia. In respiratory alkalosis, there's increased elimination of carbon dioxide (CO_2); therefore, pH is greater than 7.45 and partial pressure of arterial carbon dioxide ($Paco_2$) is less than 35 mm Hg. The condition may be acute, resulting from a sudden increase in ventilation, or chronic, which may be difficult to identify because of renal compensation.

CAUSES AND PATHOPHYSIOLOGY

Any clinical condition that increases the respiratory rate or depth can cause the lungs to eliminate, or blow off, CO_2. Because CO_2 is an acid, eliminating it causes a decrease in $Paco_2$ along with an increase in pH—alkalosis.

The most common cause of acute respiratory alkalosis is hyperventilation stemming from anxiety or panic attack. It may also occur when overzealous rescuers perform cardiopulmonary resuscitation and hyperventilate at 30 to 40 breaths per minute. Pain, which also causes an increased respiratory rate, can have the same effect. Hyperventilation is an early sign of salicylate intoxication and also occurs with the use of nicotine and xanthines such as aminophylline (Truphylline).

Hypermetabolic states—such as fever, liver failure, and sepsis (especially gram-negative sepsis)—can lead to respiratory alkalosis. Certain drugs can also stimulate an increase in respiratory drive.

Conditions that affect the respiratory control center in the medulla are also a danger. For example, the higher progesterone levels of pregnancy may stimulate this center, while stroke or trauma may injure it, both resulting in respiratory alkalosis.

Acute hypoxia secondary to high altitude, pulmonary disease, severe anemia, pulmonary embolus, or hypotension can cause respiratory alkalosis. Such conditions may overstimulate the respiratory center and make the patient breathe faster and deeper. Overventilation during mechanical ventilation causes the lungs to blow off more CO_2, resulting in respiratory alkalosis.

Assessment findings

An increase in the rate and depth of respirations is a primary sign of respiratory alkalosis. It's also common for the patient to have tachycardia. The patient may appear anxious and restless as well as complain of muscle weakness or difficulty breathing. (See *How respiratory alkalosis develops,* pages 188 and 189.)

In extreme alkalosis, confusion or syncope may occur. Because of the lack of CO_2 in the blood and its effect on cerebral blood flow and the respiratory center, you may see alternating periods of apnea and hyperventilation. The patient may complain of tingling in the fingers and toes.

You may see electrocardiogram (ECG) changes, including a prolonged PR interval, a flattened T wave, a prominent U wave, and a depressed ST segment. (For more information, see chapter 6, Potassium imbalances.)

Symptoms worsen as calcium levels drop because of vasoconstriction of peripheral and cerebral vessels resulting from hypoxia. You may see

(Text continues on page 190.)

Pathophysiology

- ✦ Clinical conditions that increase respiratory rate or depth cause lungs to eliminate CO_2
- ✦ Decreased CO_2 causes decreased $Paco_2$ and increased pH (alkalosis)

Causes

- ✦ Hyperventilation from anxiety or panic attack (most common cause of acute respiratory alkalosis)
- ✦ Salicylate intoxication
- ✦ Nicotine
- ✦ Hypermetabolic states
- ✦ Pregnancy
- ✦ Stroke
- ✦ Trauma
- ✦ Acute hypoxia
- ✦ Overventilation during mechanical ventilation

Assessment findings

- ✦ Increased rate and depth of respirations (primary finding)
- ✦ Tachycardia
- ✦ Anxiousness and restlessness
- ✦ Muscle weakness
- ✦ Difficulty breathing
- ✦ ECG changes (prolonged PR interval, flattened T wave, prominent U wave, depressed ST segment)

Respiratory alkalosis development

Step 1

- When pulmonary ventilation increases above amount needed to maintain CO_2 levels, lungs exhale excess CO_2
- Loss of excess CO_2 causes hypocapnia, leading to reduced H_2CO_3 production, reduced H^+ and HCO_3^-, and increased pH

Step 2

- In defense against rising pH, H^+ pulled out of cells and into blood in exchange for K^+
- H^+ entering blood combines with HCO_3^- to form H_2CO_3, lowering pH

Step 3

- Hypercapnia stimulates carotid and aortic bodies and medulla, causing increased heart rate without increased blood pressure

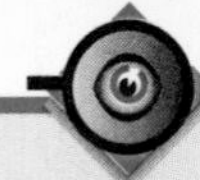

CLOSER LOOK

How respiratory alkalosis develops

This series of illustrations shows how respiratory alkalosis develops at the cellular level.

STEP 1

When pulmonary ventilation increases above the amount needed to maintain normal carbon dioxide (CO_2) levels, excessive amounts of CO_2 are exhaled. This causes hypocapnia (a fall in partial pressure of arterial carbon dioxide [$Paco_2$]), which leads to a reduction in carbonic acid (H_2CO_3) production, a loss of hydrogen ions (H^+) and bicarbonate ions (HCO_3^-), and a subsequent rise in pH. *Look for a pH level above 7.45, a $Paco_2$ level below 35 mm Hg, and a bicarbonate level below 22 mEq/L.*

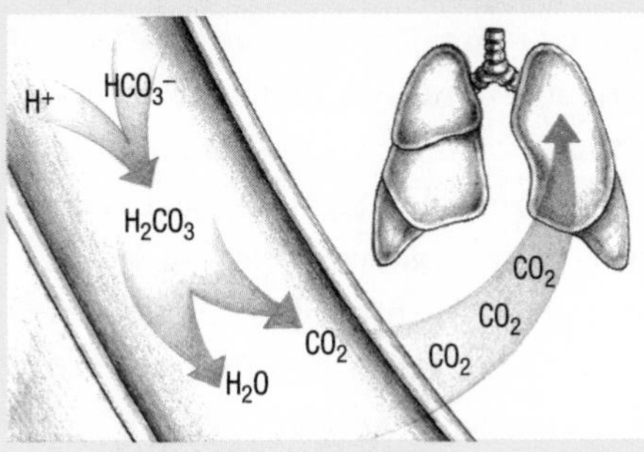

STEP 2

In defense against the rising pH, H^+ are pulled out of the cells and into the blood in exchange for potassium ions (K^+). The H^+ entering the blood combine with HCO_3^- to form H_2CO_3, which lowers the pH. *Look for a further decrease in bicarbonate levels, a fall in pH, and a fall in serum potassium levels (hypokalemia).*

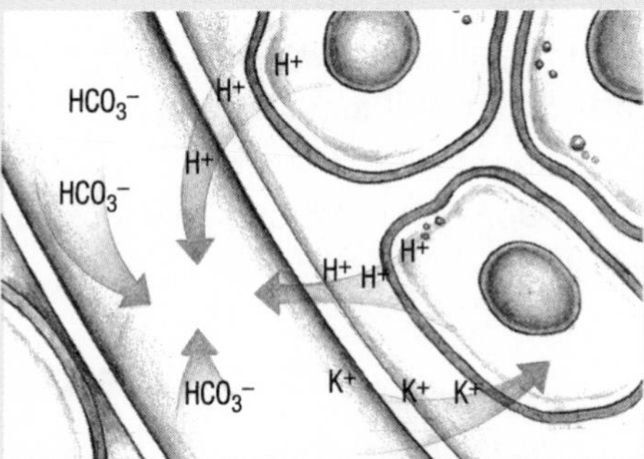

STEP 3

Hypocapnia stimulates the carotid and aortic bodies and the medulla, which causes an increase in heart rate without an increase in blood pressure. *Look for angina, electrocardiogram changes, restlessness, and anxiety.*

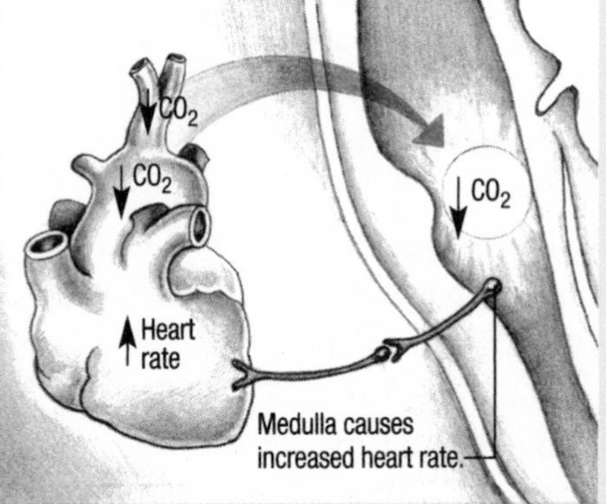

STEP 4

Simultaneously, hypocapnia produces cerebral vasoconstriction, which prompts a reduction in cerebral blood flow. Hypocapnia also overexcites the medulla, pons, and other parts of the autonomic nervous system. *Look for increasing anxiety, diaphoresis, dyspnea, alternating periods of apnea and hyperventilation, dizziness, and tingling in the fingers or toes.*

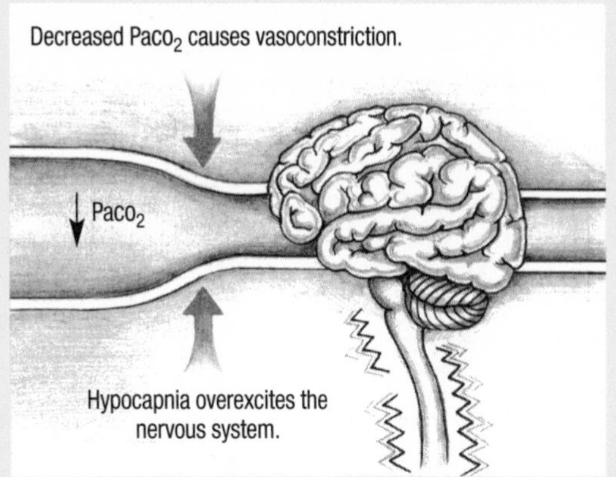

STEP 5

When hypocapnia lasts more than 6 hours, the kidneys increase secretion of HCO_3^- and reduce excretion of H^+. Periods of apnea may result if the pH remains high and the $Paco_2$ remains low. *Look for slowing of the respiratory rate, hypoventilation, and Cheyne-Stokes respirations.*

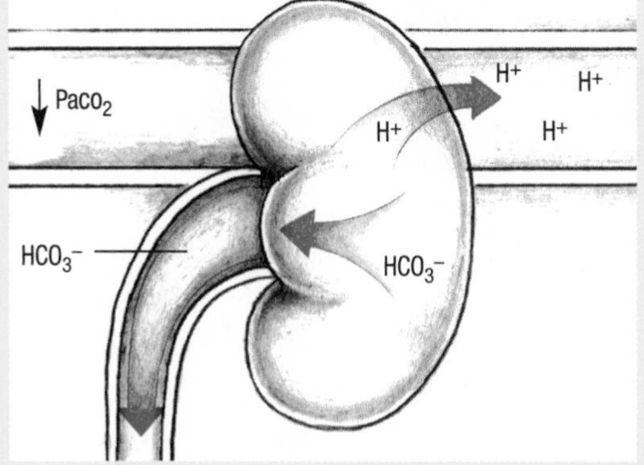

STEP 6

Continued low $Paco_2$ increases cerebral and peripheral hypoxia from vasoconstriction. Severe alkalosis inhibits calcium (Ca^{++}) ionization, which in turn causes increased nerve excitability and muscle contractions. Eventually, the alkalosis overwhelms the central nervous system and the heart. *Look for decreasing level of consciousness, hyperreflexia, carpopedal spasm, tetany, arrhythmias, seizures, and coma.*

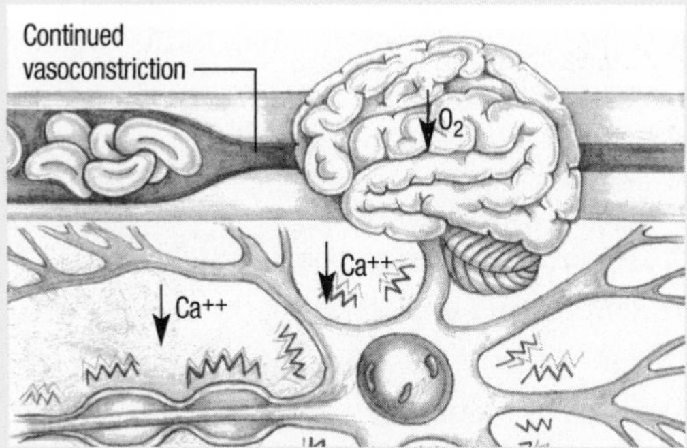

Respiratory alkalosis development *(continued)*

Step 4

- Simultaneously, hypocapnia produces cerebral vasoconstriction, prompting reduced cerebral blood flow

Step 5

- When hypocapnia lasts longer than 6 hours, kidneys increase secretion of HCO_3^- and reduce excretion of H^+

Step 6

- Continued low $Paco_2$ increases cerebral and peripheral hypoxia from vasoconstriction
- Severe alkalosis inhibits Ca^{++} ionization, causing increased nerve excitability and muscle contractions
- Eventually, alkalosis overwhelms central nerves system and heart

ABG results in respiratory alkalosis

This chart shows typical arterial blood gas (ABG) findings in uncompensated and compensated respiratory acidosis.

	UNCOMPENSATED	COMPENSATED
pH	> 7.45	Normal
$Paco_2$ (mm Hg)	< 35	< 35
HCO_3^- (mEq/L)	Normal	< 22

hyperreflexia, carpopedal spasm, tetany, arrhythmias, a progressive decrease in the patient's level of consciousness (LOC), seizures, or coma.

Diagnostic test results
- ABG analysis: pH > 7.45, $Paco_2$ < 35 mm Hg

Diagnostic test results

Typical laboratory findings for a patient with respiratory alkalosis include:

- arterial blood gas (ABG) analysis is the key diagnostic test for identifying respiratory alkalosis. Typically, the pH is above 7.45, and the $Paco_2$ level is below 35 mm Hg. Bicarbonate level may be normal (22 to 26 mEq/L) when the alkalosis is acute but usually falls below 22 mEq/L when chronic. (See *ABG results in respiratory alkalosis.*)
- serum electrolyte levels may point to a metabolic disorder that could be causing compensatory respiratory alkalosis. Hypokalemia may be evident by decreased LOC. The ionized serum calcium level may be decreased in those with severe respiratory alkalosis.
- ECG findings may indicate arrhythmias or the changes associated with hypokalemia or hypocalcemia.
- toxicology screening may reveal salicylate poisoning.

Treatment
- Focused on correction of underlying disorder
- For hyperventilation — Have patient breath into paper bag or cupped hands

Treatment

Treatment focuses on correcting the underlying disorder, which may require removing the causative agent, such as a salicylate or other drug, or taking steps to reduce fever and eliminate the source of sepsis.

If acute hypoxemia is the cause, oxygen therapy is initiated. If anxiety is the cause, the patient may receive a sedative or an anxiolytic.

Hyperventilation can be counteracted by having the patient breathe into a paper bag or into cupped hands, which forces the patient to

CHARTING CHECKLIST

Documenting respiratory alkalosis

If your patient has respiratory alkalosis, make sure you document:

- ❏ vital signs
- ❏ intake and output
- ❏ I.V. therapy
- ❏ interventions, including measures taken to alleviate anxiety
- ❏ patient's response to interventions
- ❏ serum electrolyte levels and arterial blood gas results
- ❏ safety measures
- ❏ time you notified the physician
- ❏ patient teaching provided and the patient's response.

breathe exhaled CO_2, thereby raising the CO_2 level. If a patient's respiratory alkalosis is iatrogenic, mechanical ventilator settings may be adjusted by decreasing the tidal volume or the number of breaths per minute.

Nursing interventions

Monitor all patients at risk for developing respiratory alkalosis. For your patients who have respiratory alkalosis, follow these measures:

✦ Allay anxiety whenever possible to prevent hyperventilation. Recommend activities that promote relaxation. Help the patient breath into a paper bag or cupped hands, if necessary.

✦ Monitor vital signs. Report changes in neurologic, neuromuscular, or cardiovascular functioning.

✦ Monitor ABG and serum electrolyte levels, and immediately report any variations. Remember, twitching and cardiac arrhythmias may be associated with alkalosis and electrolyte imbalances.

✦ If the patient is receiving mechanical ventilation, check ventilator settings frequently. Monitor ABG levels after making changes in settings.

✦ Provide undisturbed rest periods after the patient's respiratory rate returns to normal; hyperventilation may result in severe fatigue.

✦ Stay with the patient during periods of extreme stress and anxiety. Offer reassurance, and maintain a calm, quiet environment.

✦ Institute safety measures and seizure precautions as needed. Document all care. (See *Documenting respiratory alkalosis.*)

Key nursing interventions

- ✦ Allay anxiety whenever possible
- ✦ Monitor vital signs
- ✦ Monitor ABG and serum electrolyte levels
- ✦ Check ventilator settings for patient receiving mechanical ventilation
- ✦ Provide undisturbed rest periods

Patient teaching
- ✦ Description of disorder
- ✦ Warning signs and symptoms
- ✦ Anxiety-reducing techniques
- ✦ Controlled-breathing exercises
- ✦ Medications

Patient teaching

Be sure to cover these topics and then evaluate your patient's learning:

- ✦ description of respiratory alkalosis and its treatment
- ✦ warning signs and symptoms and when to report them
- ✦ anxiety-reducing techniques, if appropriate
- ✦ controlled-breathing exercises, if appropriate
- ✦ prescribed medications.

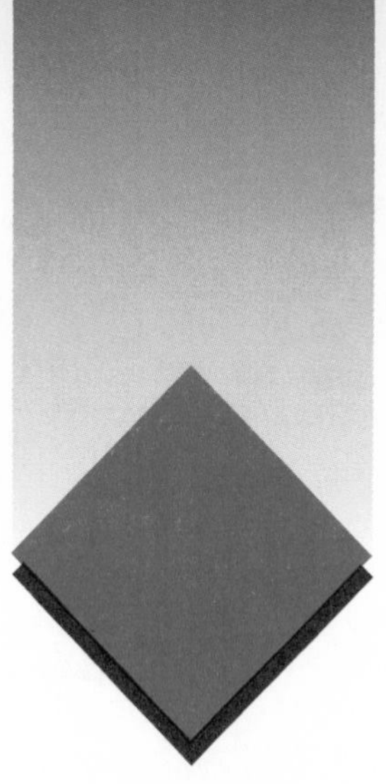

Part three

Disorders causing imbalances

Heat syndromes

Heat syndromes
- ✦ Major cause of preventable deaths worldwide
- ✦ Develop when body can't offset rising temperature, ultimately causing hyperthermia

UNDERSTANDING HEAT SYNDROMES

Heat syndromes are a major cause of preventable deaths worldwide, especially in regions with high temperatures. They develop when the body can't offset its rising temperature, thus retaining too much heat and, ultimately, causing hyperthermia. When the body gets too hot too quickly (temperature above 99° F [37.2° C]), heat syndromes occur.

Although the body initially tries to cool itself down when it's exposed to excessive heat, the mechanisms that regulate body heat can fail if the stress becomes too extreme. Normally, the body adjusts to excessive temperatures through complex cardiovascular and neurologic changes coordinated by the hypothalamus. Heat loss offsets heat production to regulate body temperature.

Types of heat transfer
- ✦ Conduction — transfer of heat through direct physical contact
- ✦ Convection — transfer of heat from body to air and water vapor surrounding body

TYPES OF HEAT TRANSFER

Heat transfer to and from the body occurs in four ways:

✦ conduction — the transfer of heat through direct physical contact (accounts for 2% of the body's heat loss)

✦ convection — the transfer of heat from the body to the air and water vapor surrounding the body (accounts for 10% of the body's heat loss);

when air temperature is higher than body temperature, the body gains heat energy

✦ radiation — the transfer of heat via electromagnetic waves (accounts for most heat loss); when the air temperature is less than the body temperature, 65% of the body's heat is lost by radiation

✦ evaporation — the transfer of heat by changing a liquid into a vapor (accounts for 30% of the body's heat loss).

In hot temperatures, the body loses heat mainly by radiation and evaporation. However, when air temperature is higher than 95° F (35° C), radiation of heat from the body stops and evaporation becomes the only means of heat loss.

When air temperatures increase and a person is exercising, he can sweat 1 to 2 L every hour. However, if humidity reaches 100%, evaporation of sweat is no longer possible and the body loses its ability to lose heat.

Causes and pathophysiology

Sweat is the body's main way to rid itself of extra heat. When a person sweats, water evaporates from the skin. The heat that makes this evaporation possible is created by blood flowing through the skin. As long as blood is flowing properly, extra heat from the core of the body is "pumped" to the skin and removed by sweat evaporation.

The effectiveness of sweat sometimes depends on the weather. Humidity inhibits sweat evaporation. In dry air, the body efficiently rids itself of excess heat through sweating and subsequent sweat evaporation.

Because the evaporation that occurs during sweating causes water loss, it's important for a person to drink water when sweating. If the body doesn't have enough water, dehydration can occur. This condition makes it harder for the body to cool itself because less water is available for the body to use in evaporation.

Heat syndromes result when the body's production of heat increases at a faster rate than the body's ability to dissipate it, causing heat loss. Heat production increases with exercise, fever, infection, and the use of certain drugs, such as amphetamines. Heat loss decreases with high temperatures or humidity, lack of acclimatization, lack of air conditioning or proper ventilation, excess clothing, obesity, decreased fluid intake, dehydration, extensive burns, cardiovascular disease, skin diseases, sweat gland dysfunction, endocrine disorders (such as hyperthyroidism, diabetes, and

Types of heat *(continued)*

✦ Radiation — transfer of heat via electromagnetic waves
✦ Evaporation — transfer of heat by changing liquid into vapor

Pathophysiology

✦ Sweat — body's main way to eliminate extra heat; extra heat from body's core pumped to skin and removed by evaporation

Causes

Increased heat production

✦ Exercise
✦ Fever
✦ Infection
✦ Medications

Decreased heat loss

✦ High temperatures or humidity
✦ Lack of acclimatization
✦ Lack of air conditioning or proper ventilation
✦ Excess clothing
✦ Obesity
✦ Decreased fluid intake
✦ Dehydration
✦ Extensive burns
✦ Cardiovascular disease
✦ Skin diseases
✦ Sweat gland dysfunction
✦ Endocrine disorders
✦ Alcohol
✦ Medication

Drugs causing heat syndromes

These drugs may cause decreased heat loss:

- anticholinergics
- antihistamines
- beta-adrenergic blockers
- cyclic antidepressants
- diuretics
- ethanol
- lithium (Lithane)
- phenothiazines
- salicylates
- sympathomimetics; for example, cocaine and amphetamines, which cause vasodilation.

pheochromocytoma), ingestion of alcohol, and use of certain medications. (See *Drugs causing heat syndromes*.)

When the body uses all its mechanisms and still can't keep its temperature down, the excess heat is retained and heat syndromes can develop.

Types of heat syndromes

Heat cramps

- Muscle contractions that typically occur in gastrocnemius or hamstring muscles
- Caused by deficiency of water and sodium
- Generally attributed to dehydration and poor conditioning
- Usually occur after exertion in high temperatures with profuse sweating and water intake without electrolyte replacement
- Symptoms usually improve with rest, water consumption, and cool environment

TYPES OF HEAT SYNDROMES

Heat syndromes cause three types of conditions: heat cramps, heat exhaustion, and heatstroke.

Heat cramps

Heat cramps are muscle contractions that typically occur in the gastrocnemius or hamstring muscles. These painful contractions are caused by a deficiency of water and sodium and are generally attributed to dehydration and poor conditioning. Cramps usually occur after exertion in high temperatures (greater than 100° F [37.7° C]) with profuse sweating and water intake without adequate electrolyte replacement. Heat cramps are common in manual laborers, athletes, and skiers who overdress for the cold as well as in those who aren't used to hot, dry climates in which excessive sweating is almost undetected because of rapid evaporation. Symptoms usually improve with rest, water consumption, and a cool environment.

Heat exhaustion

Heat exhaustion is caused by heat and fluid loss from excessive sweating without fluid replacement. Rest, water, ice packs, and a cool environment may help in mild heat exhaustion. More severely exhausted patients may need I.V. fluids, especially if vomiting keeps them from drinking enough. Circulatory collapse may occur if this condition isn't promptly treated.

Heatstroke

Heatstroke is the most severe form of heat syndrome. It's also known as *sunstroke, thermic fever,* or *siriasis,* and commonly occurs in patients who exercise in hot weather. Elderly patients and patients taking certain medications are also at risk for heatstroke in hot weather, even in the absence of exercise. Signs to look for include warm, flushed skin, and lack of sweating. Athletes who have heatstroke after vigorous exercise in hot weather may still sweat considerably.

Whether exercise-related or not, a person with heatstroke usually has a very high temperature (104° F or higher [40° C]) and may be delirious or unconscious or having seizures.

Patients suffering from heatstroke need to have their temperature reduced quickly, usually with ice packs, and must also be given I.V. fluids for rehydration. Because many body organs can fail in heatstroke, patients are typically hospitalized for observation. The body's attempt to regulate its temperature during heat syndromes causes a loss of excessive amounts of water and electrolytes. These must be replaced to avoid the continuation of hyperthermia. Extremely high body temperature may damage tissues, including muscle and brain tissues, and may lead to permanent disability and even death.

Types of heat syndromes *(continued)*

Heat exhaustion

- ✦ Caused by heat and fluid loss from excessive sweating without fluid replacement
- ✦ Rest, water, ice packs, and cool environment may help improve mild heat exhaustion
- ✦ I.V. fluids may be needed for more severe heat exhaustion
- ✦ May result in circulatory collapse if not promptly treated

Heatstroke

- ✦ Most severe form of heat syndrome
- ✦ Indicated by warm, flushed skin; lack of sweating; very high temperature; altered level of consciousness; and seizures
- ✦ Requires rapid temperature reduction, usually with ice packs and I.V. fluids for dehydration

Assessment findings

Your patient's signs and symptoms for heat syndromes vary by the severity of the syndrome. (See *Classifying heat syndromes,* page 198.)

Diagnostic test results

Typical laboratory findings for a patient with heat syndrome include:

- ✦ increased body temperatures, resulting in hyperthermia
- ✦ decreased serum sodium levels, resulting in hyponatremia
- ✦ decreased serum potassium levels, resulting in hypokalemia
- ✦ increased urine specific gravity

Diagnostic test results

- ✦ Increased body temperatures
- ✦ Decreased serum sodium levels
- ✦ Decreased serum potassium levels
- ✦ Increased urine specific gravity
- ✦ Elevated hepatic transaminase levels

Classifying heat syndromes

Heat syndromes may be classified as mild, causing heat cramps; moderate, causing heat exhaustion; or critical, causing heatstroke. This table highlights the major assessment findings associated with each classification.

CLASSIFICATION	ASSESSMENT FINDINGS
Mild hyperthermia Heat cramps	✦ Mild agitation (central nervous system findings otherwise normal) ✦ Mild hypertension ✦ Moist, cool skin and muscle tenderness; involved muscle groups possibly hard and lumpy ✦ Muscle twitching and spasms ✦ Nausea, abdominal cramps ✦ Report of prolonged activity in a very warm or hot environment, without adequate salt intake ✦ Tachycardia ✦ Temperature ranging from 99° to 102° F (37.2° to 38.9° C)
Moderate hyperthermia Heat exhaustion	✦ Dizziness ✦ Headache ✦ Hypotension ✦ Muscle cramping ✦ Nausea, vomiting ✦ Oliguria ✦ Pale, moist skin ✦ Rapid, thready pulse ✦ Syncope or confusion ✦ Temperature elevated up to 104° F (40° C) ✦ Thirst ✦ Weakness
Critical hyperthermia Heatstroke	✦ Atrial or ventricular tachycardia ✦ Confusion, combativeness, delirium ✦ Fixed, dilated pupils ✦ Hot, dry, reddened skin ✦ Loss of consciousness ✦ Seizures ✦ Tachypnea ✦ Temperature greater than 106° F (41.4° C)

✦ elevated hepatic transaminase levels, which is almost universal in heatstroke.

Other laboratory tests are used to detect end-organ damage, especially in patients with heatstroke, or to rule out other disorders.

Risks of heat syndromes

The presence of certain fluid and electrolyte imbalances is associated with increased risk of heat syndromes. These imbalances include dehydration, hyponatremia, and hypokalemia.

Dehydration

Signs and symptoms of dehydration include thirst; dry mucous membranes; hot, dry skin; decreased urine output; confusion; dizziness; postural hypotension; tachycardia; and eventually anhidrosis or absence of sweating.

Hypokalemia

Signs and symptoms of decreased hypokalemia, which reflect decreased serum levels, include fatigue, paresthesia, hypoactive reflexes, ileus, cardiac arrhythmias, and electrocardiogram changes, such as flattened T waves, development of U waves, ST depression, and prolonged PR interval.

Hyponatremia

Signs of hyponatremia, which causes decreased serum sodium levels, include lethargy, nausea and vomiting, muscle cramps and weakness, muscle twitching, and seizures.

At-risk patients

Patients who are most at risk for fluid and electrolyte loss with heat syndrome include elderly people, young children, people with chronic and debilitating diseases, those not acclimated to heat, alcoholics, and people taking certain medications, such as tranquilizers, anticholinergics, diuretics, and beta-adrenergic blockers. Fluid and electrolyte loss also occurs in healthy people who work or exercise in extreme heat and humidity and in those who don't increase their fluid intake accordingly. Football players are prone to heat illnesses because their uniforms cover nearly all of the body and practice usually begins in late summer, when the temperature outside is highest. Athletes should, therefore, pay careful attention to the amount of fluids they drink and lose and should wear lightweight clothing when possible.

AGE ALERT *Elderly patients are at increased risk for heat syndromes, especially during hot summer days, due to the decreasing thirst mechanism and ability to sweat that accompany the aging process. Neonates are also at increased risk for heat syndrome due to their bodies' poorly developed heat-regulating*

Risks of heat syndromes

- Dehydration, hyponatremia, and hypokalemia associated with increased risk

Signs and symptoms of dehydration

- Thirst
- Dry mucous membranes
- Hot, dry skin
- Decreased urine output
- Confusion
- Dizziness
- Tachycardia

Signs and symptoms of hypokalemia

- Fatigue
- Paresthesia
- Hypoactive reflexes
- ECG changes (flattened T waves, development of U waves, ST depression, and prolonged PR interval)

Signs and symptoms of hyponatremia

- Lethargy
- Nausea and vomiting
- Muscle cramps and weakness
- Muscle twitching
- Seizures

At-risk patients

- Elderly people
- Young children
- People with chronic and debilitating diseases
- People not acclimatized to heat
- Alcoholics
- People taking certain medications (tranquilizers, anticholinergics, diuretics, and beta-adrenergic blockers)

abilities. In addition, their body surface areas are larger, which increases the amount of heat loss.

Treatment

- Goal is to lower patient's body temperature as quickly as possible

Heat cramps

- Rest
- Electrolyte-rich fluids and salty foods
- Removal or loosening of clothing
- Direct pressure on cramped muscles

Heat exhaustion

- Rest in a cool location
- Water, slightly salty fluids, or electrolyte-rich sports drinks
- Removal or loosening of clothing
- Foot elevation

Heatstroke

- Hospitalization or immediate medication attention
- Ice packs
- Removal of clothing
- Sponge baths, tepid water spray, or other means to keep patient wet
- Fan to blow cool air over patient
- Cool I.V. fluids

TREATMENT

The goal of treatment for heat syndromes is to lower the patient's body temperature as quickly as possible. As in most illnesses, elderly patients may require more aggressive treatment and should be evaluated for even the mildest cases of heat cramps and heat exhaustion.

Hospitalization for heat cramps is rare, and the symptoms are usually self-limiting. Symptoms are treated with rest, intake of electrolyte-rich fluids (sports drinks), and ingestion of salty foods. Clothing can be removed or loosened and stretching or direct pressure on the muscles may decrease cramping. If the patient can't eat or drink, an I.V. infusion of normal saline solution may be necessary.

Hospitalization usually isn't necessary for heat exhaustion. It's typically treated by having the patient rest in a cool location and drink water, slightly salty fluids, or electrolyte-rich sports drinks every few minutes. Clothing can be removed or loosened and the feet can be elevated 12″ (30.5 cm). For severe cases, isotonic I.V. fluids may be given if available and if necessary. Rarely, cardiac stimulants and plasma volume expanders (such as albumin and dextran) are given; these should be used cautiously to avoid volume overload. Untreated heat exhaustion may lead to heatstroke.

Hospitalization or immediate medical attention is required for patients with heatstroke. Treatment focuses on cooling the body as quickly as possible. Ice packs should be placed on the patient's neck, armpits, and groin. Keep the patient undressed and wet by sponging him with water, spraying him with tepid water, or dabbing him with wet towels. A fan may also be used to blow cool air over the patient. This causes evaporative cooling—the best cooling method for patients with heatstroke. Cool I.V. fluids are also necessary. Other ways to support the cooling process may include oxygen therapy and, in severe cases, endotracheal intubation. Diazepam (Valium) and barbiturates may be given I.V. if seizures are uncontrollable.

Other options for cooling the patient include covering him with ice and immersing him in an ice bath. Although effective at rapidly lowering body temperature, these methods can create complications such as peripheral vasoconstriction, which can lead to less heat dissipation. These techniques are also uncomfortable for the patient, limit the ability to monitor the patient's vital signs and cardiac status, may result in hypothermia, and eventually may cause the patient to shiver. Shivering slows the cooling process because it increases core body temperature.

For all types of heat syndromes, avoid using salicylates to decrease body temperature because they increase the risk of coagulopathy. Also avoid administering acetaminophen because it doesn't reduce body temperature during heat syndromes and may actually worsen existing hepatic damage because it's metabolized by the liver.

Treatment *(continued)*

- For all heat syndromes, salicylates and acetaminophen contraindicated

Nursing interventions

Treatment of heat syndromes requires frequent monitoring of laboratory values, such as central venous and pulmonary wedge pressures, instituting rehydration measures, replacing sodium and potassium, and starting cooling measures to decrease body temperature. Also institute these nursing interventions:

- Replace fluid and electrolytes by encouraging fluid intake with a balanced electrolyte drink; give salt tablets.
- Loosen the patient's clothing.
- Ask the patient to lie down in a cool place.
- Massage his muscles.
- If heat cramps are severe, start an I.V. infusion with normal saline solution.
- If the patient has heat exhaustion, oxygen administration may be necessary. (See *Documenting heat syndromes,* page 202.)
- Initiate the ABCs (airway, breathing, and circulation) of life support.
- Quickly lower the patient's body temperature using hypothermia blankets and ice packs on arterial pressure points.
- Monitor the patient's temperature continuously. Temperatures shouldn't be allowed to fall below 101° F (38.3° C) to prevent hypothermia.
- Replace fluids and electrolytes I.V.
- When necessary, give diazepam to control seizures, chlorpromazine (Thorazine) I.V. to reduce shivering, or mannitol (Osmitrol) I.V. to maintain urine output.
- Insert a nasogastric tube to prevent aspiration.
- Monitor temperature, intake, output, and cardiac status. Assist with the insertion of a central venous catheter or a pulmonary artery catheter. Give dobutamine (Dobutrex) I.V. to correct cardiogenic shock. Vasoconstrictors shouldn't be used.

Key nursing interventions

- Replace fluids and electrolytes
- Loosen patient's clothing
- Ask patient to lie down in cool place
- If heat cramps are severe, start I.V. infusion with normal saline solution
- Quickly lower patient's body temperature using hypothermia blankets and ice packs on arterial pressure points

CHARTING CHECKLIST

Documenting heat syndromes

If your patient has a heat syndrome, make sure you document:

- ❑ vital signs, especially body temperature
- ❑ skin color
- ❑ degree of sweating
- ❑ mental status
- ❑ signs and symptoms, such as cramping or shivering
- ❑ serum electrolyte levels and urine specific gravity
- ❑ amount of oxygen administered, if necessary
- ❑ intake and output, including I.V. fluids
- ❑ medications administered
- ❑ measures taken to reduce body temperature and the patient's response
- ❑ patient teaching and the patient's response.

✦ Avoid stimulants and sedatives.
✦ Encourage bed rest for a few days.
✦ Warn the patient that his temperature may fluctuate for weeks.

Patient teaching
✦ Prevention techniques
✦ Risk factors
✦ Residual hypersensitivity

Patient teaching

Be sure to cover these topics and then evaluate your patient's learning:
✦ Advise patients to take the following precautions in hot, humid weather: rest frequently, avoid hot places, drink adequate fluids (especially when sweating), and wear loose-fitting, lightweight clothing.
✦ Advise patients who are obese, elderly, or taking drugs that impair heat regulation to avoid overheating.
✦ Tell patients who have had heat cramps or heat exhaustion to increase their salt and water intake. They should also refrain from exercising until symptoms resolve and only resume exercises gradually with plenty of electrolyte-containing fluids to drink. Advise them to take precautions to prevent overheating.
✦ Warn patients with heatstroke that residual hypersensitivity to high temperatures may persist for several months.
✦ Parents should be aware that young children and infants are at risk for overheating in hot weather.

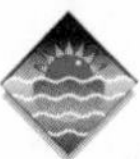

AGE ALERT *To help prevent heatstroke in your elderly patients, provide them with these instructions:*
✦ Reduce activity in hot weather, especially outdoor activity.

✦ Wear lightweight, loose-fitting clothing during hot weather; when outdoors, wear a hat and sunglasses and avoid wearing dark colors that absorb sunlight.
✦ Drink plenty of fluids, especially water, and avoid tea, coffee, and alcohol because they can cause dehydration.
✦ Use air conditioning or open windows (making sure that a secure screen is in place), and use a fan to help circulate air. (If the patient doesn't have air conditioning at home, suggest that during periods of excessive heat he go to community resources that have air conditioning, such as senior centers, libraries, and churches. Some community centers may even provide transportation for the patient.)

Age alert

✦ Teach elderly patients to reduce activity; wear lightweight, loose-fitting clothing; drink fluids; and ensure proper air circulation

Heart failure

Heart failure

- Clinical syndrome of myocardial function that causes diminished cardiac output
- Occurs when heart can't pump enough blood to meet body's metabolic needs
- Heart's ventricles function depending on interaction among preload (volume), afterload (pressure), contractility, and heart rate

Cardiac cycle

- Made up of two periods, diastole and systole
- Diastole — portion of cycle when heart is at rest, filling ventricles with blood
- Systole — portion of cycle when ventricles contract, ejecting their volume of blood

UNDERSTANDING HEART FAILURE

Heart failure is a clinical syndrome of myocardial dysfunction that causes diminished cardiac output. From the subtle loss of normal ventricular function to the presence of symptoms that no longer respond to medical treatment, heart failure occurs when the heart can't pump enough blood to meet the body's metabolic needs.

The heart's ventricles function depending on the interaction among four factors that regulate cardiac output and include preload (volume), afterload (pressure), contractility, and heart rate. Two periods — diastole and systole — make up the normal cardiac cycle. *Diastole* is the portion of the cycle during which the heart is at rest, filling the ventricles with blood. *Systole* is the portion of the cycle during which the ventricles contract, ejecting their volume of blood.

When any of the four interrelated factors are altered, cardiac output may be affected. For example, when the preload delivered to the ventricles during diastole is inadequate, cardiac output may be compromised, and diastolic heart failure may result. Further, when the afterload against which the ventricles must contract is elevated during systole, cardiac output may be compromised and systolic heart failure may result.

This ventricular dysfunction may occur in either the left or right ventricle.

Causes and pathophysiology

A wide range of pathophysiologic processes can cause heart failure, including conditions that directly damage the heart, such as myocardial infarction (MI), myocarditis, myocardial fibrosis, and ventricular aneurysm. The damage from these disorders causes a subsequent decrease in the contractility of the heart.

Ventricular overload can also cause heart failure. This overload may be caused by increased blood volume in the heart, called *increased preload,* as a result of aortic insufficiency or a ventricular septal defect. Systemic or pulmonary hypertension or an elevation in pressure against which the heart must pump, called *increased afterload,* as a result of aortic or pulmonic stenosis may also cause this overload.

Restricted ventricular diastolic filling, characterized by the absence of enough blood for the ventricle to effectively pump, can also cause heart failure. Such diastolic filling is triggered by constrictive pericarditis or cardiomyopathy, tachyarrhythmias, cardiac tamponade, or mitral or aortic stenosis and usually occurs in older patients.

Risk factors

Certain conditions can predispose a person to heart failure, especially if he has an underlying disease. Such conditions include:

- ✦ anemia, which causes the heart rate to speed up to maintain tissue oxygenation
- ✦ pregnancy and thyrotoxicosis, which increase the demand for cardiac output
- ✦ infections, which increase metabolic demands and further burden the heart
- ✦ increased physical activity, emotional stress, greater sodium or water intake, or failure to comply with the prescribed treatment regimen for underlying heart disease
- ✦ pulmonary embolism, which elevates pulmonary arterial pressures and can cause right-sided heart failure.

Pathophysiology of heart failure

Normally, the pumping actions of the right and left sides of the heart complement each other, producing a synchronized and continuous blood flow. With an underlying disorder, though, one side may fail while the other continues to function normally for some time. Because of the pro-

Causes

- ✦ Conditions that directly damage heart (MI, myocarditis, myocardial fibrosis, ventricular aneurysm)
- ✦ Ventricular overload
- ✦ Restricted ventricular diastolic filling

Risk factors

- ✦ Anemia
- ✦ Pregnancy and thyrotoxicosis
- ✦ Infections
- ✦ Increased physical activity
- ✦ Emotional stress
- ✦ Greater sodium or water intake
- ✦ Failure to comply with prescribed treatment regimen for underlying heart disease
- ✦ Pulmonary embolism

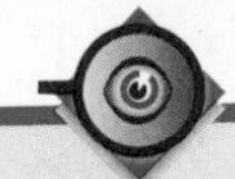

CLOSER LOOK

How left-sided heart failure develops

This illustration shows what happens when left-sided heart failure develops. The left side of the heart normally receives oxygenated blood returning from the lungs and then pumps it through the aorta to all tissues. Left-sided heart failure causes blood to back up in the lungs, which results in such respiratory symptoms as tachypnea and shortness of breath.

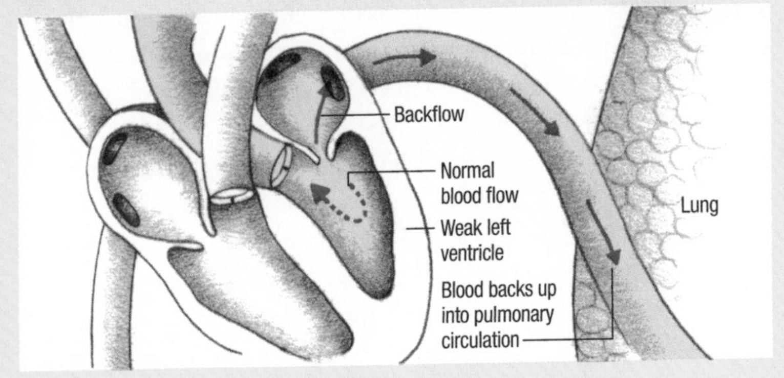

longed strain, the functioning side eventually fails, resulting in total heart failure.

Left-sided heart failure

In heart failure, typically, the heart's left side fails first. Left-sided heart failure commonly leads to and is the main cause of right-sided heart failure. It occurs when diminished left ventricular function allows blood to pool in the ventricle and atrium and eventually to back up in the pulmonary veins and capillaries. (See *How left-sided heart failure develops.*)

As the pulmonary circulation becomes engorged, rising capillary pressure pushes sodium and water into the interstitial space, causing pulmonary edema. The right ventricle becomes stressed because it's pumping against greater pulmonary vascular resistance and left ventricular pressure.

Right-sided heart failure

As the right ventricle starts to fail, symptoms worsen. Blood pools in the right ventricle and the right atrium. The backed-up blood causes pressure and congestion in the venae cavae and systemic circulation. (See *How right-sided heart failure develops.*)

Pathophysiology

Left-sided heart failure

- Heart's left side typically fails first and commonly leads to right-sided heart failure
- Diminished left ventricular function allows blood to pool in ventricle and atrium
- Blood eventually back up in pulmonary veins and capillaries
- Rising capillary pressure pushes sodium and water into interstitial space, causing pulmonary edema
- Right ventricle becomes stressed because it's pumping against greater pulmonary vascular resistance and left ventricular pressure

Right-sided heart failure

- Blood pools in right ventricle and right atrium
- Backed-up blood causes pressure and congestion in venae cavae and systemic circulation

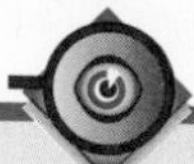

CLOSER LOOK

How right-sided heart failure develops

This illustration shows what happens when right-sided heart failure develops. The right side of the heart normally receives deoxygenated blood returning from the tissues and then pumps that blood through the pulmonary artery into the lungs. Right-sided heart failure causes blood to back up past the vena cava and into the systemic circulation. This, in turn, causes enlargement of the abdominal organs and tissue edema.

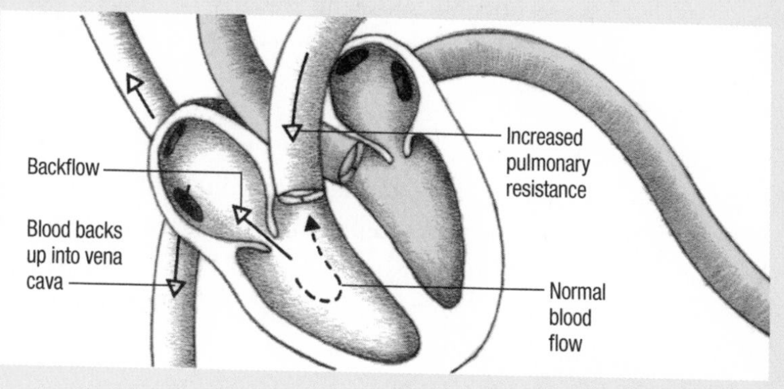

Blood also distends the visceral veins, especially the hepatic vein. As the liver and spleen become engorged, their function is impaired. Rising capillary pressure forces excess fluid from the capillaries into the interstitial space. This causes tissue edema, especially in the lower extremities and abdomen.

Compensatory responses

When the heart begins to fail, the body responds with three compensatory mechanisms to maintain blood flow to the tissues. These mechanisms include sympathetic nervous system activation, increased preload, and hypertrophy of the cardiac cells. Initially, the compensatory mechanisms serve to increase the cardiac output. However, these mechanisms will eventually contribute to heart failure.

Sympathetic nervous system

Diminished cardiac output activates the sympathetic nervous system, causing an increased heart rate and increased contractility. These increases initially stimulate cardiac output. However, both increased heart rate and increased contractility raise the heart's demand for oxygen, thereby

Pathophysiology *(continued)*

Right-sided heart failure

- Blood also distends visceral veins, especially hepatic vein
- Liver and spleen become engorged, impairing their functionality
- Tissue edema develops, especially in lower extremities and abdomen

Compensatory responses

- Three compensatory responses maintain blood flow to tissues: sympathetic nervous system activation, increased preload, and hypertrophy of cardiac cells

Sympathetic nervous system

- Activation causes increased heart rate and increased contractility; over time, contributes to heart failure, rather than compensating for it

increasing the work that the heart must do to meet this demand. Over time, this contributes to heart failure, rather than compensating for it.

With increased demand, blood then shunts away from areas of low priority, such as the skin and kidneys, to areas of high priority, such as the heart and brain.

Pulmonary congestion, a complication of heart failure, can lead to pulmonary edema, a life-threatening condition. Decreased perfusion to major organs, particularly the brain and kidneys, may cause these organs to fail, necessitating dialysis for kidney failure. The patient's level of consciousness may decrease, possibly leading to coma. MI may occur because myocardial oxygen demands can't be sufficiently met.

Increased preload

When blood is shunted away from areas of low priority, the kidneys, sensing a reduced renal blood flow, activate the renin-angiotensin-aldosterone system. This results in sodium and water retention, which increases blood volume or preload. Again, initially this serves to increase the cardiac output. However, over time, the heart can't pump this increased volume effectively, and heart failure results.

Cardiac hypertrophy

When the heart is under strain, it responds by increasing its muscle mass, a condition called *cardiac hypertrophy.* As the cardiac wall thickens, the heart's demand for blood and oxygen grows. The patient's heart may be unable to meet this demand, further accelerating heart failure.

When pressure inside the chambers, usually the left ventricle, rises for a sustained period, the heart compensates by stretching, a condition called *cardiac dilation.* Eventually, stretched muscle fibers become overstrained, reducing the heart's ability to pump.

HEART FAILURE IMBALANCES

Several imbalances may result from the heart's failure to pump blood and perfuse tissues adequately. Imbalances may also result from stimulation of the renin-angiotensin-aldosterone system or from certain treatments such as diuretic therapy. Fluid, electrolyte, and acid-base imbalances associated with heart failure include:

- ✦ hypervolemia and hypovolemia
- ✦ hyperkalemia and hypokalemia
- ✦ hypochloremia, hypomagnesemia, hyponatremia

Compensatory mechanisms *(continued)*

Increased preload

- ✦ Kidneys, sensing reduced renal blood flow, activate renin-angiotensin-aldosterone system
- ✦ Results in sodium and water retention, increasing blood volume or preload
- ✦ Over time, heart can't pump increased volume effectively and heart failure results

Cardiac hypertrophy

- ✦ Heart's response to stress
- ✦ As cardiac wall thickens, heart's demand for blood and oxygen grows
- ✦ When pressure inside heart's chambers, usually left ventricle, rises for sustained period, heart stretches (cardiac dilation)
- ✦ Stretched muscle fibers eventually become overstrained, reducing heart's ability to pump

Heart failure imbalances

- ✦ Result from heart's failure to adequately pump blood and perfuse tissues
- ✦ May also be caused by stimulation of renin-angiotensin-aldosterone system or from certain treatments (diuretic therapy)

✦ metabolic acidosis and alkalosis
✦ respiratory acidosis and alkalosis.

Fluid imbalances

Hypervolemia — the most common fluid imbalance associated with heart failure — results from the heart's failure to propel blood forward, consequent vascular pooling, and sodium and water reabsorption triggered by the renin-angiotensin-aldosterone system. Excess extracellular fluid volume commonly causes peripheral edema. Hypovolemia is usually associated with overly aggressive diuretic therapy and can be especially dangerous in elderly patients because it causes confusion and hypotension.

Electrolyte imbalances

Hyponatremia may result from sodium loss due to diuretic abuse. In some cases, it may result from a dilutional effect that occurs when water reabsorption is greater than sodium reabsorption.

In patients with heart failure, prolonged use of a diuretic without adequate potassium replacement can cause hypokalemia. Likewise, use of a potassium-sparing diuretic can cause hyperkalemia.

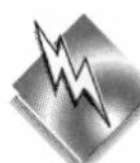

DANGER *Hypokalemia and hyperkalemia can lead to life-threatening arrhythmias. Therefore, carefully monitor potassium levels whenever a patient receives any kind of diuretic, oral or I.V.*

Hypomagnesemia may accompany hypokalemia, particularly if the patient is receiving a diuretic because many diuretics cause the kidneys to excrete magnesium. Hypochloremia may also result from excessive diuretic therapy.

Acid-base imbalances

When cells don't receive enough oxygen, they produce more lactic acid. Poor tissue perfusion in the patient with heart failure allows lactic acid to accumulate, which in turn leads to metabolic acidosis. Metabolic alkalosis may be caused by excessive diuretic use, which causes bicarbonate retention.

In the early stages of heart failure, as the respiratory rate increases, more carbon dioxide (CO_2) is blown off from the lungs, which raises pH and leads to respiratory alkalosis. As heart failure progresses, gas exchange is further impaired and CO_2 accumulates, resulting in respiratory acidosis.

Heart failure imbalances *(continued)*

Fluid imbalances

✦ Hypervolemia — results from heart's failure to propel blood forward, vascular pooling, and sodium and water reabsorption
✦ Hypovolemia — usually associated with overly aggressive diuretic therapy

Electrolyte imbalances

✦ Hyponatremia — may result from sodium loss due to diuretic abuse or from dilutional effect
✦ Hypokalemia — may result from prolonged use of diuretic without adequate potassium replacement
✦ Hyperkalemia — may result from use of potassium-sparing diuretic
✦ Hypomagnesemia — may accompany hypokalemia, especially if patient is receiving diuretic therapy
✦ Hypochloremia — may result from excessive diuretic therapy

Acid-base imbalances

✦ Metabolic acidosis — may result from poor tissue perfusion in patient with heart failure that allows lactic acid accumulation
✦ Metabolic alkalosis — may be caused by excessive diuretic use
✦ Respiratory alkalosis — may develop when lungs blow off CO_2 and pH is increased due to increased respiratory rate
✦ Respiratory acidosis — may develop when gas exchange is further impaired and CO_2 accumulates

Assessment findings

Left-sided heart failure
- With tissue hypoxia: fatigue, weakness, orthopnea, exertional dyspnea, and paroxysmal nocturnal dyspnea
- Pink, frothy sputum as pulmonary edema develops
- Kidney disorders and oliguria as cardiac output decreases

Right-sided heart failure
- Venous engorgement
- Distended, rigid neck veins with exaggerated pulsations
- Edema
- Weight gain
- Enlarged, slightly tender liver

Advanced heart failure
- Diminished pulse pressure
- Cool, clammy skin
- Palpitations
- Chest tightness
- Arrhythmias
- Cardiac arrest

ASSESSMENT FINDINGS

Signs and symptoms of heart failure vary according to the site of the failure and the stage of the disease. Expect to encounter a combination of these assessment findings.

Left-sided heart failure

If your patient has left-sided heart failure and tissue hypoxia, then he'll probably complain of fatigue, weakness, orthopnea, and exertional dyspnea. The patient may also report paroxysmal nocturnal dyspnea.

He may use two or three pillows to elevate his head to sleep, or he may have to sleep sitting up in a chair. Shortness of breath may awaken him shortly after he falls asleep, forcing him to quickly sit upright to catch his breath. He may have dyspnea, coughing, and wheezing even when he sits up. Tachypnea may occur, and you may note crackles on inspiration. Coughing may progress to the point where the patient produces pink, frothy sputum as he develops pulmonary edema.

The patient may be tachycardic and auscultation of heart sounds may reveal third and fourth heart sounds as the myocardium becomes less compliant. Hypoxia and hypercapnia can affect the central nervous system, causing restlessness, confusion, and a progressive decrease in the patient's level of consciousness. Later, with continued decrease in cardiac output, the kidneys may be affected, and oliguria may develop.

Right-sided heart failure

Inspection of a patient with right-sided heart failure may reveal venous engorgement. When the patient sits upright, his neck veins may appear distended, feel rigid, and exhibit exaggerated pulsations. Edema may develop, and the patient may report a weight gain. The nail beds may appear cyanotic and anorexia and nausea may occur. The liver may be enlarged and slightly tender. Right-sided heart failure may progress to congestive hepatomegaly, ascites, and jaundice.

Advanced heart failure

In a patient with advanced heart failure, pulse pressure may be diminished, reflecting reduced stroke volume. Occasionally, diastolic pressure rises from generalized vasoconstriction. The skin feels cool and clammy. Progression of heart failure may lead to palpitations, chest tightness, and arrhythmias. Cardiac arrest may occur.

Diagnostic test results

Because the causes of heart failure are so varied, several tests may help confirm the diagnosis.

✦ Electrocardiograms can detect arrhythmias, MI, or the presence of coronary artery disease.

✦ Chest X-rays show cardiomegaly, alveolar edema, pleural effusion, and pulmonary edema.

✦ Echocardiograms reveal enlarged heart chambers, changes in ventricular function, and the presence of valvular disease.

✦ Hemodynamic pressure readings reveal increased central venous pressure and pulmonary artery wedge pressure.

Diagnostic test results

✦ Echocardiograms revealing enlarged heart chambers, ventricular function changes, and valvular disease

✦ Hemodynamic pressure readings revealing increased central venous pressure and pulmonary artery wedge pressure

Treatment

Heart failure is a medical emergency. Relieving dyspnea and improving arterial oxygenation are the immediate therapeutic goals. Secondary goals include minimizing or eliminating the underlying cause, reducing sodium and water retention, optimizing cardiac preload and afterload, and enhancing myocardial contractility.

Medications

One or more drugs—such as a diuretic, a vasodilator, or an inotropic agent—are usually needed to manage heart failure. Diuretic therapy, the starting point of this treatment, increases sodium and water elimination by the kidneys. By reducing fluid overload, diuretics decrease total blood volume and relieve circulatory congestion. For most diuretics to work effectively, the patient must control his sodium intake.

Diuretics include thiazide diuretics and loop diuretics, such as furosemide (Lasix) and bumetanide (Bumex). Because thiazide and loop diuretics work at different sites in the nephron, they produce a synergistic effect when given in combination. Potassium-sparing diuretics, such as spironolactone (Aldactone) and triamterene (Dyrenium), may be used. Any patient who takes a diuretic should be carefully monitored because it can disturb the electrolyte balance and lead to metabolic alkalosis, metabolic acidosis, or other complications.

Vasodilators can reduce preload or afterload by decreasing arterial and venous vasoconstriction. Reducing preload and afterload helps increase stroke volume and cardiac output.

Angiotensin-converting enzyme (ACE) inhibitors decrease both afterload and preload. Because ACE inhibitors prevent potassium loss, hyper-

Treatment

✦ Immediate therapeutic goals: relieving dyspnea and improving arterial oxygenation

✦ Secondary goals: treatment of underlying cause, reducing sodium and water retention, optimizing cardiac preload and afterload, and enhancing myocardial contractility

Medications

✦ Diuretic therapy (starting point of treatment) to increase sodium and water elimination by kidneys

✦ Vasodilators to reduce preload or afterload by decreasing arterial and venous vasoconstriction

✦ ACE inhibitors to decrease preload and afterload

Treatment
(continued)

Medications
- Nitrates (primarily vasodilators) at higher doses to dilate arterial smooth muscle
- Beta-adrenergic blockers to decrease afterload through vasodilating action
- Inotropic medications to increase contractility in failing heart muscle
- Morphine to reduce anxiety and decrease preload and afterload by dilating veins

Surgery (severe heart failure)
- Cardiomyoplasty
- Left ventriculectomy
- Intra-aortic ballon counterpulsation or other ventricular assist device (biventricular pacemaker or implantable cardioverter defibrillator)
- Heart transplantation (last resort)

kalemia may develop in patients who are also taking a potassium-sparing diuretic. For this reason, potassium levels must be closely monitored.

Nitrates, primarily vasodilators, also dilate arterial smooth muscle at higher doses. Most patients with heart failure tolerate nitrates well. They are available in several forms and I.V., oral, and topical ointment or patches are considered the most useful for heart failure therapy.

Beta-adrenergic blockers such as carvedilol (Coreg) decrease afterload through their vasodilating action. Specifically, they cause peripheral vasodilation, decreasing systemic pressure directly and cardiac workload indirectly. In addition, beta-adrenergic blocker therapy enhances longevity.

Inotropic drugs such as digoxin increase contractility in the failing heart muscle. They also slow conduction through the atrioventricular node. However, there is a narrow margin of safety between therapeutic effect and toxicity level. A concurrent electrolyte imbalance, such as hyperkalemia, may contribute to digoxin toxicity because it decreases the excretion of digoxin from the body. This may lead to fatal cardiac arrhythmias, muscle weakness, and respiratory distress.

Other drugs — such as dopamine (Intropin), dobutamine (Dobutrex), milrinone (Primacor), and inamrinone (Inocor) — may be indicated for patients with acute heart failure to increase myocardial contractility and cardiac output. Hydralazine (Apresoline) and nitroprusside (Nitopress) may also be used to treat heart failure.

Morphine (Duramorph) is commonly used in heart failure patients with acute pulmonary edema. Besides reducing anxiety, it decreases preload and afterload by dilating veins.

Surgery

Finally, for those patients with severe heart failure, surgery may be required. In cardiomyoplasty, a muscle is wrapped around the failing heart to boost its pumping action. In a left ventriculectomy, a section of nonviable myocardium is removed to reduce ventricular size, which allows the heart to pump more effectively. To help the ventricles propel blood through the vascular system, an intra-aortic balloon counterpulsation or other ventricular assist device may be implanted. Such devices include a biventricular pacemaker or an implantable cardioverter defibrillator, which is sometimes necessary because a patient with heart failure may have a concurrent life-threatening arrhythmia. Heart transplantation is the last resort.

CHARTING CHECKLIST

Documenting heart failure

If your patient has heart failure, make sure you document the following information:
- ❑ prescribed medications
- ❑ daily weight, intake, and output (any weight gain over 2 lb in less than 24 hours places the patient at risk for fluid overload)
- ❑ edema
- ❑ diet restrictions
- ❑ vital signs
- ❑ lung sounds
- ❑ heart sounds
- ❑ condition of skin
- ❑ positioning of the patient and his response
- ❑ mental status
- ❑ tolerance of activity
- ❑ time you notified the physician
- ❑ safety measures implemented
- ❑ patient teaching provided and the patient's response.

Nursing interventions

To properly care for a patient with heart failure, you'll need to perform a number of specific nursing interventions, including:

✦ Assess the patient's mental status, and report changes in vital signs or mental status immediately.

✦ Assess the patient for signs and symptoms of impending cardiac failure, such as fatigue, restlessness, hypotension, rapid respiratory rate, dyspnea, coughing, decreased urine output, liver enlargement, and a rapid, thready pulse.

✦ Assess the patient for edema. Note the amount and location of the edema and the degree of pitting, if present. (See *Documenting heart failure*.)

✦ Monitor sodium and fluid intake as prescribed. Hyponatremia and fluid volume deficit can stimulate the renin-angiotensin-aldosterone system and exacerbate heart failure. Usually, mild sodium restriction — whereby the patient uses no added salt — is prescribed.

✦ Check the patient's weight and fluid intake and output daily for significant changes to determine if he is in a state of fluid overload. If the patient's weight has increased by two or more pounds over 24 hours, additional diuretic therapy is needed.

Key nursing interventions

- ✦ Assess for signs and symptoms of impending heart failure
- ✦ Assess for edema
- ✦ Monitor sodium and fluid intake
- ✦ Check weight and fluid intake and output daily
- ✦ Monitor vital signs, including blood pressure, pulse, respirations, and heart and breath sounds

Key nursing interventions *(continued)*

- Monitor serum electrolyte levels
- Maintain continuous cardiac monitoring
- Administer prescribed medications
- Instruct patient to call physician if he develops warning signs and symptoms

Patient teaching

- Description of disorder
- Activity level
- Skin care
- Medications
- Diet
- Stress and anxiety level
- Weight monitoring
- Warning signs and symptoms
- Follow-up appointments

✦ Monitor vital signs, including blood pressure, pulse, respirations, and heart and breath sounds for abnormalities that might indicate a fluid excess or deficit.

✦ Monitor serum electrolyte levels — especially sodium and potassium — for changes that may indicate an imbalance. Remember that hypokalemia can lead to digoxin toxicity. Monitor arterial blood gas results to assess adequacy of ventilation.

✦ Maintain continuous cardiac monitoring during acute and advanced stages of disease to identify arrhythmias promptly.

✦ Administer prescribed medications — such as digoxin, diuretics, angiotensin-converting enzyme inhibitors, and potassium supplements — to support cardiac function and minimize symptoms.

✦ Administer oral potassium supplements in orange juice or with meals to promote absorption and prevent gastric irritation.

✦ Place the patient in Fowler's position, and give supplemental oxygen as ordered to help him breathe more easily.

✦ Encourage independent activities of daily living as tolerated, though bed rest may be required for some patients. Reposition the patient as needed every 1 to 2 hours. Edematous skin is prone to breakdown.

✦ Instruct the patient and his family to notify the staff of any changes in the patient's condition, such as increased shortness of breath, chest pain, or dizziness.

✦ Instruct the patient to call the physician if his pulse rate is irregular, if it measures fewer than 60 beats/minute, or if he experiences dizziness, blurred vision, shortness of breath, a persistent dry cough, palpitations, increased fatigue, nocturnal dyspnea that comes and goes, swollen ankles, or decreased urine output.

Patient teaching

Be sure to cover these topics and then evaluate your patient's learning:

- description of heart failure and its treatment
- need for adequate rest
- proper skin care
- prescribed medications
- dietary restrictions
- need to reduce stress and anxiety level
- need for regular exercise
- need for daily weights
- warning signs and symptoms and when to report them
- importance of follow-up appointments.

Respiratory failure

UNDERSTANDING RESPIRATORY FAILURE

When the lungs can't sufficiently maintain arterial oxygenation or eliminate carbon dioxide (CO_2), acute respiratory failure results. Unchecked and untreated, this condition can lead to decreased oxygenation of the body tissues and metabolic acidosis.

In patients with essentially normal lung tissue, respiratory failure usually produces hypercapnia, an excessive amount of CO_2 in arterial blood, and hypoxemia, a deficiency of oxygen in arterial blood.

In patients with chronic obstructive pulmonary disease (COPD), respiratory failure may be signaled only by an acute drop in arterial blood gas (ABG) levels and clinical deterioration. This is because some patients with COPD consistently have high partial pressure of arterial carbon dioxide ($Paco_2$) levels and low partial pressure of arterial oxygen (Pao_2) levels but are able to compensate and maintain a normal, or near-normal, pH level.

Causes and pathophysiology

In patients with acute respiratory failure, gas exchange is diminished by any combination of these factors: alveolar hypoventilation, ventilation-perfusion mismatch, and intrapulmonary shunting.

Respiratory failure
- Develops when lungs can't maintain arterial oxygenation or eliminate CO_2
- Can produce excessive amount of CO_2 in arterial blood (hypercapnia) and deficiency of oxygen in arterial blood (hypoxemia)

Pathophysiology
- With acute form, gas exchange diminished by any combination of alveolar hypoventilation, ventilation-perfusion mismatch, and intrapulmonary shunting
- Associated imbalances include hypervolemia, hypovolemia, hyperkalemia, hypokalemia, respiratory acidosis, respiratory alkalosis, and metabolic acidosis

Respiratory failure development

Alveolar hypoventilation

- Occurs when amount of oxygen brought to alveoli is diminished, causing decreased partial pressure of arterial oxygen and increased alveolar CO_2
- Prevents diffusion of adequate CO_2 from capillaries, increasing partial pressure of arterial carbon dioxide

$\dot{V}/\dot{Q}$ mismatch

- Occurs when insufficient ventilation exists with normal blood flow or when normal ventilation exists with insufficient blood flow

Intrapulmonary shunting

- Occurs when blood passes from right side of heart to left side of heart without being oxygenated

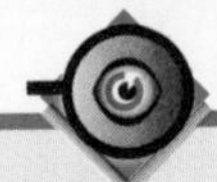

CLOSER LOOK

How acute respiratory failure develops

Three major malfunctions account for impaired gas exchange and subsequent acute respiratory failure: alveolar hypoventilation, ventilation-perfusion ($\dot{V}/\dot{Q}$) mismatch, and intrapulmonary (right-to-left) shunting.

Alveolar hypoventilation

In alveolar hypoventilation, shown here as the result of airway obstruction, the amount of oxygen brought to the alveoli is diminished, causing a drop in the partial pressure of arterial oxygen and an increase in alveolar carbon dioxide (CO_2). The accumulation of CO_2 in the alveoli prevents diffusion of adequate amounts of CO_2 from the capillaries, which increases the partial pressure of arterial carbon dioxide.

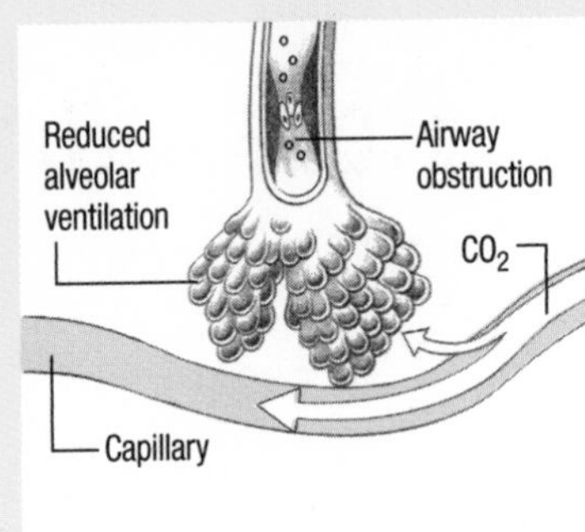

$\dot{V}/\dot{Q}$ mismatch

$\dot{V}/\dot{Q}$ mismatch, the leading cause of hypoxemia, occurs when insufficient ventilation exists with a normal flow of blood or when, as shown, normal ventilation exists with an insufficient flow of blood.

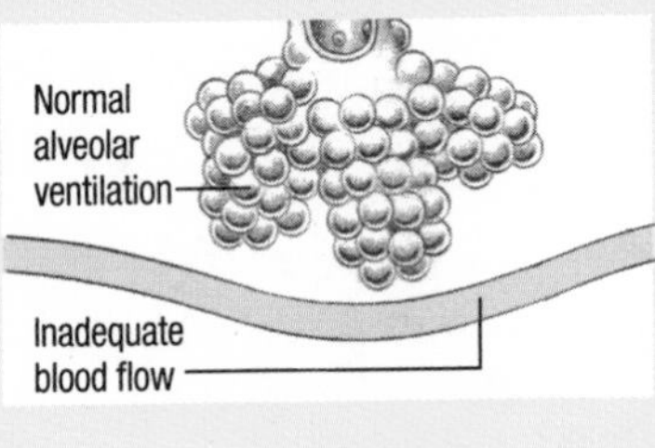

Intrapulmonary shunting

Intrapulmonary shunting occurs when blood passes from the right side of the heart to the left side without being oxygenated, as shown. Shunting can result from untreated ventilation or perfusion mismatches.

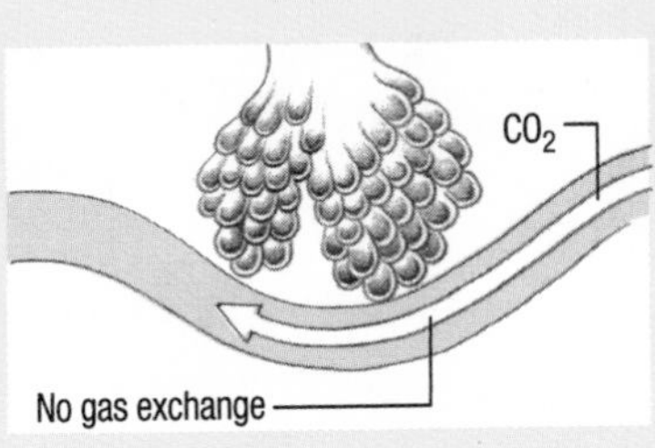

Imbalances associated with respiratory failure include hypervolemia, hypovolemia, hypokalemia, hyperkalemia, respiratory acidosis, respiratory alkalosis, and metabolic acidosis. (See *How acute respiratory failure develops.*)

Hypervolemia

Prolonged respiratory treatments, such as nebulizer use, can lead to inhalation and absorption of water vapor. Excessive fluid absorption may also result from increased lung capillary pressure or permeability, which

Causes of respiratory failure

Problems with the brain, lungs, muscles, and nerves or with pulmonary circulation can impair gas exchange and cause respiratory failure. This list contains conditions that can cause respiratory failure.

Brain
- Anesthesia
- Cerebral hemorrhage
- Cerebral tumor
- Drug overdose
- Head trauma
- Skull fracture

Lungs
- Acute respiratory distress syndrome
- Asthma
- Chronic obstructive pulmonary disease
- Cystic fibrosis
- Flail chest
- Massive bilateral pneumonia
- Sleep apnea
- Tracheal obstruction

Muscles and nerves
- Amyotrophic lateral sclerosis
- Guillain-Barré syndrome
- Multiple sclerosis
- Muscular dystrophy
- Myasthenia gravis
- Polio
- Spinal cord trauma

Pulmonary circulation
- Heart failure
- Pulmonary edema
- Pulmonary embolism

typically occurs in acute respiratory distress syndrome. The excessive fluid absorption may precipitate pulmonary edema.

Hypovolemia

Because the lungs remove water daily through exhalation, an increased respiratory rate can promote excessive loss of water. Excessive loss can also occur with fever or any other condition that increases the metabolic rate and thus the respiratory rate. (See *Causes of respiratory failure.*)

Hyperkalemia

In acidosis, excess hydrogen ions (H^+) moves into the cell. Potassium ions then move out of the cell and into the blood to balance the positive charges between the two fluid compartments and hyperkalemia may result.

Hypokalemia

If a patient begins to hyperventilate and alkalosis results, H^+ will move out of the cells and potassium ions will move from the blood into the cells. That shift can cause hypokalemia.

Primary causes of respiratory failure

- Acute respiratory distress syndrome
- Chronic obstructive pulmonary disease
- Heart failure
- Pulmonary edema
- Drug overdose
- Spinal cord trauma
- Pulmonary embolism
- Tracheal obstruction

Metabolic acidosis

Conditions that cause hypoxia induce cells to use anaerobic metabolism. That metabolism creates an increase in the production of lactic acid, which can lead to metabolic acidosis.

Respiratory acidosis

Respiratory acidosis, which is due to hypoventilation, results from the inability of the lungs to eliminate sufficient quantities of CO_2. The excess CO_2 combines with water to form carbonic acid. Increased carbonic acid levels result in decreased pH, which contributes to respiratory acidosis.

Respiratory alkalosis

Respiratory alkalosis develops from an excessively rapid respiratory rate, or *hyperventilation*, and causes excessive CO_2 elimination. Loss of CO_2 decreases the blood's acid-forming potential and results in respiratory alkalosis.

Assessment findings

Hypoxemia and hypercapnia, which are characteristic of acute respiratory failure, stimulate strong compensatory responses from all body systems, especially the respiratory, cardiovascular, and central nervous systems (CNS).

Respiratory response

When the body senses hypoxemia or hypercapnia, the respiratory center responds by increasing respiratory depth and then respiratory rate. Signs of labored breathing — flared nostrils, pursed-lip exhalation, and the use of accessory breathing muscles, among others — may signify respiratory failure.

As respiratory failure worsens, muscle retractions between the ribs, above the clavicle, and above the sternum may also occur. The patient is dyspneic and may become cyanotic. Auscultation of the chest reveals diminished or absent breath sounds over the affected area. You may also hear wheezes, crackles, or rhonchi. Respiratory arrest may occur.

Cardiovascular response

The sympathetic nervous system usually compensates by increasing the heart rate and constricting blood vessels in an effort to improve cardiac output. The patient's skin may become cool, pale, and clammy. Eventually, as myocardial oxygenation diminishes, cardiac output, blood pressure, and heart rate drop. Arrhythmias develop, and cardiac arrest may occur.

Assessment findings

Respiratory

- Signs of labored breathing (flared nostrils, pursed-lip exhalation, use of accessory breathing muscles)
- Muscle retractions between ribs, above clavicle, and above sternum
- Dyspnea
- Cyanosis
- Diminished or absent breath sounds
- Wheezes
- Crackles
- Rhonchi
- Respiratory arrest

Cardiovascular

- Cool, pale, clammy skin
- Decreased cardiac output
- Decreased blood pressure
- Decreased heart rate
- Arrhythmias
- Cardiac arrest

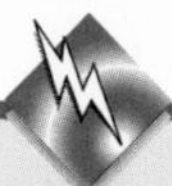

DANGER

Recognizing worsening respiratory failure

These assessment findings commonly occur in patients with worsening respiratory failure:
- ✦ arrhythmias
- ✦ bradycardia
- ✦ cyanosis
- ✦ diminished or absent breath sounds over affected area; wheezes, crackles, or rhonchi may also be heard
- ✦ dyspnea
- ✦ hypotension
- ✦ muscle retractions.

CNS response

Even a slight disruption in oxygen supply and carbon dioxide elimination can affect brain function and behavior. Hypoxia initially causes anxiety and restlessness, which can progress to marked confusion, agitation, and lethargy. The primary indicator of hypercapnia, headache, occurs as cerebral vessels dilate in an effort to increase the brain's blood supply. If the CO_2 level continues to rise, the patient is at risk for seizures and coma. (See *Recognizing worsening respiratory failure.*)

Diagnostic test results

Typical laboratory findings for a patient with respiratory failure include:
- ✦ ABG changes indicating respiratory failure. (Always compare ABG results with your patient's baseline values. For a patient with previously normal lungs, the pH is usually less than 7.35, the $Pa{O_2}$ less than 50 mm Hg, and the $Pa{CO_2}$ greater than 50 mm Hg. In a patient with COPD, an acute drop in the $Pa{O_2}$ level of 10 mm Hg or more indicates respiratory failure. Keep in mind that patients with chronic COPD have a chronically low $Pa{O_2}$, increased $Pa{CO_2}$, increased bicarbonate levels, and normal pH.)
- ✦ chest X-rays identifying an underlying pulmonary condition
- ✦ electrocardiogram (ECG) changes showing arrhythmias
- ✦ changes in serum potassium levels relating to acid-base balance.

Treatment

The underlying cause of respiratory failure must be addressed and the oxygen and carbon dioxide levels improved. Oxygen is given in con-

Assessment findings *(continued)*

CNS
- ✦ Anxiety and restlessness that progresses to marked confusion, agitation, and lethargy
- ✦ Headache
- ✦ Seizures
- ✦ Coma

Diagnostic test results

- ✦ ABG changes indicating respiratory failure (compare ABG results with patient's baseline values)
- ✦ Chest X-rays identifying underlying pulmonary condition

Treatment

- Oxygen in controlled concentrations to prevent oxygen toxicity by administering lowest dose of oxygen for shortest period of time
- Oxygen therapy should achieve oxygen saturation of 90% or more or a Pao_2 level of at least 60 mm Hg
- Intubation and mechanical ventilation if conservative treatment fails or if acidemia continues, patient becomes exhausted, or respiratory arrest occurs
- Bronchodilators (especially inhalants) to open airways
- Corticosteroids
- Antibiotics
- Chest physiotherapy, including postural drainage, chest percussion, and chest vibration
- Diuretic if patient is experiencing fluid overload

trolled concentrations, often using a Venturi mask. The goal of oxygen therapy is to prevent oxygen toxicity by administering the lowest dose of oxygen for the shortest period of time, while achieving an oxygen saturation of 90% or more or a Pao_2 level of at least 60 mm Hg.

Intubation and mechanical ventilation are indicated if conservative treatment fails to raise oxygen saturation above 90%. The patient may also be intubated and ventilated if acidemia continues, if he becomes exhausted, or if respiratory arrest occurs. Intubation provides a patent airway. Mechanical ventilation decreases the work of breathing, ventilates the lungs, and improves oxygenation.

Positive end-expiratory pressure (PEEP) therapy may be ordered during mechanical ventilation to improve gas exchange. PEEP maintains positive pressure at the end of expiration, thus preventing the airways and alveoli from collapsing between breaths.

Bronchodilators, especially inhalants, are used to open the airways. If the patient can't inhale effectively or is on a mechanical ventilator, he may receive a bronchodilator via a nebulizer. A corticosteroid, theophylline (Slo-Phyllin), and an antibiotic may also be ordered, as may be chest physiotherapy, including postural drainage, chest percussion, and chest vibration. Suctioning may be required to clear the airways. I.V. fluids may be ordered to correct dehydration and to help thin secretions. A diuretic may be used if the patient is experiencing fluid overload.

Key nursing interventions

- Assess respiratory status
- Monitor vital signs
- Monitor neurologic status
- Perform ongoing respiratory assessment (accessory muscle use, breath sounds, ABGs, secretion production and clearance, respiratory rate and pattern)
- Monitor fluid status

Nursing interventions

To care effectively for a patient with respiratory failure, follow these guidelines:

- Assess respiratory status; monitor rate, depth, and character of respirations, checking breath sounds for abnormalities.
- Monitor vital signs frequently.
- Monitor the patient's neurologic status; it may become depressed as respiratory failure worsens.
- Ongoing respiratory assessment should include accessory muscle use, changes in breath sounds, ABG analysis, secretion production and clearance, and respiratory rate, depth, and pattern. Notify the physician if interventions don't improve the patient's condition.
- Monitor fluid status by maintaining accurate fluid intake and output records. Obtain daily weights.
- Evaluate serum electrolyte levels for abnormalities that can occur with acid-base imbalances.

✦ Evaluate ECG results for arrhythmias.
✦ Monitor oxygen saturation values with a pulse oximeter.
✦ Intervene as needed to correct underlying respiratory problems and associated alterations in acid-base status.
✦ Keep a handheld resuscitation bag at the patient's bedside.
✦ Maintain patent I.V. access as ordered for medication and I.V. fluid administration.
✦ Administer oxygen as ordered to help maintain adequate oxygenation and to restore the normal respiratory rate.
✦ Use caution when administering oxygen to a patient with COPD. Increased oxygen levels can depress the breathing stimulus.
✦ Make sure the ventilator settings are at the ordered parameters.
✦ Perform chest physiotherapy and postural drainage as needed to promote adequate ventilation.
✦ If the patient is retaining carbon dioxide, encourage slow deep breaths with pursed lips. Urge him to cough up secretions. If he can't mobilize secretions, suction him when necessary.
✦ Unless the patient is retaining fluid or has heart failure, increase his fluid intake to 2 qt (2 L)/day, to help liquefy secretions.
✦ Reposition the immobilized patient every 1 to 2 hours.
✦ Position the patient for optimum lung expansion. Sit the conscious patient upright as tolerated in a supported, forward-leaning position to promote diaphragm movement. Supply an overbed table and pillows for support.
✦ If the patient isn't on a ventilator, avoid giving him an opioid analgesic or another CNS depressant, because either may further suppress respirations.
✦ Limit carbohydrate intake and increase protein intake, because carbohydrate metabolism causes more carbon dioxide production than protein metabolism.
✦ Calm and reassure the patient while giving care. Anxiety can raise oxygen demands.
✦ Pace care activities to maximize the patient's energy level and to provide needed rest. Limit his need to respond verbally. Talking may cause shortness of breath.
✦ Implement safety measures as needed to protect the patient. Reorient him if he's confused.
✦ Stress the importance of returning for routine follow-up appointments with the physician.

Key nursing interventions *(continued)*

✦ Monitor oxygen saturation with pulse oximeter
✦ Keep handheld resuscitation bag at bedside
✦ Maintain patent I.V. access
✦ Administer oxygen as ordered, using caution when administering to patient with COPD
✦ Perform chest physiotherapy
✦ Position patient for optimum lung expansion
✦ If patient isn't on ventilator, avoid opioid analgesics or other CNS depressants
✦ Pace activities to maximize patient's energy level and provide needed rest

CHARTING CHECKLIST

Documenting respiratory failure

If your patient has respiratory failure, make sure you document the following information:
- ❑ breath sounds
- ❑ lung secretions
- ❑ laboratory results
- ❑ breathing exercises and the patient's response
- ❑ color and temperature of skin
- ❑ daily weights
- ❑ intake and output
- ❑ measures taken to promote ventilation and the patient's response
- ❑ neurologic status
- ❑ time you notified the physician
- ❑ oxygen therapy
- ❑ safety measures
- ❑ patient teaching provided and the patient's response.

✦ Explain how to recognize signs and symptoms of overexertion, fluid retention, and heart failure. These may include a weight gain of 2 to 3 lb (0.9 to 1.4 kg)/day, edema of the feet or ankles, nausea, loss of appetite, shortness of breath, or abdominal tenderness.

✦ Help the patient develop the knowledge and skills he needs to perform pulmonary hygiene. Encourage adequate hydration to thin secretions—but instruct the patient to notify the physician of signs of fluid retention or heart failure.

✦ Chart all instructions given and care provided. (See *Documenting respiratory failure.*)

Patient teaching

- ✦ Description of disorder
- ✦ Pulmonary hygiene and coughing techniques
- ✦ Rest
- ✦ Smoking cessation
- ✦ Medications
- ✦ Warning signs and symptoms
- ✦ Follow-up appointments
- ✦ Diet

Patient teaching

Be sure to cover these topics and then evaluate your patient's learning:
- ✦ description of respiratory failure and its treatment
- ✦ proper pulmonary hygiene and coughing techniques
- ✦ need for proper rest
- ✦ need to quit smoking, if appropriate
- ✦ prescribed medications
- ✦ warning signs and symptoms and when to report them
- ✦ importance of follow-up appointments
- ✦ diet restrictions, if appropriate.

Excessive GI fluid losses

UNDERSTANDING EXCESSIVE GI FLUID LOSS

Normally, the GI system loses minimal fluid, because most of what's lost is reabsorbed in the intestines. However, because large amounts of fluids — isotonic and hypotonic — pass through the GI system in the course of a day, the potential for significant GI fluid loss exists.

Isotonic fluids that may be lost from the GI tract include gastric juices, bile, pancreatic juices, and intestinal secretions. The only hypotonic fluid that may be lost through the GI system is saliva, which has a lower solute concentration than other GI fluids. Understanding how and why these substances are lost from the GI system is of primary importance when caring for a susceptible patient.

Excessive GI fluid loss

- ✦ Made possible by large amounts of isotonic and hypotonic fluids that pass through GI system
- ✦ Isotonic fluids that may be lost from GI tract: gastric juices, pancreatic juices, and intestinal secretions
- ✦ Hypotonic fluid that may be lost from GI tract: saliva

CAUSES AND PATHOPHYSIOLOGY

Excessive GI fluid loss may come from the physical removal of secretions as a result of vomiting, suctioning, or increased or decreased GI tract motility. Fluids can also be excreted as waste products or secreted from the intestinal wall into the intestinal lumen, both of which can lead to fluid and electrolyte imbalances. (See *Imbalances caused by excessive GI fluid loss*, page 224.) Osmotic diarrhea, which can lead to the loss of acids

Causes

- ✦ Physical removal of secretions resulting from vomiting, suctioning, or increased or decreased GI tract motility
- ✦ Excretion as waste products
- ✦ Secretion from intestinal wall into intestinal lumen
- ✦ Osmotic diarrhea

Imbalances caused by excessive GI fluid loss

Excessive GI fluid loss can lead to various fluid, electrolyte, and acid-base imbalances.

FLUID IMBALANCES

- Hypovolemia and dehydration — Large amounts of fluid can be lost during prolonged, uncorrected vomiting and diarrhea. Hypovolemia can also result if gastric and intestinal suctioning occur without proper monitoring of intake and output to ensure that lost fluid and electrolytes are adequately replaced.

ELECTROLYTE IMBALANCES

- Hypokalemia — The excessive loss of gastric fluids rich in potassium can lead to hypokalemia.
- Hypomagnesemia — Although gastric secretions contain little magnesium, several weeks of vomiting, diarrhea, or gastric suctioning can result in hypomagnesemia. Because hypomagnesemia itself can cause vomiting, the patient's condition may be self-perpetuating.
- Hyponatremia — Prolonged vomiting, diarrhea, or gastric or intestinal suctioning can deplete the body's supply of sodium and lead to hyponatremia.
- Hypochloremia — Any loss of gastric contents causes the loss of chloride. Prolonged gastric fluid loss can lead to hypochloremia.

ACID-BASE IMBALANCES

- Metabolic acidosis — Any condition that promotes intestinal fluid loss can result in metabolic acidosis. Intestinal fluid contains large amounts of bicarbonate. With the loss of bicarbonate, pH falls, creating an acidic condition.
- Metabolic alkalosis — Loss of gastric fluids from vomiting or the use of drainage tubes in the upper GI tract can lead to metabolic alkalosis. Gastric fluids contain large amounts of acids that, when lost, lead to an increase in pH and alkalosis. Excessive use of antacids can also worsen the imbalance by adding to the alkalotic state.

and bases from the GI tract, may occur in the intestines when a high solute load in the intestinal lumen attracts water into the cavity.

Causes *(continued)*

Vomiting and suctioning

- Cause loss of hydrogen ions and electrolytes (chloride, potassium, sodium)
- Deplete fluid volume supply, resulting in hypovolemia and dehydration

Vomiting and suctioning

Vomiting or mechanical suctioning of stomach contents, as with a nasogastric (NG) tube, causes the loss of hydrogen ions and electrolytes, such as chloride, potassium, and sodium. Vomiting also depletes the patient's fluid volume supply, resulting in hypovolemia and dehydration. When assessing acid-base balance, remember that the pH of the upper GI tract is low and that vomiting causes the loss of those acids and raises the risk of alkalosis. (See *Characteristics and causes of vomiting.*)

Characteristics and causes of vomiting

Vomiting may lead to serious fluid, electrolyte, and acid-base disturbances and can occur for a variety of reasons. By carefully observing the characteristics of the vomitus, you may gain clues as to the underlying disorder. Here are descriptions of what the patient's vomitus may indicate.

BILE-STAINED, GREENISH
Obstruction below the pylorus, as from a duodenal lesion

BLOODY
Upper-GI bleeding, as from gastritis or peptic ulcer (if bright) or from gastric or esophageal varices (if dark red)

BROWN WITH A FECAL ODOR
Intestinal obstruction or infarction

BURNING, BITTER-TASTING
Excessive hydrochloric acid in gastric contents

COFFEE-GROUND CONSISTENCY
Digested blood from slowly bleeding gastric or duodenal lesions

UNDIGESTED FOOD
Gastric outlet obstruction, as from gastric tumor or ulcer

Bowel movements

An increase in the frequency and amount of bowel movements and a change in the stool to a watery consistency can cause excessive GI fluid loss, resulting in hypovolemia, dehydration, and the loss of potassium, magnesium, and sodium. Fluids lost from the lower GI tract carry a large amount of bicarbonate with them, which lowers the amount of bicarbonate available to counter the effects of acids in the body.

Laxatives and enemas

Laxatives — such as magnesium sulfate, milk of magnesia, and Fleet Phospho-soda — and enemas may be used by patients to treat constipation, or they may be given before abdominal surgery or diagnostic studies to clean the bowel. Excessive use of laxatives can cause hypermagnesemia, resulting in high magnesium levels, and hyperphosphatemia, resulting in high phosphorus levels.

Causes *(continued)*

Bowel movements
- Increase in bowel movements can result in hypovolemia, dehydration, and loss of potassium, magnesium, sodium, and bicarbonate

Laxatives and enemas
- Excessive use of laxatives can cause hypermagnesemia and hyperphosphatemia
- Excessive use of commonly prepared enemas containing sodium and phosphate can cause hypernatremia
- Excessive use of tap-water enemas can cause decreased sodium levels

Excessive use of commercially prepared enemas containing sodium and phosphate, such as Fleet enemas, can cause hypernatremia, resulting in high phosphorus and sodium levels, if the enemas are absorbed before they can be eliminated. Excessive use of tap-water enemas can cause a decrease in sodium levels because water absorbed by the colon can have a dilutional effect on sodium.

Causes *(continued)*

Other risk factors
- GI tract bacterial infections
- Antibiotic administration
- Young age
- Pregnancy
- Pancreatitis or hepatitis
- Pyloric stenosis (in young children)
- Eating disorders
- Fistulas
- GI bleeding
- Intestinal obstruction
- Tube feedings
- Postsurgical complications

Other risk factors

Excessive GI fluid loss can result from several other conditions, including bacterial infections of the GI tract, which are usually accompanied by vomiting or diarrhea; antibiotic administration, which removes normal flora and promotes diarrhea; young age, which makes the person vulnerable to diarrhea, a frequent cause of GI fluid loss in children; pregnancy, which may be accompanied by vomiting; pancreatitis or hepatitis, which may be accompanied by vomiting; or pyloric stenosis in young children, which may also be accompanied by vomiting.

Imbalances can also result from fecal impaction, poor absorption of foods, poor digestion, anorexia nervosa, and bulimia as well as excessive intake of alcoholic substances and some illicit drugs. Such disorders as anorexia nervosa and bulimia, which primarily affect young women, typically involve the use of laxatives and vomiting as a means of controlling weight.

AGE ALERT *When treating an adolescent, especially a female, for excessive GI fluid loss, assess for signs and symptoms of anorexia nervosa and bulimia. Teeth that appear yellow and worn away and a history of laxative or diet pill use are two obvious signs. Also, assess the patient for use of alternative diet therapies that speed metabolism by mimicking the effects of adrenaline on the body.*

Other disorders that can cause disturbances in fluid, electrolyte, or acid-base balance include the presence of fistulas involving the GI tract, GI bleeding, intestinal obstruction, and paralytic ileus. (See *How intestinal obstruction affects fluids and electrolytes.*)

The use of enteral tube feedings and ostomies, especially ileostomies, may also lead to imbalances. Enteral tube feedings may cause diarrhea or vomiting, depending on their composition and the patient's condition. Suctioning of gastric secretions through tubes may deplete the body of vital fluids, electrolytes, and acids. Saliva may be lost from the body when it can't be swallowed, as with dysphagia related to extensive head and neck cancer.

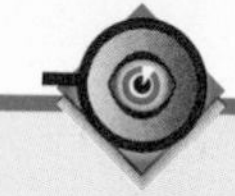

CLOSER LOOK

How intestinal obstruction affects fluids and electrolytes

An intestinal obstruction can be a partial or complete blockage of the lumen in the small or large bowel. When intestinal obstruction occurs, fluid, air, and gas collect near the site. Peristalsis increases temporarily as the bowel attempts to force its contents through the obstruction, injuring intestinal mucosa and causing distention at and above the obstruction site. This distention blocks the flow of venous blood and halts normal absorptive processes. As a result, the bowel begins to secrete water, sodium, and potassium into the fluid pooled in the lumen. This results in hypovolemia, hyponatremia, hypokalemia, distention, and the retention of enormous amounts of fluid in the gut.

An obstruction in the upper intestine results in metabolic alkalosis from dehydration and loss of gastric hydrochloric acid; a lower obstruction causes slower dehydration and loss of intestinal alkaline fluids, resulting in metabolic acidosis. Ultimately, an intestinal obstruction may lead to ischemia, necrosis, and death.

Understanding intestinal obstruction

- ✦ Fluid, air, and gas collect near site of intestinal obstruction, causing distention at and above obstruction site
- ✦ Distention blocks flow of venous blood and halts normal absorptive processes
- ✦ Bowel secretes water, sodium, and potassium into fluid pooled in lumen
- ✦ Results in hypovolemia, hyponatremia, hypokalemia, distention, and fluid pooling in gut
- ✦ Obstruction in upper intestine results in metabolic alkalosis
- ✦ Obstruction in lower intestine results in metabolic acidosis

Postsurgical complications can cause fluid and electrolyte imbalances in patients who are restricted from taking food or drink orally before, during, and after surgery. They may also have an NG tube and other drainage tubes in place, which may account for the loss of protein- and electrolyte-rich fluids. If they're on antibiotics, they may have such adverse effects as nausea, vomiting, and diarrhea.

Assessment findings

With excessive GI fluid loss, the patient may show signs of hypovolemia. This occurs as the body tries to compensate for the low blood count by increasing the heart rate. Along with tachycardia, blood pressure falls as intravascular volume is lost. The patient's skin may become cool and dry as the body shunts blood flow to major organs, and his skin turgor may be decreased or his eyeballs may appear to be sunken, as occurs with dehydration. Urine output may decrease as the kidneys try to conserve fluid and electrolytes.

Cardiac arrhythmias may occur from electrolyte imbalances, such as those related to potassium and magnesium. The patient may become weak and confused. Mental status may deteriorate as fluid, electrolyte, and acid-base imbalances progress.

Assessment findings

- ✦ Tachycardia
- ✦ Decreased blood pressure
- ✦ Cool, dry skin
- ✦ Decreased skin turgor
- ✦ Sunken eyeballs
- ✦ Decreased urine output

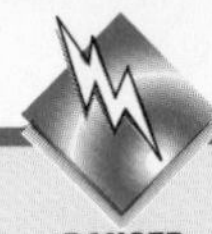

DANGER

Recognizing excessive GI fluid loss

Besides the signs and symptoms related to underlying disorders, the patient with excessive GI fluid loss may show these warning signs and symptoms of hypovolemia:

✦ changes in respirations
✦ confusion or deteriorated mental status
✦ cool, dry skin
✦ decreased skin turgor or sunken eyeballs
✦ decreased urine output
✦ falling blood pressure
✦ possible cardiac arrhythmias
✦ tachycardia
✦ weakness.

Assessment findings *(continued)*

✦ Cardiac arrhythmias
✦ Weakness
✦ Confusion
✦ Deteriorated mental status
✦ Alerted respirations

Diagnostic test results

✦ Altered ABG levels
✦ Elevated or decreased electrolyte levels
✦ Falsely elevated hematocrit
✦ Positive cultures

Respirations may change according to the type of acid-base imbalance the patient develops. For instance, acidosis will cause respirations to be deeper as the patient tries to blow off acid from the lungs.

The patient will also have signs and symptoms related to the underlying disorder — for instance, pancreatitis. (See *Recognizing excessive GI fluid loss.*)

Diagnostic test results

Typical laboratory findings for a patient with excessive GI fluid loss include:

✦ changes in arterial blood gas levels related to metabolic acidosis and metabolic alkalosis
✦ alterations in the levels of certain electrolytes such as potassium, magnesium, and sodium
✦ falsely elevated hematocrit in a volume-depleted patient
✦ bacteria responsible for the underlying disorder, as identified by cultures of body fluid samples.

Treatment

Treatment is aimed at the underlying cause of the imbalance. For instance, an antiemetic and an antidiarrheal may be given for vomiting and diarrhea, respectively. GI drainage tubes and the suction applied to them are discontinued as soon as possible.

CHARTING CHECKLIST

Documenting excessive GI fluid loss

If your patient has the potential for or is experiencing excessive GI fluid loss, make sure you document this information:
- ❑ vital signs
- ❑ intake and output
- ❑ daily weight
- ❑ presence and characteristics of vomitus, diarrhea, or GI fluid drainage
- ❑ skin turgor
- ❑ correct placement of GI tube, if present, including care related to the tube
- ❑ interventions used to decrease GI fluid loss
- ❑ I.V. or oral fluid and electrolyte replacement therapy and the patient's response
- ❑ patient teaching given and the patient's response.

The patient should also receive I.V. or oral fluid replacement, depending on his tolerance and the cause of fluid loss. Electrolytes should also be replaced if serum levels are decreased. Long-term parenteral nutrition may be needed. An antibiotic may be administered if infection is the underlying cause of the fluid loss.

To minimize the risk of fluid and electrolyte complications after surgery, correct preoperatively any fluid or electrolyte imbalances that may exist, provide I.V. fluids until the patient is able to tolerate oral fluids, and replace fluid and electrolyte losses from gastric or intestinal suctioning or drainage tubes to maintain daily requirements.

Treatment
- ✦ Antiemetic and antidiarrheal for vomiting and diarrhea
- ✦ Removal of GI drainage tubes and suction applied to them
- ✦ I.V. or oral fluid replacement
- ✦ Electrolyte replacement
- ✦ Antibiotics

Nursing interventions

A patient with a condition that alters fluid and electrolyte balance through GI losses must be closely monitored. An increase in the amount of drainage from GI tubes or an increase in the frequency of vomiting or diarrhea should be reported. Follow these nursing interventions when caring for a patient with GI fluid losses:

✦ Measure and record the amount of fluid lost through vomiting, diarrhea, or gastric or intestinal suctioning. Remember to include GI losses as part of the patient's total output. A significant increase in GI loss places the patient at greater risk for fluid and electrolyte imbalances and metabolic alkalosis or acidosis. (See *Documenting excessive GI fluid loss.*)

Key nursing interventions
- ✦ Measure and record amount of fluid lost through vomiting, diarrhea, or gastric or intestinal suctioning

Key nursing interventions (continued)
- Monitor intake and output, daily weight, and skin turgor
- Administer oral fluids containing water and electrolytes
- Administer I.V. replacement fluids
- Irrigate suction tube with isotonic normal saline solution
- Restrict amount of ice chips given by mouth when patient is connected to gastric suction
- Evaluate serum electrolyte levels and pH

Patient teaching
- Description of disorder
- Warning signs and symptoms
- Avoidance of enemas and laxatives
- Gastric tube irrigation technique
- I.V. infusion monitoring

✦ Assess the patient's fluid status by monitoring intake and output, daily weight, and skin turgor.

✦ Assess vital signs and report changes that may indicate fluid deficits, such as decreased blood pressure or increased heart rate.

✦ Report vomiting to keep imbalances from becoming severe and to initiate prompt treatment.

✦ Administer oral fluids containing water and electrolytes, such as Gatorade or Pedialyte, if the patient can tolerate fluids.

✦ Maintain patent I.V. access, as ordered. Administer I.V. replacement fluids as prescribed. Monitor the infusion rate and volume to prevent hypervolemia.

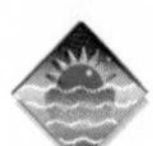

AGE ALERT *Elderly patients can develop heart failure if I.V. fluids are infused too rapidly. Therefore, use caution when administering I.V. fluids to replace fluid losses in these patients.*

✦ If the patient is undergoing gastric suctioning, check GI tube placement often to prevent fluid aspiration.

✦ Irrigate the suction tube with isotonic normal saline solution as ordered. Remember never to use plain water for irrigation because it draws more gastric secretions into the stomach in an attempt to make the fluid isotonic for absorption. Also, the fluid is suctioned out of the stomach, causing further depletion of fluids and electrolytes.

✦ When the patient is connected to gastric suction, restrict the amount of ice chips given by mouth and explain the reason for the restriction. Gastric suctioning of ice chips can deplete fluid and electrolytes from the stomach.

✦ Administer medications, such as an antiemetic or an antidiarrheal, as prescribed, to control the patient's underlying condition.

✦ Evaluate serum electrolyte levels and pH to detect abnormalities and to monitor the effectiveness of therapy.

Patient teaching

Be sure to cover these topics and then evaluate your patient's learning:

✦ description of excessive GI fluid loss and its treatment

✦ need to report prolonged vomiting or diarrhea

✦ importance of avoiding repeated use of enemas and laxatives

✦ proper technique for irrigating a gastric tube, if appropriate

✦ proper technique for monitoring I.V. infusion, if appropriate.

Renal failure

UNDERSTANDING RENAL FAILURE

The kidneys play a major role in regulating fluids, electrolytes, acids, and bases. They respond to fluid excesses by excreting a more dilute urine, which rids the body of fluid and conserves electrolytes. If they don't function properly, the body has difficulty controlling fluid balance.

Renal failure occurs when there's a disruption of normal kidney function. When the kidneys can't rid the body of fluid and conserve electrolytes, acute or chronic renal failure results. Acute renal failure occurs suddenly and is usually reversible. Conversely, chronic renal failure occurs slowly and is irreversible.

Renal failure

- Kidneys play major role in regulating fluids, electrolytes, acids, and bases
- Renal failure occurs when disrupted kidneys can't eliminate bodily fluids or conserve electrolytes
- Acute renal failure — occurs suddenly and is usually reversible
- Chronic renal failure — occurs slowly and is irreversible

CAUSES AND PATHOPHYSIOLOGY

Acute and chronic renal failure affect the kidneys' functional unit, the nephron, which forms urine. Imbalances occur as the kidneys lose the ability to excrete water, electrolytes, wastes, and acid-base products through the urine. Patients may also develop hypertension, anemia, and uremia as well as renal osteodystrophy, which includes softening of bones and a reduction of bone mass.

Causes of acute renal failure

- ✦ Intrarenal conditions that damage kidneys
- ✦ Prerenal conditions that cause diminished blood flow to kidneys
- ✦ Obstructive postrenal conditions that cause urine to back up into kidneys

Pathophysiology of acute renal failure

Oliguric-anuric phase

- ✦ First clinical sign: Decrease in urine output to < 400 ml/ 24 hours
- ✦ Kidney failure results in nitrogenous waste accumulation, causing increased BUN and serum creatinine levels
- ✦ Generally lasts 1 to 2 weeks, but can last longer

Diuretic phase

- ✦ Starts with gradual increase in daily urine output from 400 ml/ 24 hours to 1 to 2 L/24 hours
- ✦ BUN level stabilizes
- ✦ Lasts about 10 days

Recovery phase

- ✦ Begins when fluid and electrolyte values start to stabilize, indicating return to normal kidney function
- ✦ Lasts a few months; patient may experience slightly reduced kidney function for rest of life

Acute renal failure

About 5% of patients in health care facilities develop acute renal failure at some point during their stay. It may stem from intrarenal conditions, which damage the kidneys themselves; from prerenal conditions such as heart failure, which causes a diminished blood flow to the kidneys; or from obstructive postrenal conditions such as prostatitis, which can cause urine to back up into the kidneys. (See *Causes of acute renal failure.*) Regardless of cause, acute renal failure normally passes through three distinct phases: oliguric-anuric, diuretic, and recovery.

Oliguric-anuric phase

A decrease in urine output is the first clinical sign of the oliguric-anuric phase. Typically, as the glomerular filtration rate (GFR) decreases, the patient's urine output decreases to less than 400 ml during a 24-hour period.

When the kidneys fail, nitrogenous waste products accumulate, causing an elevation in blood urea nitrogen (BUN) and serum creatinine levels. The result is uremia. Electrolyte imbalances, metabolic acidosis, and other effects follow as the patient becomes increasingly uremic, and renal dysfunction disrupts other body systems. Left untreated, the condition is fatal.

The oliguric-anuric phase generally lasts 1 to 2 weeks but may last for several more. The longer the patient remains in this phase, the poorer the prognosis for a return to normal renal function.

Diuretic phase

The diuretic phase starts with a gradual increase in daily urine output from 400 ml/24 hours to 1 to 2 L/24 hours as well as the stabilization of the BUN level. Although urine output begins to increase in this phase, a potential for fluid and electrolyte imbalances still exists as glomerular filtration increases.

The diuretic phase lasts about 10 days.

Recovery phase

The recovery or convalescent phase begins when fluid and electrolyte values start to stabilize, indicating a return to normal kidney function. The patient may experience a slight reduction in kidney function for the rest of his life, so he'll still be at risk for fluid and electrolyte imbalances.

The recovery phase generally lasts a few months.

Causes of acute renal failure

The causes of acute renal failure can be divided into three categories: prerenal, intrarenal, and postrenal. Prerenal causes involve conditions that diminish blood flow to the kidneys. Intrarenal causes involve conditions that damage the kidneys themselves. Postrenal causes involve conditions that obstruct urine outflow, which causes urine to back up into the kidneys.

PRERENAL CAUSES

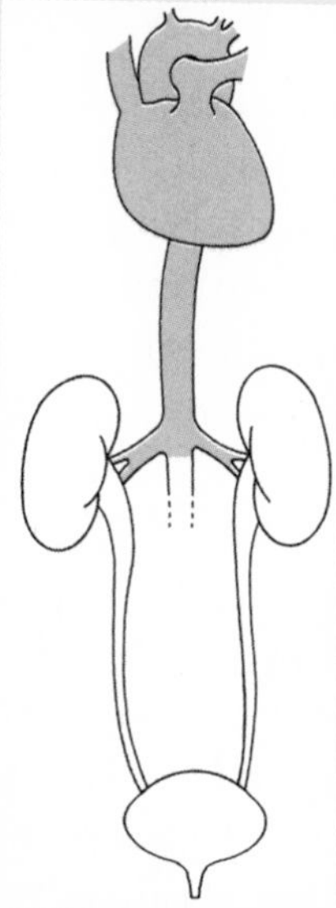

- Hypovolemia
- Peripheral vasodilation
- Renal vascular obstruction
- Serious cardiovascular disorders
- Severe vasoconstriction
- Trauma

INTRARENAL CAUSES

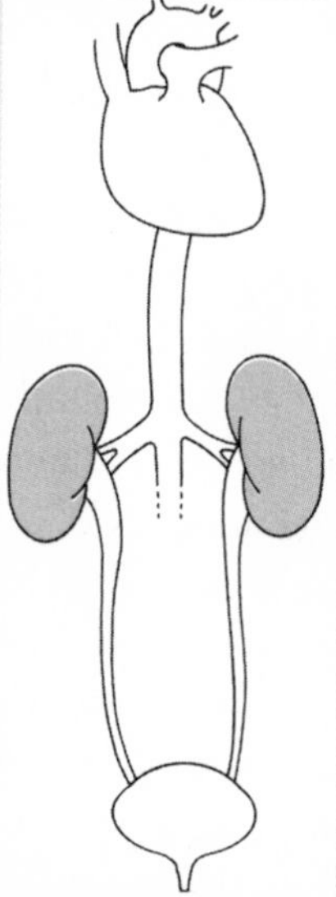

- Acute tubular necrosis
- Aminoglycosides or nonsteroidal anti-inflammatory drugs
- Crush injury, myopathy, sepsis, or transfusion reaction
- Eclampsia, postpartum renal failure, or uterine hemorrhage
- Heavy metals
- Ischemic damage from poorly treated renal failure
- Nephrotoxins
- Trauma

POSTRENAL CAUSES

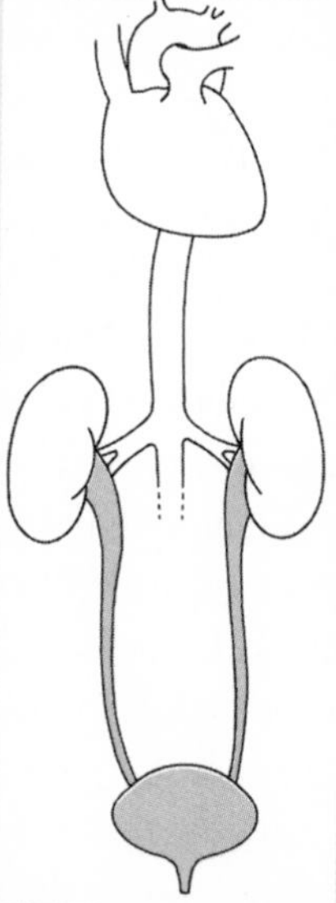

- Bladder obstruction
- Trauma
- Ureteral obstruction
- Urethral obstruction

Causes of chronic renal failure

- Chronic glomerular disease
- Chronic infections
- Congenital anomalies
- Vascular disease
- Obstructions
- Collagen diseases
- Long-term therapy with nephrotoxic drugs
- Endocrine diseases

Staging chronic renal failure

- Progression staged by degree of kidney function
- Reduced renal reserve: GFR 40 to 70 ml/minute
- Renal insufficiency: GFR 20 to 40 ml/minute
- Renal failure: GFR 10 to 20 ml/minute
- End-stage renal disease: GFR < 10 ml/minute

Imbalances caused by renal failure

Fluid

- Hypervolemia results when urine output decreases and body retains fluid or when fluid intake exceeds urine output
- Hypovolemic water losses usually occur during diuretic phase of acute renal failure

Chronic renal failure

Chronic renal failure, which has a more insidious onset than acute renal failure, may result from chronic glomerular disease, such as glomerulonephritis; chronic infections, such as chronic pyelonephritis or tuberculosis; congenital anomalies, such as polycystic kidney disease; vascular diseases, such as renal nephrosclerosis or hypertension; obstructions, such as those from calculi; collagen diseases, such as systemic lupus erythematosus; long-term therapy with nephrotoxic drugs, such as aminoglycosides; and endocrine diseases, such as diabetes mellitus.

Staging chronic renal failure

Because chronic renal failure has a slow onset and the rate at which kidney function deteriorates depends on the underlying disorder, identifying specific time frames for its stages may be difficult. It's possible, however, to stage progression of the disease by the degree of kidney function.

Chronic renal failure can be divided into four basic stages:

- reduced renal reserve (GFR 40 to 70 ml/minute)
- renal insufficiency (GFR 20 to 40 ml/minute)
- renal failure (GFR 10 to 20 ml/minute)
- end-stage renal disease (GFR less than 10 ml/minute).

The kidneys have great functional reserve. Few symptoms develop until more than 75% of glomerular filtration is lost. The remaining functional nephrons then deteriorate progressively; symptoms worsen as renal function diminishes. Failing kidneys can't regulate fluid balance or filter solutes or participate effectively in acid-base balance. If chronic renal failure continues unchecked, uremic toxins accumulate and produce potentially fatal physiologic changes in all major organ systems.

Imbalances caused by renal failure

Renal failure — acute or chronic — can cause a number of fluid, electrolyte, and acid-base imbalances, including hypervolemia, hypovolemia, hyperkalemia, hyperphosphatemia, hypocalcemia, hyponatremia, hypernatremia, hypermagnesemia, metabolic acidosis, and metabolic alkalosis.

Fluid imbalances

When urine output decreases, especially with the sudden onset of acute renal failure, the body retains fluid, which can lead to hypervolemia. That condition may also occur if fluid intake exceeds urine output. The resulting fluid overload can lead to hypertension, peripheral edema, heart failure, or pulmonary edema.

Hypovolemic water losses usually occur during the diuretic phase of acute renal failure and can result in hypotension or circulatory collapse.

Potassium imbalances

As the kidneys' ability to excrete potassium is impaired, serum potassium levels increase, resulting in hyperkalemia. Additional stressors — such as infection, GI bleeding, trauma, and surgery — can also lead to high serum potassium levels. Keep in mind that hyperkalemia may develop more suddenly in patients with acute renal failure than in patients with chronic renal failure because of their lower tolerance for high potassium levels.

Metabolic acidosis, which occurs with renal failure, causes potassium to move from intracellular fluid into the extracellular fluid. This is problematic because the release of potassium from any necrotic or injured cell worsens hyperkalemia.

Calcium and phosphorus imbalances

Serum calcium and phosphorus have an inverse relationship, so when one goes out of balance, the other follows suit. For example, when the kidneys lose the ability to excrete phosphorus, hyperphosphatemia develops. This increase in serum phosphorus causes a decrease in serum calcium, because of their inverse relationship.

Decreased activation of vitamin D by the kidneys results in decreased GI absorption of calcium — another cause for low serum calcium levels. When serum calcium levels are low, hyperphosphatemia develops.

Sodium imbalances

Sodium levels may be either abnormally high or unusually low during renal failure. Hyponatremia can occur with acute renal failure because a decreased GFR and damaged tubules increase water and sodium retention. This dilutional hyponatremic state can also be caused by the intracellular-extracellular exchange between sodium and potassium during metabolic acidosis.

Hypernatremia can occur with chronic renal failure, and it can worsen with subsequent progressions in the degree of kidney failure that cause less sodium to be excreted.

Magnesium imbalances

The patient with renal failure may retain magnesium as a result of a decreased GFR and destruction of the tubules. However, a high serum magnesium level usually isn't recognized unless the patient receives external

Imbalances caused by renal failure *(continued)*

Potassium

- Hyperkalemia results from impaired kidney excretion of potassium
- Worsened by metabolic acidosis that causes potassium to move from intracellular fluid into extracellular fluid

Calcium and phosphorus

- Hyperphosphatemia develops when kidneys lose ability to excrete phosphorus
- As serum potassium levels increase, serum calcium levels decrease
- Hyperphosphatemia may also develop due to decreased kidney activation of vitamin D (results in decreased serum calcium)

Sodium

- Hyponatremia can occur (in acute renal failure) because decreased GFR and damaged tubules increase water and sodium retention
- Hyponatremia can also be caused by intracellular-extracellular exchange between sodium and potassium during metabolic acidosis
- Hypernatremia can occur in chronic renal failure due to decreased sodium excretion

Magnesium

- Hypermagnesemia may result from decreased GFR and tubular destruction

Imbalances caused by renal failure *(continued)*

Acid-base
- Metabolic acidosis (most common) develops due to impaired kidney secretion of hydrogen ions in urine; exacerbated by kidney failure to hold onto bicarbonate

sources of magnesium, such as laxatives, antacids, I.V. solutions, or hyperalimentation solutions.

Acid-base imbalances

Metabolic acidosis is the most common acid-base imbalance occurring with renal failure. It develops as the kidneys lose the ability to secrete hydrogen ions — an acid — in the urine. The imbalance is also exacerbated as the kidneys fail to hold onto bicarbonate — a base.

Patients with chronic renal failure have more time to compensate for this acid-base imbalance than patients with acute renal failure. The lungs try to compensate for the excess acid by increasing the depth and rate of respirations in an attempt to blow off carbon dioxide.

Metabolic alkalosis rarely occurs with renal failure. When it does, it usually results from excessive intake of bicarbonate, given in an effort to correct metabolic acidosis.

Assessment findings

Key early
- Dry mouth
- Fatigue
- Nausea
- Hypotension
- Loss of skin turgor
- Listlessness

Key late
- Decreased, dilute urine output with casts or crystals
- Muscle irritability followed by muscle weakness, irregular pulse, and life-threatening cardiac arrhythmias
- Fluid overload
- Palpable edema
- Weight gain

Cardiovascular
- Hypertension
- Irregular pulse
- Tachycardia

ASSESSMENT FINDINGS

The patient's health history may reveal a disorder that can cause renal failure; it may also uncover a recent episode of fever; chills; GI problems, such as anorexia, nausea, vomiting, diarrhea, or constipation; and central nervous system problems such as headache.

Signs and symptoms vary, depending on the length of time in which renal failure develops. Fewer signs and symptoms may appear in patients with acute renal failure because of the condition's shorter clinical course. In patients with chronic renal failure, however, almost all body systems are affected. (See *Recognizing renal failure.*)

In cases of renal failure in which the kidneys are unable to retain salt, hyponatremia may occur. The patient may complain of dry mouth, fatigue, and nausea. You may note hypotension, loss of skin turgor, and listlessness that progresses to somnolence and confusion.

Later, as the number of functioning nephrons decreases, so does the kidney's capacity to excrete sodium and potassium. Urine output decreases and it may be dilute, with casts or crystals present. Accumulation of potassium causes muscle irritability and then muscle weakness, irregular pulse, and life-threatening cardiac arrhythmias. Sodium retention causes fluid overload, and edema becomes palpable. The patient gains weight from fluid retention. Metabolic acidosis can also occur.

When the cardiovascular system is involved, you'll find hypertension, an irregular pulse and, possibly, tachycardia. Signs of a pericardial rub,

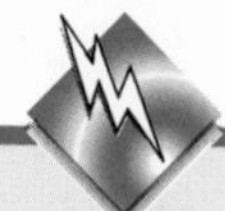

Recognizing renal failure

These signs and symptoms are associated with renal failure and involve several body systems. Your patient may develop some or all of them.

CARDIOVASCULAR
- Anemia
- Cardiac arrhythmias
- Heart failure
- Hypertension
- Hypotension
- Irregular pulse
- Pericardial rub
- Tachycardia
- Weight gain with fluid retention

GASTROINTESTINAL
- Ammonia smell to the breath
- Anorexia
- Bleeding
- Constipation or diarrhea
- Dry mouth
- Inflammation and ulceration of GI mucosa
- Metallic taste in the mouth
- Nausea and vomiting
- Pain on abdominal palpation and percussion

GENITOURINARY
- Amenorrhea in women
- Anuria or oliguria
- Changes in urinary appearance or patterns
- Decreased libido
- Dilute urine with casts and crystals
- Impotence in men
- Infertility

INTEGUMENTARY
- Dry, brittle hair that may change color or fall out easily
- Dry, scaly skin with ecchymoses, petechiae, and purpura
- Dry mucous membranes
- Loss of skin turgor
- Severe itching
- Thin, brittle fingernails with lines
- Uremic frost (in later stages)
- Yellow-bronze skin color

MUSCULOSKELETAL
- Bone and muscle pain
- Gait abnormalities or loss of ambulation
- Muscle cramps
- Muscle weakness
- Pathologic fractures

NEUROLOGIC
- Burning, itching, and pain in the legs and feet
- Coma
- Confusion
- Fatigue
- Hiccups
- Irritability
- Listlessness and somnolence
- Muscle irritability and twitching
- Seizures
- Shortened attention span and memory

RESPIRATORY
- Crackles
- Decreased breath sounds, if pneumonia is present
- Dyspnea
- Kussmaul's respirations

Assessment findings *(continued)*

Respiratory
- Kussmaul's respirations (with metabolic acidosis)

GI
- Gum ulceration and bleeding
- Metallic taste in mouth
- Ammonia smell to breath

Integumentary
- Yellow-bronze skin color
- Uremic frost
- Thin, brittle fingernails with characteristic lines
- Complaints of severe itching

Neurologic
- Mild behavior changes
- Shortened memory and attention span
- Apathy
- Drowsiness
- Irritability
- Confusion
- Coma
- Seizures

Neuromuscular
- Muscle cramps and twitching
- Pain, burning, and itching in legs and feet

related to pericarditis, may be heard, especially in patients with chronic renal failure. Crackles at the lung bases may be heard, and peripheral edema may be palpated if heart failure occurs.

Respiratory changes include reduced pulmonary macrophage activity with increased susceptibility to infection. If pneumonia is present, breath sounds may decrease over areas of consolidation. Crackles at the lung bases occur with pulmonary edema. Kussmaul's respirations occur with metabolic acidosis.

With inflammation and ulceration of GI mucosa, inspection of the mouth may reveal gum ulceration and bleeding. The patient may complain of hiccups, a metallic taste in the mouth, anorexia, nausea, and vomiting caused by esophageal, stomach, or bowel involvement. You may note an ammonia smell to the patient's breath. Abdominal palpation and percussion may cause pain.

Integumentary changes include skin that typically reveals a yellow-bronze color. It's dry and scaly with purpura, ecchymoses, and petechiae that form as a result of thrombocytopenia and platelet dysfunction caused by uremia. In later stages, the patient may experience uremic frost, which produces powdery deposits on the skin as a result of urea and uric acid being excreted in sweat, and thin, brittle fingernails with characteristic lines. Mucous membranes are dry. Hair is dry and brittle and may change color and fall out easily. The patient usually complains of severe itching.

The patient may have a history of pathologic fractures and complain of bone and muscle pain, which may be caused by an imbalance in calcium and phosphorus or in the amount of parathyroid hormone produced. You may note gait abnormalities or, possibly, that the patient is no longer able to ambulate.

With chronic renal failure, the patient may have a history of infertility and decreased libido. Women may have amenorrhea, and men may be impotent.

You may note that the patient has changes in his level of consciousness that progress from mild behavior changes, shortened memory and attention span, apathy, drowsiness, and irritability to confusion, coma, and seizures. The patient may complain of muscle cramps and twitching caused by muscle irritability, as well as pain, burning, and itching in the legs and feet that may be relieved by voluntarily shaking, moving, or rocking them. Symptoms may eventually progress to paresthesia and motor nerve dysfunction.

Laboratory results associated with acute renal failure

In patients with acute renal failure, keep alert for these early signs:
- ✦ urine output below 400 ml over 24 hours
- ✦ increased blood urea nitrogen level
- ✦ increased serum creatinine level.

Diagnostic test results

Typical laboratory findings for a patient with renal failure include:

✦ elevated serum BUN, creatinine, potassium, and phosphorus levels (See *Laboratory results associated with acute renal failure.*)

✦ arterial blood gas (ABG) results that indicate metabolic acidosis—specifically, a low pH and bicarbonate level

✦ low hematocrit, low hemoglobin level, and mild thrombocytopenia

✦ urinalysis showing casts, cellular debris, decreased specific gravity, and proteinuria

✦ electrocardiogram (ECG) showing tall, peaked T waves; a widened QRS complex; and disappearing P waves if hyperkalemia is present

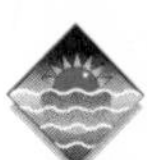

AGE ALERT *As people age, nephrons are lost and kidneys decrease in size. These changes decrease renal blood flow and may result in BUN levels that double in older patients.*

✦ other studies, such as kidney-ureter-bladder radiography and kidney ultrasonography, may also be performed to determine the cause of renal failure.

Diagnostic test results
- ✦ Elevated BUN, creatinine, potassium, and phosphorus levels
- ✦ Urinalysis showing casts, cellular debris, decreased specific gravity, and proteinuria

Treatment

Treatment of renal failure aims to correct specific symptoms and to alter the disease process. Dietary changes can play an important role. The patient should be put on a low-protein diet, which will reduce end products of protein metabolism that the kidneys are unable to excrete. If he must have protein, it should be in the form of such foods as eggs, milk, poultry and meat, all of which contain the essential amino acids that prevent the breakdown of body protein.

In addition to a low-protein diet, intake of sodium and potassium should be restricted and the patient should be placed on a high-calorie

Treatment
- ✦ Low-protein, high-calorie diet with restricted sodium and potassium intake

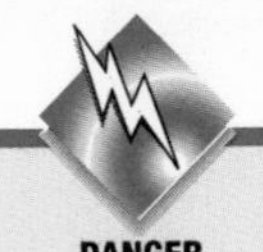

DANGER

Emergency treatment of hyperkalemia

In patients with hyperkalemia, emergency treatment is required. Treatment includes dialysis and administration of 50% hypertonic glucose I.V., regular insulin, calcium gluconate I.V., and sodium bicarbonate I.V. In addition, Kayexalate may also be administered.

Treatment
(continued)

- ✦ Loop diuretics and fluid restriction to reduce fluid retention
- ✦ Phosphate-binding antacid to lower serum phosphorus levels
- ✦ Synthetic erythropoietin to stimulate bone marrow production of RBCs
- ✦ Hemodialysis and peritoneal dialysis

diet that meets daily requirements and prevents breakdown of body protein.

Maintaining fluid balance requires careful monitoring of vital signs, weight changes, and urine output. Fluid retention can be reduced, if some renal function remains, with the use of a loop diuretic such as furosemide (Lasix) and with fluid restriction.

Careful monitoring of serum potassium levels is necessary to detect hyperkalemia. If the patient develops this condition, emergency treatment should be initiated. (See *Emergency treatment of hyperkalemia*.) A phosphate-binding antacid may be given to lower serum phosphorus levels.

In patients with chronic renal failure, kidney production of erythropoietin is diminished. This hormone controls the rate of red blood cell (RBC) production in bone marrow and functions as a growth factor and differentiating factor. Treatment includes administration of synthetic erythropoietin (Procrit) to stimulate bone marrow to produce RBCs.

Hemodialysis and peritoneal dialysis are used in acute and chronic renal failure. By assuming the function of the kidneys, these measures help correct fluid and electrolyte disturbances and relieve some of the symptoms of renal failure.

Nursing interventions

Caring for a patient with renal failure requires careful monitoring, administration of various medications and therapeutic regimens, and empathic ministering to the patient and family. Use these nursing interventions in your care:

✦ Assess the patient carefully to determine the type and severity of fluid, electrolyte, and acid-base imbalances.

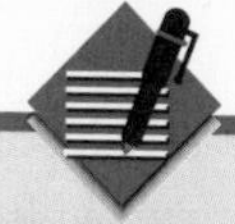

CHARTING CHECKLIST

Documenting renal failure

If your patient has renal failure, make sure you document this information:

- ❑ assessment findings, such as those related to fluid, electrolyte, or acid-base imbalances
- ❑ vital signs, including breath sounds and central venous pressure readings, if available
- ❑ daily weight
- ❑ laboratory test results
- ❑ intake and output
- ❑ administration of I.V. or oral electrolyte replacement therapy
- ❑ dialysis and care of the vascular access site
- ❑ notification of the physician
- ❑ performance of patient and family teaching and the patient's response.

✦ Maintain accurate fluid intake and output records. (See *Documenting renal failure.*)

✦ Weigh the patient daily, and compare the results with the 24-hour intake and output record.

✦ Monitor vital signs, including breath sounds and central venous pressure when available, to detect changes in fluid volume. Report hypertension, which may occur as a result of fluid and sodium retention.

✦ Observe the patient for signs and symptoms of fluid overload, such as edema, bounding pulse, and shortness of breath.

✦ Monitor serum electrolyte and ABG levels for abnormalities. Report significant changes to the physician.

✦ Observe the patient for signs and symptoms that may indicate an electrolyte or acid-base imbalance — such as tetany, paresthesia, muscle weakness, tachypnea, or confusion.

✦ Monitor ECG readings to detect electrolyte imbalances.

✦ Monitor hemoglobin levels and hematocrit.

✦ If the patient requires dialysis, check the vascular access site every 2 hours for patency and signs of clotting, and feel for a bruit. Check the site for bleeding after dialysis.

✦ Restrict fluids as prescribed.

✦ Administer prescribed diuretics if the patient's kidneys can still excrete excess fluid.

Key nursing interventions

- ✦ Maintain accurate fluid intake and output records
- ✦ Weigh patient daily
- ✦ Observe for signs and symptoms of fluid overload
- ✦ Monitor serum electrolyte and ABG levels for abnormalities
- ✦ Monitor ECG readings
- ✦ If patient requires dialysis, check vascular access site every 2 hours for patency, signs of clotting, and bruits; check site for bleeding after dialysis
- ✦ Restrict fluids as prescribed
- ✦ Administer prescribed diuretics

Key nursing interventions *(continued)*

- Provide diet high in calories and low in protein, sodium, and potassium
- Don't use arm prepared for dialysis with shunt or fistula for measuring blood pressure, drawing blood, or inserting I.V. catheters

- Administer other prescribed medications, such as oral or I.V. electrolyte replacement to correct electrolyte imbalances and vitamin supplements to correct nutritional deficiencies.
- Know the route of excretion for medications being given. Drugs excreted through the kidney or removed during dialysis will need dosage adjustments.
- Expect to administer sodium bicarbonate I.V. to control acute acidosis and orally to control chronic acidosis. Remember that sodium bicarbonate has a high sodium content. Multiple doses of the drug may result in hypernatremia, which could contribute to the onset of heart failure and pulmonary edema.
- Maintain the patient's nutritional status. Provide a diet high in calories and low in protein, sodium, and potassium. Restrict electrolyte intake, especially potassium and phosphorus, if ordered. Initiate a nutritional consultation as needed.
- Be prepared to initiate dialysis when electrolyte or acid-base imbalances don't respond to drug therapy or when fluid removal isn't possible.
- If a shunt or fistula for dialysis has been placed in the patient's arm, don't use that extremity for measuring blood pressure, drawing blood, or inserting I.V. catheters.
- Provide emotional support to the patient and his family.

Patient teaching

- Description of disorder
- Medications
- Diet
- Weight monitoring
- Warning signs and symptoms
- Activity level
- Counseling services
- Vascular access device care
- Peritoneal dialysis

Patient teaching

Be sure to cover these topics and then evaluate your patient's learning:

- description of renal failure and its treatment
- prescribed medications
- avoidance of high-sodium and high-potassium foods
- importance of weighing himself daily
- warning signs and symptoms and when to report them
- need for frequent rest for the patient with anemia
- referrals to counseling services, if indicated
- proper methods of caring for the shunt, fistula, or vascular access device
- proper method of performing peritoneal dialysis at home, if appropriate.

Burns

BURN INJURIES

A major burn is a horrifying injury, requiring painful treatment with a long period of rehabilitation. Burns can cause the destruction of the epidermis, dermis, or subcutaneous layers of the skin — injuries that can be permanently disfiguring and incapacitating, both emotionally and physically, and possibly life-threatening.

Burns, like any injury to the skin, interfere with the skin's ability to help keep out infectious organisms, maintain fluid balance, and regulate body temperature. Burn injuries cause major changes in the body's fluid and electrolyte balance. Many of those imbalances change over time as the initial injury progresses.

The extreme heat from a burn can be severe enough to completely destroy cells. Even with a lesser injury, normal cell activity is disrupted. The patient's prognosis depends on the size and severity of the burn and its cause, as well as the presence of preexisting medical conditions and the patient's age.

Burn injuries

- ✦ Interfere with skin's ability to help keep out infectious organisms, maintain fluid balance, and regulate body temperature
- ✦ Prognosis depends on burn size and severity, its cause, presence of preexisting medical conditions, and patient's age

CAUSES AND PATHOPHYSIOLOGY

Several factors determine the severity of a burn, including the cause, degree, and extent of the burn as well as the part of the body involved. They can result from thermal, mechanical, or electrical injuries as well as from exposure to chemicals or radiation.

Causes

- ✦ Can result from thermal, mechanical, or electrical injuries as well as from exposure to chemicals or radiation

Causes
(continued)

- Thermal burns—most common type of burn injury; result from exposure to dry heat (flames) or moist heat (steam, hot liquids)
- Mechanical burns—result from friction or abrasion that occurs when skin is rubbed harshly against course surface
- Electrical burns—result from contact with faulty wiring, high-voltage power lines, or immersion in electrified water; also from lightning strikes
- Chemical burns—result from direct contact, ingestion, inhalation, or injection of acids, alkali, or vesicants
- Radiation burns—typically associated with sunburn or radiation treatment

Thermal burns

Thermal burns, the most common type of burn injury, result from exposure to dry heat, such as flames, or moist heat, such as steam and hot liquids. They commonly occur with residential fires, motor vehicle accidents, childhood accidents, exposure to improperly stored gasoline, exposure to space heaters, electrical malfunctions, and arson. Other causes may include the improper handling of firecrackers, contact with scalding liquids, and kitchen accidents.

Because its effects are similar to those of thermal burn, frostbite is included in this category.

Mechanical burns

Mechanical burns are caused by the friction or abrasion that occurs when the skin is rubbed harshly against a coarse surface. A motorcycle accident in which a person experiences "road rash" is an example of this type of burn.

Electrical burns

Electrical burns commonly occur after contact with faulty electrical wiring, high-voltage power lines, or immersion in water that has been electrified. Lightning strikes can also cause these injuries.

DANGER *When caring for a patient with an electrical burn, keep in mind that he may have internal damage; check him for entrance and exit wounds. Tissue damage from an electrical burn is difficult to assess because internal destruction along the conduction pathway is usually greater than the surface burn indicates.*

An electrical burn that ignites the patient's clothing may cause thermal burns as well.

Chemical and radiation burns

Chemical burns result from the direct contact, ingestion, inhalation, or injection of acids, alkali, or vesicants. The chemical destroys protein in tissues, leading to necrosis. The type and extent of damage caused depends on the properties of the particular chemical.

Radiation burns are typically associated with sunburn or radiation treatment for cancer. These burns tend to be superficial, involving the outer layer of the skin.

Classification of burns

Burn thickness affects cell function. Therefore, classifying the degree of a burn helps to determine the type of nursing intervention necessary.

First-degree burns

First-degree burns, or partial-thickness burns, affect the superficial layer of the epidermis. These burns are usually pink or red and dry and painful. No blistering occurs, but some edema may be present.

First-degree burns aren't classified as severe because the epidermis remains intact and continues to prevent water loss from the skin, so they don't affect fluid and electrolyte balance. Regrowth of the epidermis occurs, and healing is generally rapid without scarring.

Second-degree burns

Second-degree burns, or deep partial-thickness burns, affect the epidermis and dermis. These burns are caused by prolonged exposure—usually longer than 10 seconds—to intense heat or by prolonged contact with hot liquids or objects.

To identify a second-degree burn, look for the area to be painful, swollen, and red, with blister formation. When pressure is applied to the burn, it blanches and refills.

In second-degree burns, regeneration of the epithelial layer may occur and the amount of scarring varies. Fluid and electrolyte imbalances are associated with second-degree burns that cover significant areas of the body.

Third-degree burns

Third-degree burns, or full-thickness burns, affect the epidermis, dermis, and tissues below the dermis. These burns look dry and leathery, are painless—because nerve endings are destroyed—and don't blanch when pressure is applied. The color of the burned area varies from white to black or charred.

Full-thickness burns require skin grafting and carry the greatest risk of fluid and electrolyte imbalance.

Extent of burns

Assessment tools, such as the Rule of Nines or the Lund-Browder classification, are used to estimate the percentage of body surface area involved in a burn. (See *Estimating the extent of burns,* pages 246 and 247.) The

(Text continues on page 248.)

Classification of burns

First-degree

- Also known as *partial-thickness burns*
- Affect superficial layer of epidermis
- Typically pink or red and dry and painful
- Edema without blistering may be present

Second-degree

- Also known as *deep partial-thickness burns*
- Affect epidermis and dermis
- Painful
- Appear swollen and red with blister formation
- Blanch and refill when pressure applied
- Amount of scarring varies
- Associated with fluid and electrolyte imbalances if burn covers significant body surface

Third-degree

- Also known as *full-thickness burns*
- Affect epidermis, dermis, and tissues below dermis
- Painless
- Appear dry and leathery
- No blanching when pressure applied
- Color of burned area varies from white to black or charred
- Require skin grafting
- Carry greatest risk of fluid and electrolyte imbalance

Extent of burns

- Rule of Nines or Lund-Browder classification used to estimate percentage of body surface area involved in burn

Estimating the extent of burns

You can quickly estimate the extent of an adult patient's burns by using the Rule of Nines. This method divides an adult's body surface areas into percentages.

To use this method, match your adult patient's burns to the body chart shown below. Then add up the corresponding percentages for each burned section. The total — a rough estimate of the extent of your patient's burns — enters into the formula to determine his initial fluid replacement needs.

An infant or a child's body-section percentages differ from those of an adult. For instance, an infant's head accounts for a greater percentage of his total body surface area when compared with an adult's. For an infant or child, use the Lund-Browder classification, as shown at right.

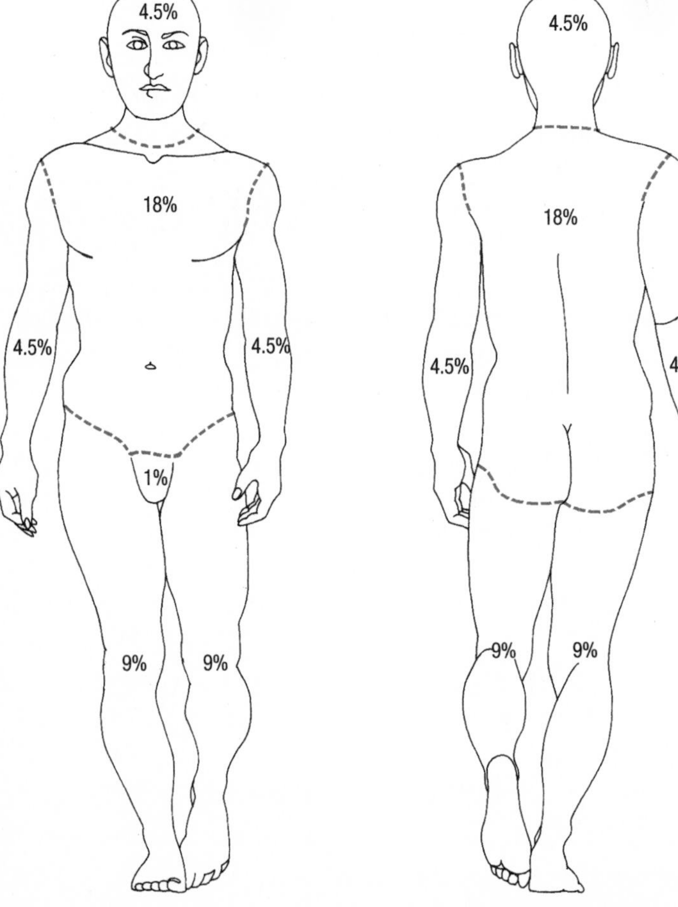

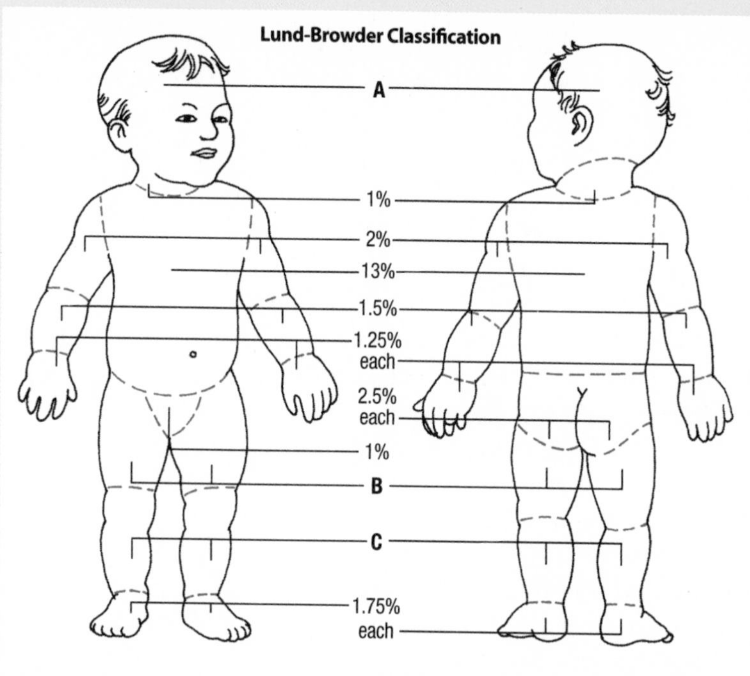

Relative percentages of areas affected by growth

AT BIRTH	1 TO 4 YRS	5 TO 9 YRS	10 TO 14 YRS	15 YRS	ADULT
A: Half of head					
9.5%	8.5%	6.5%	5.5%	4.5%	3.5%
B: Half of thigh					
2.75%	3.25%	4%	4.25%	4.5%	4.75%
C: Half of leg					
2.5%	2.5%	2.75%	3%	3.25%	3.5%

Extent of burns *(continued)*

Major
- Second-degree burns on more than 25% of adult's body surface or more than 20% of child's
- Third-degree burns on more than 10% of body surface area, regardless of body size
- Burns of hands, face, eyes, ears, feet, or genitalia
- All inhalation burns
- All Electrical burns
- Burns complicated by fractures or other major trauma
- All burns in high-risk patients (children younger than age 2, adults older than age 60, patients who have preexisting medical conditions)

Moderate
- Third-degree burns on 2% to 10% of body surface area, regardless of body size
- Second-degree burns on 15% to 25% of adult's body surface area or 10% to 20% of child's

Minor
- Third-degree burns on less than 2% of body surface area, regardless of body size
- Second-degree burns on less than 15% of adult's body surface area or 10% of child's

severity of a burn can be estimated by correlating its depth and size and is characterized as major, moderate, or minor.

Major burns

Major burns require care in a specialized burn care facility and include:
- second-degree burns on more than 25% of an adult's body surface area or on more than 20% of a child's
- third-degree burns on more than 10% of the body surface area, regardless of body size
- burns of the hands, face, eyes, ears, feet, or genitalia
- all inhalation burns
- all electrical burns
- burns complicated by fractures or other major trauma
- all burns in high-risk patients, such as children younger than age 2, adults older than age 60, and patients who have preexisting medical conditions such as heart disease.

Moderate burns

Moderate burns usually require care in either a burn care facility or a general health care facility and include:
- third-degree burns on 2% to 10% of the body surface area, regardless of body size
- second-degree burns on 15% to 25% of an adult's body surface area and 10% to 20% of a child's.

Minor burns

Minor burns can be treated on an outpatient basis and include:
- third-degree burns on less than 2% of the body surface area, regardless of body size
- second-degree burns on less than 15% of an adult's body surface area and 10% of a child's.

Phases of burns

Burns affect many body systems and can lead to several serious fluid and electrolyte balances, which vary depending on the burn's phase. Burn phases, which include the fluid accumulation, fluid remobilization, and convalescent phases, describe the physiologic changes that occur after a burn.

Fluid accumulation phase

The fluid accumulation phase lasts for 36 to 48 hours after a burn injury. During this phase, fluid shifts from the vascular compartment to the interstitial space, a process known as *third-space shift.* This shift of fluids causes edema and typically reaches its maximum extent within 8 hours after the injury. Severe edema may compromise circulation and diminish pulses. Fluid imbalances, respiratory problems, muscle and tissue injury, GI problems, and electrolyte imbalances occur during this phase.

Fluid imbalances

Because of the burn injury, capillary damage alters the permeability of the vessels. Plasma — the liquid and protein part of blood — also escapes from the vascular compartment into the interstitium. Because less fluid is available to dilute the blood, it becomes hemoconcentrated and the patient's hemoglobin level and hematocrit rise.

Because of the third-space shift — the loss of fluids from the vascular compartment — hypovolemia occurs, causing decreased cardiac output, tachycardia, and hypotension. The patient may also develop shock or cardiac arrhythmias or his mental status may decrease.

With the burn's damage to the skin surface, the skin's ability to prevent water loss is also decreased. As a result, the patient can lose up to 8 L of fluid per day, or 400 ml/hour.

Diminished kidney perfusion causes decreased urine output. In response to a burn, the body produces and releases stress hormones, such as aldosterone and antidiuretic hormone, which cause the kidneys to retain sodium and water.

Respiratory problems

Depending on the type of burn, a patient may have a compromised, edematous airway. Look for burns of the head or neck, singed nasal hairs, soot in the mouth or nose, coughing, voice changes, mucosal burns, and stridor. You may hear crackles or wheezes over the lung fields. The patient may breathe rapidly or pant. Circumferential burns and edema of the neck or chest can restrict respirations and cause shortness of breath.

Muscle and tissue injury

Injured tissue causes the release of acids that can cause a drop in the pH level of blood and subsequent metabolic acidosis. Damage to muscle tissue in full-thickness burns causes a release of myoglobin, which can

Fluid accumulation phase

- Lasts for 36 to 48 hours after burn injury
- Fluid shifts from vascular compartment to interstitial space (third-space shift), causing edema
- Fluid imbalances, respiratory problems, muscle and tissue injury, GI problems, and electrolyte imbalances occur

Fluid imbalances

- Hemoglobin and hematocrit rise
- Hypovolemia occurs, causing decreased cardiac output, tachycardia, hypotension and, possibly, shock, cardiac arrhythmias, or decreased mental status
- Loss of up to 8/L of fluid/day or 400 ml/hour
- Decreased urine output
- Production and release of stress hormones (aldosterone, antidiuretic hormone)

Respiratory problems

- Edematous airway
- Coughing
- Voice changes
- Mucosal burns
- Stridor
- Crackles or wheezes over lung fields
- Rapid or panting respirations

Muscle and tissue injury

- Drop in pH of blood and subsequent metabolic acidosis
- Myoglobin release gives urine darkened appearance

Fluid accumulation phase
(continued)

GI problems
- Paralytic ileus
- Curling's ulcers

Electrolyte imbalances
- Hyperkalemia
- Hyponatremia
- Hypernatremia
- Hypocalcemia
- Metabolic acidosis
- Respiratory acidosis

cause renal damage and acute tubular necrosis. Myoglobin gives urine a darkened appearance.

GI problems

Hypovolemia can cause a decrease in circulation to the GI system, resulting in paralytic ileus, which is evidenced by decreased or absent peristalsis and bowel sounds.

Curling's ulcers, or stress ulcers, can develop in the antrum of the stomach or in the duodenum as a result of the intense physiological stress associated with burn trauma. They're probably caused during the fluid accumulation phase as a result of decreased blood flow to the stomach along with reflux of duodenal contents and release of large amounts of pepsin. The combined ischemia, pepsin, and acid leads to ulceration. Endoscopy allows for observation of these ulcers approximately 72 hours after injury.

Signs of Curling's ulcers include bloody or coffee-ground emesis and occult blood in the stool. The lesions typically heal after the patient recovers from the acute injury.

The body's metabolic needs also increase due to the burn injury, usually proportional to the size of the burn wound. Additionally, a negative nitrogen balance can occur after a burn injury due to tissue destruction, protein loss, and the body's stress response.

Electrolyte imbalances

Many electrolyte imbalances can occur during the fluid accumulation phase due to hypermetabolic needs and the priority that fluid replacement takes over nutritional needs during the emergency phase.

Hyperkalemia can result from massive cellular trauma, metabolic acidosis, or renal failure. The condition develops as potassium is released into the extracellular fluid in the initial days after the burn injury.

Hyponatremia can result from the increased loss of sodium and water from the cells. Large amounts of sodium become trapped in edematous fluid during the fluid accumulation phase. Aqueous silver nitrate dressings may also contribute to this electrolyte imbalance.

Hypernatremia can occur as a result of the aggressive use of hypertonic sodium solutions during fluid replacement therapy.

Hypocalcemia can occur because calcium travels to the damaged tissue and becomes immobilized at the burn site 12 to 24 hours after the burn injury. It may also occur due to an inadequate dietary intake of calcium or inadequate supplementation during treatment.

Metabolic acidosis can develop as a result of the accumulation of acids released from the burned tissue. It can also occur due to decreased tissue perfusion from hypovolemia.

Respiratory acidosis can result from inadequate ventilation, as happens in inhalation burns.

Fluid remobilization phase

The fluid remobilization phase, also known as the *diuresis stage,* starts about 48 hours after the initial burn. During this phase, fluid shifts back to the vascular compartment. Edema at the burn site decreases, and blood flow to the kidneys increases, which increases urine output. Sodium is lost through the increase in diuresis, and potassium either moves back into the cells or is lost through the urine.

Fluid and electrolyte imbalances present during the initial phase after a burn can change during the fluid remobilization phase. These imbalances include:

- ✦ hypokalemia, which develops as potassium shifts from the extracellular fluid back into the cells (The condition usually occurs 4 to 5 days after a major burn.)
- ✦ hypervolemia, which occurs as fluid shifts back to the vascular compartment (Excessive administration of I.V. fluids may exacerbate the condition.)
- ✦ hyponatremia, which occurs when sodium is lost during diuresis.

Fluid remobilization phase

- ✦ Also known as *diuresis stage*
- ✦ Starts about 48 hours after initial burn
- ✦ Fluid shifts back to vascular compartment, edema at burn site decreases, and blood flow to kidneys increases, increasing urine output
- ✦ Hypokalemia, hypervolemia, and hyponatremia may occur

Convalescent phase

The convalescent phase begins after the first two phases have been resolved and is characterized by the need to focus on the healing or reconstruction of the burn wound. Although the major fluid shifts have been resolved, further fluid and electrolyte imbalances may continue as a result of inadequate dietary intake. Anemia commonly develops at this time because severe burns typically destroy RBCs

Convalescent phase

- ✦ Begins after first two phases have resolved
- ✦ Characterized by need to focus on healing or reconstruction of burn wound
- ✦ Major fluid shifts resolved, but further fluid and electrolyte imbalances may continue as result of inadequate dietary intake
- ✦ Anemia commonly develops because of RBC destruction

ASSESSMENT FINDINGS

Overall assessment provides a general idea of burn severity. Assessment findings will vary according to the classification of burn injury (first-, second-, or third-degree), as well as the phase of burn injury (fluid accumulation phase, fluid remobilization phase, or convalescent phase).

Assessment findings

- ✦ Vary by burn classification and phase

Diagnostic test results
- Increased hemoglobin levels and hematocrit
- Increased serum potassium levels
- Increased BUN and creatinine levels (renal failure)
- Low pH and bicarbonate levels (metabolic acidosis)
- Increased carboxyhemoglobin levels (smoke inhalation)
- ECG changes reflecting electrolyte imbalances or myocardial damage

Treatment
- Restoration of ABCs (priority)
- Prevention of hypoxia for patient with severe facial burns or inhalation injury (ET intubation, oxygen administration)
- Fluid resuscitation

Diagnostic test results

Typical laboratory findings in a patient with burns include:
- increased hemoglobin levels and hematocrit
- increased serum potassium levels
- decreased serum sodium levels
- increased blood urea nitrogen (BUN) and creatinine levels, indicating renal failure
- low pH and bicarbonate levels, indicating metabolic acidosis
- increased carboxyhemoglobin levels, indicating smoke inhalation
- ECG changes reflecting electrolyte imbalances or indicating myocardial damage
- myoglobin in the urine.

Treatment

Priorities in treating a patient with burns include the ABCs — airway, breathing, and circulation. For a patient with severe facial burns or suspected inhalation injury, treatment to prevent hypoxia includes endotracheal (ET) intubation, administration of high concentrations of oxygen, and positive-pressure ventilation. Be aware that acute respiratory distress syndrome may develop from the body's immune response to injury and the leakage of fluid across the alveolocapillary membrane.

Fluid resuscitation is also a vital part of treatment. Several formulas have been created to guide initial treatment for the patient with burns. The Parkland formula is commonly used. (See *Using the fluid replacement formula.*)

Initial treatment includes administration of lactated Ringer's solution through a large-bore I.V. line to expand vascular volume. This balanced isotonic solution supplies water, sodium, and other electrolytes; it can help correct metabolic acidosis because the lactate in the solution is quickly metabolized into bicarbonate.

Hypertonic solutions called *colloids* may be used to increase blood volume. They draw water from the interstitial space into the vasculature. However, the use of colloids in the immediate postburn period is controversial because they increase colloid osmotic pressure in the interstitial space, which may worsen edema at the burn site. Examples of colloid solutions are plasma, albumin, and dextran.

A solution of dextrose 5% in water may be used to replace normal insensible water loss as well as water loss associated with damage to the skin

Using the fluid replacement formula

The Parkland formula is a commonly used formula for calculating fluid replacement in patients with burns. Always base the volume of fluid replacement on the patient's response, especially his urine output. Urine output of 30 to 50 ml/hour is a sign of adequate renal perfusion.

The Parkland formula

Over 24 hours, 4 ml of lactated Ringer's solution per kilogram of body weight per percentage of body surface area burned.

Use this example to calculate the formula — for a 68 kg person with 27% body surface area burns: 4 ml × 68 kg × 27 = 7,344 ml over 24 hours. Give one-half of the total over the first 8 hours after the burn and the remainder over the next 16 hours.

barrier. Central and peripheral I.V. lines are inserted as necessary. Potassium may be added to I.V. fluids 48 to 72 hours after the burn injury.

An indwelling urinary catheter permits accurate monitoring of urine output. Administration of morphine (Duramorph) I.V. alleviates pain and anxiety. The patient may need a nasogastric (NG) tube to prevent gastric distention from paralytic ileus, along with histamine blockers and antacids to prevent Curling's ulcers.

All patients with burns need a booster of 0.5 ml of tetanus toxoid given I.M. Most burn care facilities don't recommend administering a prophylactic antibiotic because overuse of antibiotics fosters the development of resistant bacteria.

Burn wound treatment

Treatment of the burn wound includes:

- ✦ initial debridement by washing the surface of the wound area with mild soap
- ✦ sharp debridement of loose tissue and blisters because blister fluid contains vasospastic agents that can worsen tissue ischemia
- ✦ coverage of the wound with an antibacterial agent, such as silver sulfadiazine (Silvadene), and an occlusive cotton gauze dressing
- ✦ removal of eschar, called an *escharotomy,* if the patient is at risk for vascular, circulatory, or respiratory compromise — for example, if the patient has a circumferential burn that circles around an extremity, the chest cavity, or the abdomen. Skin grafts may be required.

Parkland formula

- ✦ Over 24 hours, 4 ml of lactated Ringer's solution per kilogram of body weight per percentage of body surface area burned

Treatment *(continued)*

- ✦ Indwelling urinary catheter for accurate monitoring of urine output
- ✦ NG tube to prevent gastric distention from paralytic ileus
- ✦ Histamine blockers and antacids to prevent Curling's ulcers
- ✦ Booster of 0.5 ml of tetanus toxoid given I.M.

Burn wound treatment

- ✦ Initial debridement with mild soap
- ✦ Sharp debridement of loose tissue and blisters
- ✦ Coverage of wound with antibacterial agent and occlusive cotton gauze dressing
- ✦ Removal of eschar
- ✦ Skin grafts, if required

Key nursing interventions

Emergency care

- ✦ Maintain head and spinal alignment
- ✦ Give emergency treatment for electric shock, if needed
- ✦ Make sure patient has adequate airway and effective breathing and circulation
- ✦ Take steps to control bleeding
- ✦ Remove smoldering clothing; if clothing is stuck to patient's skin, soak it in saline solution
- ✦ Remove rings, jewelry, and other constricting items
- ✦ Assess skin for location, depth, and extent of burn
- ✦ Start I.V. therapy at once
- ✦ Insert indwelling urinary catheter as ordered
- ✦ Monitor intake and output every 15 to 30 minutes

Nursing interventions

For the patient with burns, proper nursing care can make the difference between life and death. The priority during the emergency phase is to provide immediate, aggressive burn treatment to increase the patient's chance for survival. Later, the priority shifts to providing supportive measures and using strict aseptic technique to minimize the risk of infection. For handling burns outside the health care facility, see *Emergency burn care.*

Emergency care

✦ Maintain head and spinal alignment until head and spinal cord injuries have been ruled out.

✦ Give emergency treatment for electric shock if needed. If an electric shock caused ventricular fibrillation and subsequent cardiac and respiratory arrest, begin cardiopulmonary resuscitation at once. Try to obtain an estimate of the voltage that caused the injury.

✦ Make sure the patient has an adequate airway and effective breathing and circulation. If needed, assist with ET intubation. The patient may have a tracheostomy tube inserted if ET intubation isn't possible. Administer 100% oxygen as ordered, and adjust the flow to maintain adequate gas exchange. Draw blood for arterial blood gas (ABG) analyses as ordered.

✦ Assess vital signs every 15 minutes. Assess breath sounds, and watch for signs of hypoxia and pulmonary edema.

✦ Take steps to control bleeding, and remove clothing that's still smoldering. If clothing is stuck to the patient's skin, soak it in saline solution. Remove rings, jewelry, and other constricting items.

✦ Assess the skin for the location, depth, and extent of the burn.

✦ Assist with the insertion of a central venous line and additional arterial and I.V. lines.

✦ Start I.V. therapy at once to prevent hypovolemic shock and maintain cardiac output. Follow the Parkland formula or another fluid resuscitation formula, as ordered by the physician.

✦ Insert an indwelling urinary catheter as ordered, and monitor intake and output every 15 to 30 minutes.

✦ Maintain adequate pulmonary hygiene by turning the patient and performing postural drainage regularly.

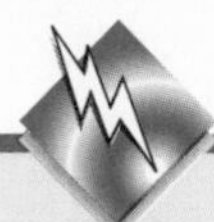

Emergency burn care

If you encounter a person who has just been burned, follow these steps:

- ✦ Extinguish any remaining flames on the patient's clothing.
- ✦ Don't directly touch the patient if he's still connected to live electricity. Unplug or disconnect the electrical source if possible.
- ✦ Assess the ABCs (airway, breathing, circulation), and initiate cardiopulmonary resuscitation if necessary.
- ✦ Send for emergency medical assistance.
- ✦ Assess the scope of the burns and other injuries.
- ✦ Remove the patient's clothing, but don't pull at clothing that sticks to the skin.
- ✦ Irrigate areas of chemical burns with copious amounts of water.
- ✦ Remove from the patient jewelry or other metal objects that can retain heat and constrict patient movement.
- ✦ Cover the patient with a blanket.

Assessment and monitoring

✦ Watch for signs of decreased tissue perfusion, increased confusion, and agitation. Assess peripheral pulses for adequacy.

✦ Assess the patient's heart and hemodynamic status for changes that might indicate fluid imbalances, such as hypervolemia or hypovolemia.

✦ Watch for signs and symptoms of pulmonary edema, which can result from fluid replacement therapy and the shift of fluid back to the vascular compartment.

✦ Observe the pattern of third-space shifting, which causes generalized edema, ascites, and pulmonary or intracranial edema, and document your findings.

✦ Monitor potassium levels, and watch for signs and symptoms of hyperkalemia, such as cardiac rhythm strip changes, weakness, diarrhea, and a slowed, irregular heart rate.

✦ Monitor sodium levels, and watch for signs and symptoms of hyponatremia, such as increasing confusion, twitching, seizures, abdominal pain, nausea, and vomiting.

✦ Watch for signs and symptoms of metabolic acidosis, such as headache, disorientation, drowsiness, nausea, vomiting, and rapid, shallow breathing.

✦ Monitor ABG results.

✦ Monitor other laboratory results.

Key nursing interventions *(continued)*

Assessment and monitoring

- ✦ Watch for signs of decreased tissue perfusion, increased confusion, and agitation
- ✦ Assess patient's heart and hemodynamic status
- ✦ Watch for signs of pulmonary edema
- ✦ Observe pattern of third-space shifting
- ✦ Monitor potassium levels
- ✦ Monitor sodium levels
- ✦ Watch for signs of metabolic acidosis
- ✦ Monitor ABG results

Key nursing interventions *(continued)*

Assessment and monitoring
- ✦ Monitor ECG results for arrhythmias
- ✦ Monitor for temperature changes
- ✦ Insert an NG tube, if ordered
- ✦ Take and record daily weights

Burn wound care
- ✦ Use strict aseptic technique
- ✦ Observe for signs of infection
- ✦ Administer analgesic 30 minutes before wound care
- ✦ Cover burns with dry, sterile dressing
- ✦ Maintain joint function with physical therapy and use of support garments and splints

✦ Monitor ECG results for arrhythmias.

✦ Anticipate the need to administer maintenance I.V. replacement fluids, based on daily assessment of fluid, electrolyte, acid-base, and nutritional status.

✦ Monitor the patient for temperature changes because skin impairment leads not only to body temperature alterations and chills but also to infection.

✦ Maintain core body temperature by covering the patient with a sterile blanket and exposing only small areas of his body at a time.

✦ Insert an NG tube, if ordered, to decompress the stomach. Avoid aspiration of stomach contents during the procedure.

✦ Obtain a preburn weight from the patient or from a family member or friend. If bowel sounds are present, provide a diet high in potassium, protein, vitamins, fats, nitrogen, and calories to maintain the patient's preburn weight. If necessary, feed the patient enterally until he can tolerate oral feedings. If he can't tolerate oral or enteral feedings, administer hyperalimentation as ordered.

✦ Weigh the patient every day at the same time with the same amount of linen, clothes, and dressings.

Burn wound care

✦ Use strict aseptic technique for all patient care, including routinely washing your hands and using protective isolation clothing.

✦ Observe the patient for signs of infection, such as fever, tachycardia, and purulent wound drainage. Blisters, charring, and scarring may appear, depending on the type and age of the burn. Burn patients have an increased risk of infection from destruction of the skin barrier and the loss of nutrients.

✦ Administer an analgesic 30 minutes before wound care.

✦ Culture burn wounds before applying a topical antibiotic for the first time.

✦ Cover burns with a dry, sterile dressing. Never cover large burns with saline-soaked dressings because they can drastically lower body temperature. A topical ointment and an antibiotic may be applied as appropriate. Silver nitrate and mafenide (Sulfamylon) can cause electrolyte imbalances and metabolic alterations.

✦ Maintain joint function with physical therapy and use of support garments and splints.

CHARTING CHECKLIST

Documenting burn care

If your patient has a burn injury, make sure you document this information:
- ❑ assessment findings
- ❑ depth, extent, and severity of burn injury
- ❑ extent of edema
- ❑ pertinent laboratory results
- ❑ I.V. therapy
- ❑ support made available to the patient and family
- ❑ other interventions, such as wound care and physical therapy
- ❑ patient and family teaching that was provided along with the patient's response.

✦ Notify the physician of significant changes in the patient's condition or pertinent laboratory test results.

Communicating with the patient

✦ Explain all procedures to the patient before performing them. Speak calmly and clearly to help alleviate anxiety. Encourage the patient to participate in self-care as much as possible.

✦ Provide opportunities for the patient to voice concerns, especially about altered body image. If appropriate, arrange a meeting with another patient with similar injuries. When possible, reinforce how bodily functions are improving. If necessary, refer the patient for mental health counseling.

✦ Document all care given, all teaching done, and the patient's reaction to each. (See *Documenting burn care.*)

Patient teaching

Be sure to cover these topics and then evaluate your patient's learning:
✦ burn basics and treatment
✦ the patient's particular plan of treatment and wound management
✦ warning signs and symptoms and when to report them
✦ long-term care issues, such as home care follow-up and rehabilitation.

Key nursing interventions *(continued)*

Patient communication
- ✦ Explain all procedures before performing them
- ✦ Speak calmly and clearly to help alleviate anxiety
- ✦ Encourage patient to participate in self-care
- ✦ Provide opportunities for patient to voice concerns, especially about altered body image

Patient teaching

- ✦ Burn basics and treatment, including patient's particular plan of treatment and wound management
- ✦ Warning signs and symptoms
- ✦ Long-term care issues

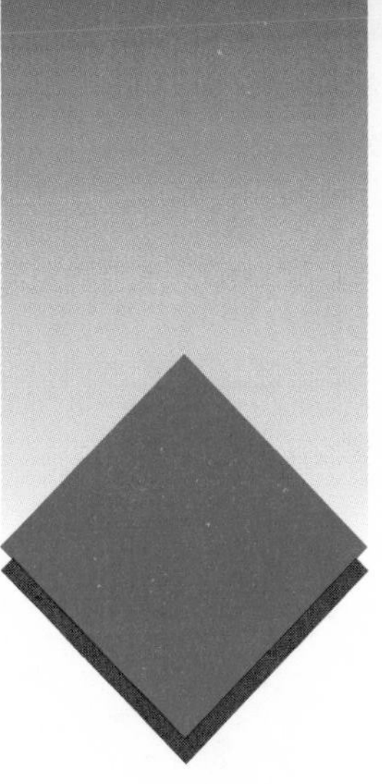

Part four

Treatment

I.V. fluid replacement therapy

I.V. fluid replacement therapy

- I.V. route preferred for administering fluids, electrolytes, and medications in emergencies

Advantages

- Offers immediate, predictable therapeutic effects
- Allows for fluid intake when patient has GI malabsorption
- Permits accurate dosage titration for analgesics and other medications

Disadvantages

- Possible medication and solution incompatibility
- Adverse reactions
- Infection

UNDERSTANDING I.V. FLUID REPLACEMENT THERAPY

To maintain health, the balance of fluids and electrolytes in the body's intracellular and extracellular spaces needs to remain relatively constant. Whenever a person experiences an illness or a condition that prevents normal fluid intake or causes excessive fluid loss, I.V. fluid replacement may be necessary.

ADVANTAGES

I.V. therapy that provides the patient with life-sustaining fluids, electrolytes, and medications offers the advantages of immediate and predictable therapeutic effects. The I.V. route is, therefore, the preferred route, especially for administering fluids, electrolytes, and medications in emergency situations. The I.V. route also allows for fluid intake when a patient has GI malabsorption. I.V. therapy permits accurate dosage titration for analgesics and other medications.

DISADVANTAGES

Potential disadvantages associated with I.V. therapy include medication and solution incompatibility, adverse reactions, infection, and other complications.

TYPES OF I.V. SOLUTIONS

Solutions used for I.V. fluid replacement fall into the broad categories of crystalloids, which may be isotonic, hypotonic, or hypertonic, and colloids, which are always hypertonic.

CRYSTALLOIDS

Crystalloids are solutions with small molecules that flow easily from the bloodstream into cells and tissues. Isotonic crystalloids contain about the same concentration of osmotically active particles as extracellular fluid, so fluid doesn't shift between the extracellular and intracellular areas.

Hypotonic crystalloids are less concentrated than extracellular fluid, so they move from the bloodstream into the cell, causing the cell to swell. In contrast, hypertonic crystalloids are more highly concentrated than extracellular fluid, so fluid is pulled into the bloodstream from the cell, causing the cell to shrink. (See *Comparing fluid tonicity*, page 262.)

Isotonic solutions

Isotonic solutions, such as dextrose 5% in water, have an osmolality, or concentration, of 275 to 295 mOsm/L. The dextrose metabolizes quickly, however, acting like a hypotonic solution and leaving water behind. Large amounts of the solution may cause hyperglycemia.

Normal saline solution, another isotonic solution, contains only the electrolytes sodium and chloride. Other isotonic solutions are more similar to extracellular fluid. For instance, Ringer's solution contains sodium, potassium, calcium, and chloride. Lactated Ringer's solution contains those electrolytes plus lactate, which the liver converts to bicarbonate.

Hypotonic solutions

Hypotonic solutions, such as half-normal saline solution, 0.33% sodium chloride solution, and dextrose 2.5% in water, are fluids that have an osmolality less than 275 mOsm/L. They should be given cautiously because fluid moves from the extracellular space into cells, causing them to swell. That fluid shift can cause cardiovascular collapse from vascular fluid depletion. It can also cause increased intracranial pressure (ICP) from fluid shifting into brain cells.

Types of I.V. solutions

- Crystalloids — may be isotonic, hypotonic, or hypertonic
- Colloids — always hypertonic

Crystalloids

- Solutions with small molecules that flow easily from bloodstream into cells and tissues

Isotonic solutions

- Contain about same concentration of osmotically active particles as extracellular fluid, thereby preventing fluid shift between extracellular and intracellular areas
- Osmolality 275 to 295 mOsm/L
- Examples include dextrose 5% in water and normal saline solution

Hypotonic solutions

- Less concentrated than extracellular fluid, so they move from bloodstream into cell, causing cell to swell
- Osmolality < 27 mOsm/L
- Examples include half-normal saline solution and dextrose 2.5 % in water
- Shouldn't be given to patients at risk for increased ICP or to patients with abnormal fluid shifts into interstitial space or body cavities

Comparing fluid tonicity

These illustrations show the effects of different types of I.V. fluids on fluid movement and cell size.

ISOTONIC

Isotonic fluids, such as normal saline solution, have a concentration of dissolved particles, or tonicity, equal to that of intracellular fluid. Osmotic pressure is therefore the same inside and outside the cells, so they neither shrink nor swell with fluid movement.

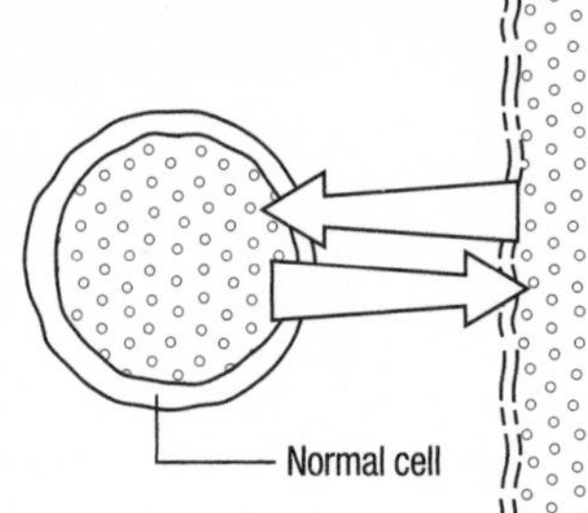

HYPERTONIC

Hypertonic fluid has a tonicity greater than that of intracellular fluid, so osmotic pressure is unequal inside and outside the cells. Dehydration or rapidly infused hypertonic fluids, such as 3% saline or 50% dextrose, draws water out of the cells into the more highly concentrated extracellular fluid.

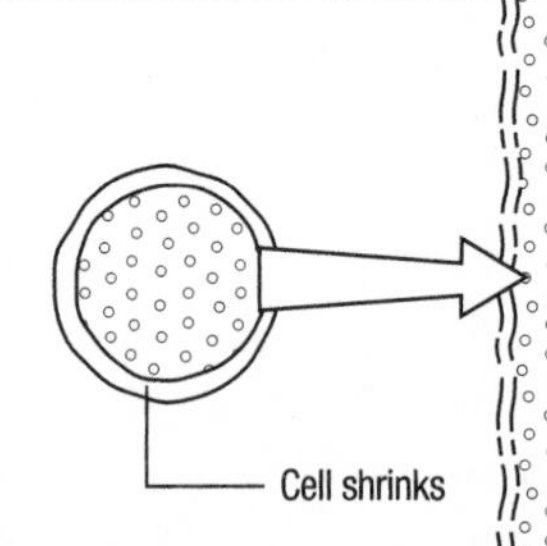

HYPOTONIC

Hypotonic fluids, such as half-normal saline solution, have a tonicity less than that of intracellular fluid, so osmotic pressure draws water into the cells from the extracellular fluid. Severe electrolyte losses or inappropriate use of I.V. fluids can make body fluids hypotonic.

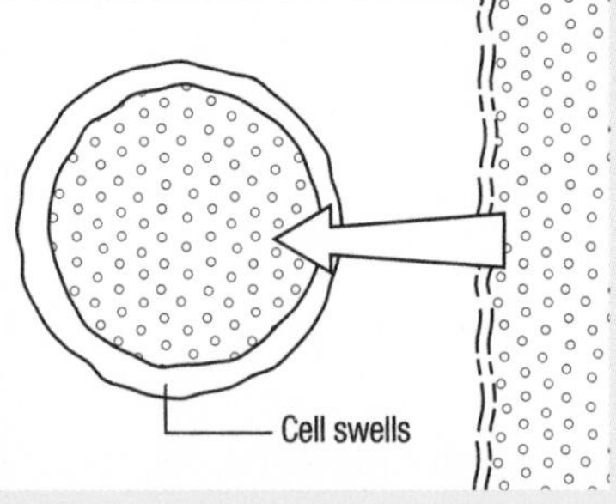

DANGER *Hypotonic solutions shouldn't be given to a patient at risk for increased ICP—for example, those who have had a stroke, head trauma, or neurosurgery. Signs of increased ICP include a change in the patient's level of consciousness, motor or sensory deficits, and changes in the size, shape, or response to light in the pupils. Hypotonic solutions also shouldn't be used for patients who suffer from abnormal fluid shifts into the interstitial space or the body cavities—such as from liver disease, a burn, or trauma.*

Hypertonic solutions

Hypertonic solutions, such as dextrose 5% in half-normal saline solution, dextrose 5% in normal saline solution, dextrose 5% in lactated Ringer's solution, and dextrose 10% in water, are fluids that have an osmolality greater than 295 mOsm/L. They draws fluids from the intracellular space, causing cells to shrink and the extracellular space to expand. Patients with cardiac or renal disease may be unable to tolerate extra fluid. Watch for fluid overload and pulmonary edema.

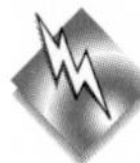

DANGER *Because hypertonic solutions draw fluids from cells, patients at risk for cellular dehydration, such as those with diabetic ketoacidosis, shouldn't receive them.* *(See* Comparing I.V. solutions, *pages 264 and 265.)*

Crystalloids *(continued)*

Hypertonic solutions
- More highly concentrated than extracellular fluid, so fluid is pulled into bloodstream from cell, causing cell to shrink
- Osmolality > 295 mOsm/L
- Examples include dextrose 5% in half-normal saline solution and dextrose 10% in water

COLLOIDS

The use of colloids over crystalloids is controversial. Still, the physician may prescribe a colloid—or *plasma expander*—if your patient's blood volume doesn't improve with crystalloids. Examples of colloids that may be given include albumin (available in 5% solutions, which are osmotically equal to plasma, and 25% solutions, which draw about four times their volume in interstitial fluid into the circulation within 15 minutes of administration), plasma protein fraction, dextran, and hetastarch.

Colloids pull fluid into the bloodstream. Their effects last several days if the lining of the capillaries is normal. Closely monitor the patient during a colloid infusion for increased blood pressure, dyspnea, and bounding pulse, which are all signs of hypervolemia.

If neither crystalloids nor colloids are effective in treating the imbalance, the patient may require a blood transfusion or other treatment.

Colloids
- Pull fluid into bloodstream
- Colloid infusion requires close monitoring for signs of hypervolemia (increased blood pressure, dyspnea, bounding pulse)
- Examples include albumin, plasma protein fraction, dextran, and hetastarch

I.V. DELIVERY METHODS

The choice of I.V. delivery is based on the purpose of the therapy and its duration; the patient's diagnosis, age, and health history; and the condition of the patient's veins. I.V. solutions can be delivered through a peripheral or a central vein. Catheters and tubing are chosen based on the therapy and site to be used. Choosing an I.V. site includes a peripheral or central venous line; the equipment for each type varies.

I.V. delivery methods
- Choice of method based on purpose and duration of therapy; patient's diagnosis, age, and health history; and condition of his veins

Comparing I.V. solutions

This chart shows examples of some commonly used I.V. fluid solutions and includes some of the clinical uses and special considerations associated with their use.

I.V. SOLUTION	USES	SPECIAL CONSIDERATIONS
Hypertonic		
Dextrose 5% in half-normal saline solution	✦ Diabetic ketoacidosis (DKA) after initial treatment with normal saline solution and half-normal saline solution — prevents hypoglycemia and cerebral edema (occurs when serum osmolality is reduced too rapidly)	✦ In patients with DKA, use only when glucose falls under 250 mg/dl.
Dextrose 5% in normal saline solution	✦ Addisonian crisis ✦ Hypotonic dehydration ✦ Syndrome of inappropriate antidiuretic hormone (or use 3% sodium chloride) ✦ Temporary treatment of circulatory insufficiency and shock if plasma expanders aren't available	✦ Don't use in patients with cardiac or renal disorders because of risk of heart failure and pulmonary edema.
Dextrose 10% in water	✦ Conditions in which some nutrition with glucose is required ✦ Water replacement	✦ Monitor serum glucose levels.
Hypotonic		
0.45% sodium chloride (half-normal saline solution)	✦ DKA after initial normal saline solution and before dextrose infusion ✦ Gastric fluid loss from nasogastric suctioning or vomiting ✦ Hypertonic dehydration ✦ Sodium and chloride depletion ✦ Water replacement	✦ Use cautiously; may cause cardiovascular collapse or increased intracranial pressure. ✦ Don't use in patients with liver disease, trauma, or burns.

Peripheral lines

- Peripheral I.V. therapy administered for short-term or intermittent therapy through vein in arm, hand, leg, or foot

PERIPHERAL LINES

Peripheral I.V. therapy is administered for short-term or intermittent therapy through a vein in the arm, hand, leg, or foot. Potential I.V. sites

Comparing I.V. solutions *(continued)*

I.V. SOLUTION	USES	SPECIAL CONSIDERATIONS
Isotonic		
Dextrose 5% in water	✦ Fluid loss and dehydration ✦ Hypernatremia	✦ The solution is isotonic initially and becomes hypotonic when dextrose is metabolized. ✦ Don't use for resuscitation; it can cause hyperglycemia. ✦ Use cautiously in patients with renal or cardiac disease; it can cause fluid overload. ✦ It doesn't provide enough daily calories for prolonged use and may cause eventual protein breakdown.
0.9% sodium chloride (normal saline solution)	✦ Blood transfusions ✦ Fluid challenges ✦ Fluid replacement in patients with DKA ✦ Hypercalcemia ✦ Hyponatremia ✦ Metabolic alkalosis ✦ Resuscitation ✦ Shock	✦ Because this replaces extracellular fluid, don't use in patients with heart failure, edema, or hypernatremia; it can lead to overload.
Lactated Ringer's solution	✦ Acute blood loss ✦ Burns ✦ Dehydration ✦ Hypovolemia due to third-space shifting ✦ Lower GI tract fluid loss ✦ Mild metabolic acidosis ✦ Salicylate overdose	✦ Electrolyte content is similar to serum but doesn't contain magnesium. ✦ It contains potassium; don't use in patients with renal failure because it can cause hyperkalemia. ✦ Don't use in patients with liver disease because they can't metabolize lactate (a functional liver converts it to bicarbonate); don't give if patient's pH is more than 7.5.

include the metacarpal, cephalic, basilic, median cubital, and greater saphenous veins. Using veins in the leg or foot is unusual because of the risk of thrombophlebitis. However, veins in the foot are commonly used in neonates and infants.

Peripheral lines *(continued)*

Site selection
- ✦ Place I.V. catheters in hand or lower arm so site can be moved upward as needed
- ✦ Use patient's nondominant hand, if possible
- ✦ For patient suffering from trauma or cardiac arrest, use large vein in antecubital area for rapid access (avoid antecubital area in mobile patient)
- ✦ Avoid using veins over joints
- ✦ Avoid using veins in injured arm or arm with loss of sensation or arteriovenous fistula
- ✦ Don't use veins in arm on same side where mastectomy or axillary node removal was performed
- ✦ Don't use veins in arm affected by stroke

Catheter selection
- ✦ Steel scalp-vein (winged-infusion) needles—easily inserted, but infiltration common
- ✦ Indwelling catheters—inserted over steel needle; easy to use and more comfortable for patient
- ✦ Plastic catheters—inserted through hollow needle; difficult to use

Needle size selection
- ✦ Higher needle gauge means smaller needle diameter
- ✦ For administering a lot of fluid over short time period, use lower-gauge, shorter-length needles
- ✦ For routine I.V. fluid administration, use higher-gauge catheters

Site selection

Choose a site that meets the patient's need for fluids, while keeping him as comfortable as possible. Place I.V. catheters in the hand or the lower arm so sites can be moved upward as needed. Use the patient's nondominant hand, if possible. For a patient who has suffered trauma or cardiac arrest, use a large vein in the antecubital area to gain rapid access. Avoid the antecubital site in a mobile patient because the catheter may kink with movement or cause other discomfort. Avoid using veins over joints. Catheters in those veins are uncomfortable and awkward and can be easily displaced.

Also avoid using veins in the patient with an injured arm or in an arm with loss of sensation or an arteriovenous fistula. Don't use veins in an arm on the same side where a mastectomy or axillary node removal was performed, or that was affected by a stroke.

Catheter selection

Three main types of catheters are used for insertion into a peripheral vein:

✦ Steel scalp-vein, or winged-infusion, needles are inserted easily, but infiltration is common. These catheters are small, nonflexible, and used when access with another device proves unsuccessful. The catheters are also used for short-term therapy in adults, especially for giving medications by I.V. push through a syringe over a short period of time.

✦ Indwelling catheters inserted over a steel needle are easy to use and less likely to infiltrate. When in place, these catheters are more comfortable for the patient. They're also more difficult to insert than a scalp-vein needle.

✦ Plastic catheters inserted through a hollow needle are longer and are more commonly used for central-vein infusions. The catheter must be threaded through the vein for a greater distance, which makes these catheters more difficult to use.

Needle size selection

Choosing the right diameter, or gauge, needle or catheter is important for ensuring adequate flow and patient comfort. The higher the needle gauge you choose, the smaller the diameter of the needle.

If you want to give a lot of fluid over a short period of time or need to transfuse blood, use a catheter with a lower gauge, such as 14G, 16G, or 18G, and a shorter length, which offers less resistance to fluid flow and won't damage blood cells. For routine I.V. fluid administration, use higher-gauge catheters, such as a 20G or 22G. French catheters are the exception to the needle-gauge rule: the higher the number the greater the diameter.

AGE ALERT *In children and elderly patients, generally, a smaller size catheter is needed for their smaller veins. For these age-groups, use 22G to 24G needles or catheters.*

Central venous therapy

Central venous therapy involves administering solutions through a catheter placed in a central vein, typically the subclavian or internal jugular vein; less commonly, the femoral vein. This type of I.V. therapy is used for patients who have inadequate peripheral veins, need access for blood sampling, require a large volume of fluid, need a hypertonic solution to be diluted by rapid blood flow in a larger vein, or need a high-calorie nutritional supplement.

Catheter selection

Three main types of catheters are used for short- and long-term central venous therapy:

✦ The traditional central venous catheter is a multilumen catheter typically used for short-term therapy. Although the lumen size may vary, a multilumen catheter provides multiple I.V. access using one insertion site.

✦ A peripherally inserted central catheter is now commonly used in health care facilities and in home care. A certified nurse can insert this catheter through a vein in the antecubital area, at the bedside. Fewer, less-severe adverse effects occur with these catheters than with traditional central venous catheters. Also, the catheters can be left in place for several months, making them ideal for long-term therapy.

✦ For extended long-term therapy, the patient may receive a vascular access port implanted in a pocket surgically constructed in the subcutaneous tissue or a tunneled catheter, such as a Hickman, Broviac, or Groshong. Some of these catheters have multiple lumens and are used in the health care facility and at home.

Tubing systems

The mechanics of infusing a solution require an I.V. tubing system that can deliver medication at the correct infusion rate. I.V. tubing is available principally in microdrip sets, which are designed so that 60 gtt

Age alert

✦ Use smaller size needles or catheters (22G to 24G) for children and elderly patients because of their smaller veins

Central venous therapy

✦ Involves administering solutions through catheter placed in central vein

Functions

✦ For patient with inadequate peripheral veins
✦ Access for blood sampling
✦ Large fluid requirements
✦ Dilution of hypertonic solution by rapid blood flow in larger vein
✦ High-calorie nutritional supplementation

Catheter selection

✦ Traditional central venous catheter — multilumen catheter typically used for short-term therapy
✦ Peripherally inserted central catheter — ideal for long-term therapy; can be left in place for several months
✦ Vascular access port implantation or tunneled catheter — for extended long-term therapy

Tubing systems

Microdrip sets
- Designed so 60 gtt equal 1 ml
- Useful for infusion rates < 100 m/hour

Macrodrip sets
- Designed so 10 to 15 gtt equal 1 ml, depending on manufacturer's instructions
- Preferred for infusion rates > 100 ml/hour

Needleless systems
- Minimize exposure to contaminated needles
- Examples include blunt metal cannulas, needles that recess into plastic housing, and blunt plastic cannulas

Infusion pumps
- Deliver fluids at precisely controlled infusion rates
- Each machine requires own type of tubing

equal 1 ml. Microdrip sets are useful for infusion rates lower than 100 ml/hour—for instance, when using a solution to keep a vein open.

A macrodrip set, on the other hand, is designed so that 10 to 15 gtt equal 1 ml, depending on the manufacturer's instructions. Macrodrip sets are preferred for infusion rates greater than 100 ml/hour—for instance, when treating a patient with shock.

Needleless systems

The Occupational Safety and Health Administration requires health care facilities to initiate controls to isolate or remove hazardous blood-borne pathogens from the workplace. Several products now available are designed to minimize exposure to contaminated needles. These products include blunt metal cannulas, needles that recess into a plastic housing, and blunt plastic cannulas.

Infusion pumps

Electronic infusion pumps deliver fluids at precisely controlled infusion rates. Because each machine requires its own type of tubing, check the manufacturer's directions before use.

Most tubings contain back-check valves to prevent drugs from mixing inside piggyback systems, where one I.V. line is plugged into another at a piggyback port. Filters on some tubing eliminate particulate matter, bacteria, and air bubbles. Other types of tubing are available specifically for administering individual medications or for piggybacking multiple medications.

COMPLICATIONS OF I.V. THERAPY

Caring for a patient with an I.V. line requires careful monitoring as well as a clear understanding of what the possible complications are, what to do if they arise, and how to deal with flow issues.

Infiltration, infection, phlebitis, and thrombophlebitis are the most common complications of I.V. therapy. Other complications include extravasation, a severed catheter, an allergic reaction, an air embolism, speed shock, and fluid overload.

Air embolism

An air embolism occurs when air enters the vein and can cause a decrease in blood pressure, an increase in the pulse rate, respiratory distress, an increase in intracranial pressure (ICP), and a loss of consciousness.

Nursing interventions

If the patient develops an air embolism, notify the physician, and clamp off the I.V. Place the patient on his left side, and lower his head to allow the air to enter the right atrium, where it can disperse more safely by way of the pulmonary artery. Monitor him, and administer oxygen. To avoid this serious complication, prime all tubing completely, tighten all connections securely, and use an air detection device on an I.V. pump.

Allergic reaction

A patient may suffer an allergic reaction to the fluid, medication, I.V. catheter, or even the latex port in the I.V. tubing. However, the source of the reaction may be unknown. Look for a red streak extending up the arm, rash, itching, watery eyes and nose, and wheezing.

Nursing interventions

Left untreated, an allergic reaction may progress rapidly to anaphylaxis. Nursing measures for allergic reaction include stopping the I.V. immediately, notifying the physician, monitoring the patient, and giving oxygen and medications as ordered.

Extravasation

Extravasation, similar to infiltration, is the leakage of fluid into surrounding tissues. It results when medications — such as dopamine (Intropin), calcium solutions, and chemotherapeutic agents — seep through veins and produce blistering and, eventually, necrosis. Initially, the patient may experience discomfort, burning, or pain at the I.V. site. Look also for skin tightness, blanching, and lack of blood return. Delayed reactions include inflammation and pain within 3 to 5 days and ulcers or necrosis within 2 weeks.

Nursing interventions

When administering medications that may extravasate, know your facility's policy. Nursing actions include stopping the infusion, notifying the physician, infiltrating the site with an antidote as ordered — this is typi-

Air embolism

- Occurs when air enters vein
- Signs and symptoms: decreased blood pressure, increased pulse rate, respiratory distress, increased ICP, and loss of consciousness

Key nursing interventions

- Notify physician
- Clamp off I.V. line
- Place patient on left side
- Lower patient's head to allow air to enter right atrium
- Monitor patient
- Administer oxygen

Allergic reaction

- Occurs from allergic reaction to fluid, medication, I.V. catheter, or latex port in I.V. tubing
- Signs and symptoms: red streak extending up arm, rash, itching, watery eyes and nose, and wheezing

Key nursing interventions

- Stop I.V. immediately
- Notify physician
- Monitor patient
- Give oxygen and medications as ordered

Extravasation

- Similar to infiltration
- Occurs when medications seep through veins, producing blistering and, eventually, necrosis
- Signs and symptoms: discomfort, burning, or pain at I.V. site; skin tightness, blanching, and lack of blood return

Key nursing interventions

- Stop infusion
- Notify physician
- Infiltrate site with antidote as ordered

Extravasation
(continued)

Key nursing interventions
- ✦ Apply ice early and warm soaks later
- ✦ Elevate extremity
- ✦ Assess circulation and limb nerve function

Fluid overload
- ✦ Signs and symptoms: neck-vein distention, increased blood pressure and respirations, shortness of breath, cough, and crackles on auscultation

Key nursing interventions
- ✦ Slow I.V. rate
- ✦ Notify physician
- ✦ Monitor vital signs
- ✦ Keep patient warm
- ✦ Keep head of bed elevated
- ✦ Give oxygen and other medications as ordered

Infection
- ✦ Occurs because I.V. therapy involves puncturing skin, body's barrier to infection
- ✦ Signs and symptoms: purulent drainage at I.V. site, tenderness, erythema, warmth, and hardness on palpation

Key nursing interventions
- ✦ Swab site for culture
- ✦ Remove catheter as ordered
- ✦ Maintain aseptic technique

Infiltration
- ✦ Occurs when access device dislodges from vein, causing fluid to leak from vein into surrounding tissue
- ✦ Signs and symptoms: coolness at site, pain, swelling, leaking, and lack of blood return

cally done through the I.V. before removing the catheter—applying ice early and warm soaks later, and elevating the extremity. Assess the patient's circulation and nerve function of the limb.

Fluid overload

Fluid overload can begin gradually or suddenly, depending on how well the patient's circulatory system can accommodate the fluid. Look for neck-vein distention, increased blood pressure, increased respirations, shortness of breath, cough, and crackles in the lungs on auscultation.

Nursing interventions

If the patient develops fluid overload, slow the I.V. rate, notify the physician, and monitor vital signs. Keep the patient warm; keep the head of the bed elevated; and give oxygen and other medications, such as a diuretic, as ordered.

Infection

I.V. therapy involves puncturing the skin, the body's barrier to infection. As a result, the patient may develop an infection. Look for purulent drainage at the I.V. site, tenderness, erythema, warmth, or hardness on palpation. Signs and symptoms that the infection has become systemic include fever, chills, and an elevated white blood cell count.

Nursing interventions

Nursing actions for an infected I.V. site include monitoring vital signs and notifying the physician. Swab the site for culture, and remove the catheter as ordered. Always maintain aseptic technique to prevent infection.

Infiltration

During infiltration, fluid may leak from the vein into surrounding tissue. This occurs when the access device dislodges from the vein. Look for coolness at the site, pain, swelling, leaking, and lack of blood return. Also, look for a sluggish flow that continues even if a tourniquet is applied above the site.

Nursing interventions

If you see infiltration, stop the infusion, elevate the extremity, and apply warm soaks. To prevent infiltration, use the smallest catheter that will accomplish the infusion, avoid placement in joint areas, and anchor the catheter in place.

Phlebitis and thrombophlebitis

Phlebitis is inflammation of the vein; *thrombophlebitis* is an irritation of the vein with the formation of a clot and is usually more painful than phlebitis. Either poor insertion technique or the pH or osmolality of the solution or medication can cause these complications. Look for pain, redness, swelling, or induration at the site; a red line streaking along the vein; fever; or a sluggish flow of the solution.

Nursing interventions

When phlebitis or thrombophlebitis occurs, remove the I.V. line, monitor the patient's vital signs, notify the physician, and apply warm soaks to the I.V. site. To prevent these complications, choose large-bore veins and change the catheter every 72 hours when infusing a medication or solution with high osmolality.

Severed catheter

A severed catheter can occur when a piece of the catheter becomes dislodged and is set free in the vein. Look for pain at the fragment site, decreased blood pressure, cyanosis, loss of consciousness, and a weak, rapid pulse.

Nursing interventions

If this extremely rare but serious complication occurs, apply a tourniquet above the site of pain, immediately notify the physician, monitor the patient, and provide support as needed. To avoid this problem altogether, don't reinsert a needle through its plastic catheter after the needle has been withdrawn.

Speed shock

Speed shock occurs when I.V. solutions or medications are given too rapidly. Almost immediately, the patient will have facial flushing, an irregular pulse, a severe headache, and decreased blood pressure. Loss of consciousness and cardiac arrest may also occur.

Infiltration *(continued)*

Key nursing interventions

- ✦ Stop infusion
- ✦ Elevate extremity
- ✦ Apply warm soaks

Phlebitis and thrombophlebitis

- ✦ Phlebitis — vein inflammation
- ✦ Thrombophlebitis — irritation of vein with clot formation; usually more painful than phlebitis
- ✦ Caused by poor insertion technique or pH osmolality of medication or solution
- ✦ Signs and symptoms: pain, redness, swelling, or induration at site; red streak along vein; fever; or sluggish flow of solution

Key nursing interventions

- ✦ Remove I.V. line
- ✦ Monitor vital signs
- ✦ Notify physician
- ✦ Apply warm soaks

Severed catheter

- ✦ Occurs when a piece of catheter dislodges and is set free in vein
- ✦ Signs and symptoms: pain at fragment site, decreased blood pressure, cyanosis, loss of consciousness, and weak, rapid pulse

Key nursing interventions

- ✦ Apply tourniquet above pain site
- ✦ Immediately notify physician
- ✦ Monitor patient
- ✦ Provide support as needed

Speed shock

- ✦ Occurs when I.V. solutions or medications given too rapidly
- ✦ Signs and symptoms: facial flushing, irregular pulse, severe headache, decreased blood pressure

Speed shock
(continued)

Key nursing interventions
- Clamp off I.V. line
- Notify physician
- Administer oxygen
- Monitor vital signs
- Administer medications as ordered

Managing I.V. therapy
- Check I.V. order for completeness and accuracy
- Measure intake and output
- Monitor infusion of solutions that contain medication
- Change site, dressing, and tubing per facility policy

Nursing interventions

If speed shock occurs, clamp off the I.V., and immediately notify the physician. Provide oxygen, obtain vital signs frequently, and administer medications as ordered. Also, keep in mind that the use of infusion control devices can prevent this complication.

MANAGING THE PATIENT RECEIVING I.V. THERAPY

Nursing care for the patient with an I.V. includes these actions:

- Check the I.V. order for completeness and accuracy. Most I.V. orders expire after 24 hours. A complete order should specify the amount and type of solution, specific additives and their concentrations, and the rate and duration of the infusion. If the order is incomplete or confusing, clarify the order before proceeding.
- Monitor daily weights to document fluid retention or loss. A 2% increase or decrease in body weight is significant. A 2.2-lb (1-kg) change corresponds to 1 qt (1 L) of fluid gained or lost.
- Measure intake and output carefully at scheduled intervals. The kidneys attempt to restore fluid balance during dehydration by reducing urine production. Urine output less than 30 ml/hour signals retention of metabolic wastes. Notify the physician if your patient's urine output falls below 30 ml/hour.
- Always carefully monitor the infusion of solutions that contain medication because rapid infusion and circulation of the medication can be dangerous.

AGE ALERT *Keep in mind the age, size, and health history of your patient when giving I.V. fluids to prevent fluid overload. For pediatric patients, use a Buretrol or other device to limit the amount of fluid the patient receives hourly and to prevent the accidental administration of excessive amounts of fluid.*

- Note the pH of the I.V. solution. The pH can alter the effect and stability of medications mixed in the I.V. bag. Consult medication literature or the physician if you have questions.
- Change the site, dressing, and tubing as often as your facility's policy requires. Solutions should be changed at least every 24 hours. Be sure to document your actions. (See *Documenting I.V. fluid replacement therapy*.)
- When changing I.V. tubing, be sure not to move or dislodge the I.V. device. If you have difficulty disconnecting the tubing, use a hemostat to

CHARTING CHECKLIST

Documenting I.V. fluid replacement therapy

If your patient is receiving I.V. fluid replacement therapy, make sure you document this information:

- ❑ date, time, and type of catheter inserted
- ❑ site of I.V. insertion and its appearance
- ❑ type and amount of I.V. fluid infused
- ❑ patient's tolerance of, and response to, I.V. fluid replacement therapy
- ❑ patient teaching provided and the patient's response.

hold the I.V. hub while twisting the tubing. Don't clamp the hemostat shut because doing so may crack the hub.

✦ Always report needle-stick injuries. Exposure to a patient's blood increases the risk of infection with blood-borne viruses such as human immunodeficiency virus (HIV), hepatitis B virus, hepatitis C virus, and cytomegalovirus. About 1 out of 300 people with occupational needle-stick injuries become HIV-seropositive.

✦ Always listen to your patient carefully. Subtle statements such as, "I just don't feel right" may be your clue to the beginning of an allergic reaction.

✦ Keep in mind that a candidate for home I.V. therapy must have a family member or friend who can safely and competently administer I.V. fluids, as well as a backup person, a suitable home environment, a telephone, available transportation, adequate reading skills, and the ability to prepare, handle, store, and dispose of equipment properly. Procedures for caring for the I.V. are the same at home as in a health care facility, except at home the patient uses clean technique instead of sterile technique.

✦ Be sure to tell the patient what to expect before, during, and after the I.V. procedure; the signs and symptoms of complications and when to report them; any activity or diet restrictions; and how to care for his I.V. line at home.

Managing I.V. therapy ***(continued)***

✦ Report needle-stick injuries
✦ Listen to patient carefully
✦ Ensure all requirements are met for patients receiving home I.V. therapy

Total parenteral nutrition

TPN therapy

- TPN — highly concentrated, hypertonic nutrient solution administered via infusion pump through large central vein

Functions

- Provides calories, restores nitrogen balance, and replaces fluids, vitamins, electrolytes, minerals, and trace elements
- Promotes tissue and wound healing and normal metabolic function
- Allows bowel to heal
- Reduces activity in gallbladder, pancreas, and small intestine
- Improves response to surgery

Indications

- Patients who can't absorb nutrients from GI tract for more than 10 days
- Debilitating illness lasting > 2 weeks
- Loss of 10% or more of pre-illness weight

TPN THERAPY

Total parenteral nutrition (TPN) is a highly concentrated, hypertonic nutrient solution administered via an infusion pump through a large central vein. For patients with high caloric and nutritional needs due to illness or injury, TPN provides crucial calories, restores nitrogen balance, and replaces essential fluids, vitamins, electrolytes, minerals, and trace elements. (See *Common TPN additives.*)

TPN also promotes tissue and wound healing and normal metabolic function; provides the bowel a chance to heal; reduces activity in the gallbladder, pancreas, and small intestine; and is used to improve a patient's response to surgery.

Patients who can't meet their nutritional needs by oral or enteral feedings may require I.V. nutritional supplementation or TPN. Generally, this treatment is prescribed for any patient who can't absorb nutrients from the GI tract for more than 10 days. More specific indications include debilitating illnesses lasting longer than 2 weeks; loss of 10% or more of pre-illness weight; serum albumin level below 3.5 g/dl; excessive nitrogen loss from a wound infection, a fistula, or an abscess; renal or hepatic failure; and nonfunction of the GI tract lasting for 5 to 7 days. (See *Using PPN,* page 276.)

Common illnesses or treatments that can trigger the need for TPN include inflammatory bowel disease, ulcerative colitis, bowel obstruction or

Common TPN additives

Common components of total parenteral nutrition (TPN) solutions—such as dextrose 10% in water ($D_{10}W$), amino acids, and other additives—are used for specific purposes. For instance, $D_{10}W$ provides calories for metabolism. This list contains other common additives and the purposes each serve. Lipids may be infused separately.

ELECTROLYTES

- Calcium promotes development of bones and teeth and aids in blood clotting.
- Chloride regulates acid-base balance and maintains osmotic pressure.
- Magnesium helps the body absorb carbohydrates and protein.
- Phosphorus is essential for cell energy and calcium balance.
- Potassium is needed for cellular activity and cardiac function.
- Sodium helps control water distribution and maintains normal fluid balance.

VITAMINS

- Folic acid is needed for deoxyribose nucleic acid formation and promotes growth and development.
- Vitamin B complex helps the final absorption of carbohydrates and protein.
- Vitamin C helps in wound healing.
- Vitamin D is essential for bone metabolism and maintenance of serum calcium levels.
- Vitamin K helps prevent bleeding disorders.

OTHER ADDITIVES

- Acetate prevents metabolic acidosis.
- Amino acids provide the proteins necessary for tissue repair.
- Micronutrients, such as zinc, cobalt, and manganese, help in wound healing and red blood cell synthesis.

resection, radiation enteritis, severe diarrhea or vomiting, acquired immunodeficiency syndrome, chemotherapy, and severe pancreatitis, all of which hinder a patient's ability to absorb nutrients. Also, patients may benefit from TPN if they've undergone major surgery or if they have a high metabolic rate due to sepsis, trauma, or burns of more than 40% of total body surface area. Infants with congenital or acquired disorders may need TPN to promote proper growth and development.

TPN has limited value for well-nourished patients with GI tracts that are healthy. The treatment also may be inappropriate for a patient with a poor prognosis or when the risks of TPN outweigh its benefits.

TPN therapy *(continued)*

Indications

- Serum albumin level < 3.5 g/dl
- Excessive nitrogen loss from wound infection, fistula, or abscess
- Renal or hepatic failure
- Nonfunction of GI tract lasting 5 to 7 days

> **Using PPN**
>
> Peripheral parenteral nutrition (PPN) is prescribed for patients who are able to take oral feedings but not enough to meet nutritional levels. PPN is infused peripherally in various combinations of lipid, or fat, emulsions and amino acid-dextrose solutions.

TPN trends

- Tailoring TPN formulas to specific needs
- Nutritional support teams (assess, prescribe for, and monitor patients receiving TPN)

TPN TRENDS

The trend of today's nutritional supplementation is to tailor TPN formulas to the patient's specific needs. As a result, standard TPN mixtures are becoming less popular. Nutritional support teams consisting of nurses, physicians, pharmacists, and dietitians assess, prescribe for, and monitor patients receiving TPN.

The solutions may consist of protein (amino acids in a 2.5% to 8.5% solution), with varying types available for patients with renal or hepatic failure; dextrose (10% to 50% solution); fat emulsions (10% to 20% solution); electrolytes; vitamins; trace element mixtures; and medications.

Lipid emulsions

- Thick emulsions that supply essential fatty acids and calories
- Assist in wound healing, red blood cell production, and prostaglandin synthesis

LIPID EMULSIONS

Lipid emulsions are thick emulsions that supply patients with both essential fatty acids and calories. These emulsions assist in wound healing, red blood cell production, and prostaglandin synthesis. Although they're typically given with TPN, they may be given alone through a peripheral or central venous line, or they may be mixed with amino acids and dextrose in one container, providing a three-in-one-system, and infused over 24 hours.

Precautions

- Should be given cautiously to patients with hepatic or pulmonary disease, anemia, coagulation disorders, and those at risk for fat embolism
- Shouldn't be given to patients with conditions that disrupt normal fat metabolism

PRECAUTIONS

Lipid emulsions should be given cautiously to patients with hepatic or pulmonary disease, anemia, or a coagulation disorder and to patients at risk for developing a fat embolism. These emulsions shouldn't be given to patients who have conditions that disrupt normal fat metabolism, such as pathologic hyperlipidemia, lipid nephrosis, and acute pancreatitis.

Make sure you report adverse reactions to the physician so the TPN regimen can be adjusted as needed. (See *Adverse reactions to lipid emulsions.*)

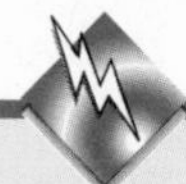

DANGER

Adverse reactions to lipid emulsions

Immediate or early adverse reactions to lipid emulsions include:

- back and chest pain
- cyanosis
- diaphoresis or flushing
- dyspnea
- headache
- hypercoagulability
- irritation at the site
- lethargy or syncope
- nausea or vomiting
- slight pressure over the eyes
- thrombocytopenia.

Delayed complications associated with prolonged administration include:

- blood dyscrasias
- fatty liver syndrome
- hepatomegaly
- jaundice
- splenomegaly.

INFUSING TPN

TPN must be infused through a central vein. As a hypertonic solution, it may be up to six times the concentration of blood and, therefore, too irritating for a peripheral vein.

TPN may be infused around the clock or for part of the day — for instance, as the patient sleeps at night. A sterile catheter made of polyurethane, polyvinyl chloride, or silicone rubber (Silastic) is inserted into the subclavian or jugular vein. A polyurethane catheter is for short-term use only because it stiffens within a short period of time and can cause thrombophlebitis. A Silastic catheter is a better alternative for therapy lasting months or years because it's more flexible and durable and is compatible with many medications and solutions.

A peripherally inserted central catheter (PICC), a variation of central venous therapy, can be used for therapy lasting longer than 3 months. The catheter is inserted through the basilic or cephalic vein and threaded so that the tip lies in the superior vena cava.

Infusing TPN

- Must be infused through central vein
- May be infused on constant or partial basis

The patient generally experiences less discomfort with a peripheral catheter, especially if he can move around easily. Movement stimulates blood flow and decreases the risk of phlebitis. PICCs are becoming the preferred choice for intermediate-term therapy, at home and in the health care facility.

Setting up

- ✦ Use infusion pump for rate control
- ✦ Flush central lines according to facility protocol
- ✦ Never add medication to TPN solution container
- ✦ Don't use three-way stopcock unless necessary
- ✦ Review patient's serum chemistry and nutritional studies, and alert physician or nutrition support team of abnormal results

Setting up

Whenever you prepare to administer TPN, make sure to follow these guidelines:

✦ In most health care facilities, central venous lines and PICCs require an order and a patient-consent form. Only a registered nurse specializing in inserting those lines should obtain the form.

✦ Use an infusion pump for rate control.

✦ Flush central lines according to your facility's protocol.

✦ If using a single-lumen central venous line, don't use the line for blood or blood products, give a bolus injection, administer simultaneous I.V. solutions, measure the central venous pressure, or draw blood for laboratory tests.

✦ Never add medications to a TPN solution container.

✦ Don't use a three-way stopcock unless absolutely necessary; add-on devices increase the risk of infection.

✦ Review the patient's serum chemistry and nutritional studies, and alert the physician or nutrition support team of abnormal results, which may indicate that the TPN fluid concentration or ingredients may need to be adjusted to meet the patient's specific needs.

✦ Explain the insertion procedure to the patient.

Starting the infusion

- ✦ Start infusion slowly — about 1,000 calories over 24 hours — and increase gradually
- ✦ Continually monitor cardiac and respiratory status

Starting the infusion

Avoid an adverse reaction by starting TPN slowly — about 1,000 calories over 24 hours — and increasing gradually. Occasionally, a patient may react adversely to specific ingredients in the TPN solution. Protein may need to be reduced if blood urea nitrogen (BUN) and creatinine levels are elevated. Continually monitor the patient's cardiac and respiratory status.

Because the TPN solution is high in glucose, starting the infusion slowly will also allow the patient's pancreatic beta cells to adapt to the glucose by increasing insulin output. Within the first 3 to 5 days of TPN administration, the typical adult can tolerate about 3 qt (3 L) of solution per day without experiencing an adverse reaction.

DANGER *When a patient is severely malnourished, starting TPN may cause refeeding syndrome, which includes a rapid drop in potassium, magnesium, and phosphorus levels. To avoid compromising cardiac function, initiate feeding slowly and monitor the patient's electrolyte levels closely until they stabilize.*

Complications of TPN administration

After you've started the infusion, watch the patient for complications of TPN administration. Signs and symptoms of electrolyte imbalances caused by TPN administration include abdominal cramps, lethargy, confusion, malaise, muscle weakness, tetany, seizures, and cardiac arrhythmias. Acid-base imbalances can also occur due to the patient's condition or the TPN content. Look for these other complications:

- ✦ heart failure or pulmonary edema from fluid and electrolyte administration, conditions that can lead to tachycardia, lethargy, confusion, weakness, and labored breathing
- ✦ hyperglycemia from dextrose infusing too quickly, a condition that may require an adjustment in the patient's insulin dosage
- ✦ adverse reactions to medications added to TPN—for example, added insulin can cause hypoglycemia, which can result in confusion, restlessness, lethargy, pallor, and tachycardia
- ✦ complications from I.V. cannulas and central venous catheters.

Complications

- ✦ Electrolyte imbalances
- ✦ Heart failure or pulmonary edema
- ✦ Hyperglycemia
- ✦ Adverse reactions to medications added to TPN
- ✦ Complications from I.V. cannulas and central venous catheters

MANAGING THE PATIENT RECEIVING TPN THERAPY

Proper management of the patient receiving TPN therapy includes assessment and monitoring, follow-up care, and patient teaching.

ASSESSMENT AND MONITORING

- ✦ Carefully monitor patients receiving TPN to detect early signs of complications, such as metabolic problems, heart failure, pulmonary edema, or allergic reactions. Adjust the TPN regimen as needed.
- ✦ Assess the patient's nutritional status, and weigh the patient at the same time each morning after he voids, in similar clothing, and on the same scale. Weight is indicative of nutritional progress and also determines fluid overload. Patients ideally should gain 1 to 2 lb (0.5 to 1 kg)/week. Weight gain greater than 1 lb/day indicates fluid retention.
- ✦ Assess the patient for peripheral and pulmonary edema. Edema is a sign of fluid overload.

Managing TPN therapy

Assessment and monitoring

- ✦ Assess nutritional status
- ✦ Weigh patient at same time each morning after morning void

Managing TPN therapy *(continued)*

Assessment and monitoring

- Monitor serum glucose levels every 6 hours initially, then once per day
- Monitor electrolyte and protein levels
- Check renal function by monitoring BUN and creatinine levels
- Assess liver function with liver function tests and bilirubin, triglyceride, and cholesterol levels
- Change I.V. administration set according to facility policy
- Don't allow TPN solutions to hang more than 24 hours
- Return TPN solution to pharmacy if you see particulate matter, cloudiness, or oily layer in bag

✦ Monitor serum glucose levels every 6 hours initially, then once per day. Watch for thirst and polyuria, indications that the patient may have hyperglycemia. Periodically confirm serum glucose meter readings with laboratory test results. Serum glucose levels should be less than 200 mg/dl. This indicates the patient's tolerance of the glucose solution.

✦ Monitor for signs and symptoms of glucose metabolism disturbance, fluid and electrolyte imbalances, and nutritional problems. Some patients may require insulin added directly to the TPN for the duration of treatment.

✦ Monitor electrolyte and protein levels daily at first, and then twice per week for serum albumin. Albumin levels may drop initially as treatment restores hydration.

✦ Check renal function by monitoring BUN and creatinine levels; increases may indicate excess amino acid intake.

✦ Assess nitrogen balance with 24-hour urine collection.

✦ Assess liver function with liver function tests and bilirubin, triglyceride, and cholesterol levels. Abnormal values may indicate intolerance.

✦ Obtain a chest X-ray to check catheter placement after insertion.

✦ Record vital signs at least every 4 hours. Temperature elevation is one of the earliest signs of catheter-related sepsis.

✦ Measure arm circumference and skinfold thickness over the triceps, if ordered.

✦ Perform site care and dressing changes at least three times per week (once per week for transparent semipermeable dressings), or whenever the dressing becomes wet, soiled, or nonocclusive. Use strict aseptic technique.

✦ Monitor the patient for signs of inflammation and infection, and document your findings. (See *Documenting TPN*.)

✦ Change the I.V. administration set according to your facility's policy — be sure to use aseptic technique. Changes of I.V. administration sets are usually done every 24 hours for TPN.

✦ Don't allow TPN solutions to hang for more than 24 hours.

✦ If you see particulate matter, cloudiness, or an oily layer in the bag when preparing to hang a TPN solution, return the bag to the pharmacy. (The TPN solution should be clear or pale yellow if multivitamins are added to the solution.)

CHARTING CHECKLIST

Documenting TPN

If your patient is receiving TPN, make sure you document this information:

- ❑ adverse reactions or catheter complications
- ❑ signs of inflammation or infection at the I.V. site
- ❑ nursing interventions, including infusion rate, and the patient's response
- ❑ time and date of solution and administration set changes
- ❑ specific dietary intake
- ❑ patient teaching and the patient's response.

Follow-up care

✦ Provide emotional support, especially if the patient's eating is restricted due to his condition.

✦ Provide frequent mouth care.

✦ While weaning the patient from TPN, document his dietary intake and total calorie and protein intake. Use percentages when recording food intake. For instance, chart that, "The patient ate 50% of a baked potato," rather than "The patient had a good appetite."

✦ When discontinuing TPN, decrease the infusion slowly, depending on current glucose intake. Slowly decreasing the infusion minimizes the risk of hyperinsulinemia and resulting hypoglycemia. Weaning usually takes place over 24 to 48 hours but can be completed in 4 to 6 hours if the patient receives sufficient oral or I.V. carbohydrates.

✦ Promptly report adverse reactions to the physician.

✦ Prepare your patient for home care.

✦ Accurately document all aspects of care, according to your facility's policy.

Patient teaching

Be sure to cover these topics and then evaluate your patient's learning:

✦ description of TPN and its specific use for the patient

✦ adverse reactions or catheter complications and when to report them

✦ basic care of a TPN line

✦ maintenance of equipment

✦ how to monitor weight, calorie count, intake and output, and glucose levels.

Managing TPN therapy *(continued)*

Follow-up care

✦ While weaning patient from TPN, document dietary intake and total calorie and protein intake

✦ When discontinuing TPN, decrease infusion slowly, depending on current glucose intake

Patient teaching

✦ Description of TPN

✦ Adverse reactions or catheter complications

✦ Care and maintenance of equipment

✦ Monitoring techniques

Blood products

Understanding blood products

- Can restore blood volume
- Can correct deficiencies in blood's oxygen-carrying capacity and coagulation components

UNDERSTANDING BLOOD PRODUCTS

Transfusion therapy can restore blood volume as well as correct deficiencies in the blood's oxygen-carrying capacity and its coagulation components. Nursing responsibilities in blood transfusion include administering blood products and monitoring patients receiving the therapy. Nurses should be knowledgeable about the various blood products available to safely transfuse blood to their patients.

Compatibility

- Affected by antigens in blood, including ABO blood group, Rh factor, and HLA blood group
- Verified by technicians who crossmatch characteristics between donor's and recipient's blood

COMPATIBILITY

Blood contains various antigens that affect how compatible one person's blood is with another's. The antigens include the ABO blood group, the rhesus (Rh) factor, and the human leukocyte antigen (HLA) blood group. Laboratory technicians crossmatch these characteristics — especially the Rh factor and the ABO blood type — to ensure compatibility between the donor's and recipient's blood before transfusion.

ABO blood group

- ABO method identifies A and B antigens on RBCs
- A person has either both A and B antigens (type AB), only one antigen (type A or type B), or neither (type O)

ABO blood group

The ABO method of typing blood identifies two antigens on red blood cells (RBCs) — A and B. A person has either both A and B antigens, type AB; only one antigen, type A or type B; or neither, type O. In the United States, 85% of the population has either type A or type O, with type O

Identifying compatible blood types

A blood transfusion most likely will be safe if the donor and recipient have compatible blood types. Use this chart as a guide to blood-type compatibility.

RECIPIENT'S BLOOD TYPE	COMPATIBLE DONOR TYPE
A	A, 0
B	B, 0
AB	A, B, AB, 0
0	0

being the most common. In the remaining 15% of the population, 10% has type B and 5% has type AB.

If a patient has A antigens, he has anti-B antibodies floating freely in his plasma. If he has B antigens, he has anti-A antibodies in his plasma. This relationship is vital to remember, because a patient may experience a blood transfusion reaction if he receives a blood type for which he has antibodies.

Patients who have type AB blood are called *universal recipients.* They don't have antibodies and, therefore, can receive blood types O, A, B, or AB without having an ABO reaction. Patients with type O blood, by contrast, are called *universal donors.* Their blood may be transfused into a person with any blood type, but because type O patients have both anti-A and anti-B antibodies, they may receive only type O blood safely.

Ideally, transfusions should be performed using the same type of blood as the patient's. If that isn't possible, patients should receive blood that's compatible with their own blood type to keep transfusion reactions to a minimum. (See *Identifying compatible blood types.*)

In an emergency, when waiting for a crossmatch would be inadvisable, blood from a universal donor or plasma volume expanders may be given. (See *Transfusing blood in a crisis,* page 284.) Perfluorocarbons — milky, white emulsions that act like plasma but carry oxygen like RBCs — may provide an alternative in some health care facilities.

Compatibility
(continued)

ABO blood group

- If patient has A antigens, his plasma has anti-B antibodies
- If patient has B antigens, his plasma has anti-A antibodies
- Universal recipients — patients with type AB blood — can receive blood types 0, A, B, or AB without having ABO reaction
- Universal donors — patients with type 0 blood — may have their blood transfused into people with any blood type, but can only receive type 0 safely

Transfusing blood in a crisis

In a crisis situation, during which it may not be possible to wait for blood cross-matching, these substitutes can be given to your patient until tested blood is available:

- artificial blood substitutes
- artificial plasma substitutes (dextran, hetastarch)
- plasma protein solution (albumin)
- type O Rh-negative blood (blood from a universal donor).

Compatibility *(continued)*

Rh factor

- Rh-positive — indicated by possession of Rh antigen (about 85% of U.S. population)
- Rh-negative — indicated by lack of Rh antigen
- Rh-negative people may develop Rh antibodies if exposed to Rh-positive blood
- First exposure to Rh-positive blood by Rh-negative person usually causes sensitization; second exposure can result in fatal hemolytic reaction
- Reactions can occur during transfusions or pregnancy

HLA blood group

- HLA located on surface of circulating platelets, WBCs, and most tissue cells
- HLA responsible for febrile reactions in patients receiving blood transfusion that contains platelets from several donors
- Antigen-antibody reaction causes platelet destruction, making patient less responsive to platelet transfusions

Rhesus factor

About 85% of the U.S. population is Rh-positive, which means possessing the Rh antigen, an antigen found on the membrane of RBCs. People who don't have the Rh antigen are said to be Rh-negative.

No natural antibodies to Rh antigens exist. However, people who are Rh-negative may develop an Rh antibody if exposed to Rh-positive blood. The first exposure usually causes sensitization, but the second exposure may result in a fatal hemolytic reaction. These reactions can occur during transfusions or pregnancy. (See *Correcting an Rh problem.*)

Human leukocyte antigen blood group

HLA is located on the surface of circulating platelets, white blood cells (WBCs), and most tissue cells. HLA is responsible for febrile reactions in patients receiving a blood transfusion that contains platelets from several donors.

In that instance, an antigen-antibody reaction causes platelet destruction. As a result, the patient becomes less responsive to platelet transfusions. Giving HLA-matched platelets greatly decreases the risk of such antigen-antibody reactions. Generally, HLA tests benefit patients who receive multiple transfusions over a long period of time or frequent transfusions during a short-term illness.

Correcting an Rh problem

If a patient who's Rh-negative is exposed to Rh-positive blood, the problem can be corrected with an injection of Rh_0(D) immune globulin, given within 72 hours of exposure. Rh_0(D) immune globulin inhibits antibody formation. Common preparations include MICRhoGAM, BayRho-D, and RhoGAM.

TYPES OF BLOOD PRODUCTS

Many blood products are available for transfusion, including whole blood, red blood cells (RBCs), packed RBCs, granulocytes, fresh frozen plasma, cryoprecipitate, albumin, and platelets. In addition, patients may also receive transfusions of their own blood through a process called *autologous blood transfusion.*

Whole blood

Whole blood is rarely used unless the patient has lost more than 25% of total blood volume. It's generally available in bags of 500 ml and may be used to treat hemorrhage, trauma, or major burns.

Whole blood should be avoided if fluid overload is a concern. Stored whole blood is also high in potassium. After 24 hours, the viability and function of RBCs decreases. ABO compatibility and Rh matching are required before administration.

Whole blood

- Rarely used unless patient has lost > 25% of total blood volume
- Indications include hemorrhage, trauma, or major burns
- ABO compatibility and Rh matching required before administration

Packed red blood cells

Packed RBCs are prepared by removing about 90% of the plasma surrounding the cells and adding an anticoagulant preservative. A 250-ml bag of packed RBCs can help restore or maintain the oxygen-carrying capacity of the blood in patients with anemic conditions or can correct blood losses during or after surgery. About 70% of the leukocytes in packed RBCs have been removed, which reduces the risk of febrile, nonhemolytic reactions. ABO compatibility and Rh matching are still required, however, for these types of blood transfusions.

Packed RBCs

- Prepared by removing about 90% of plasma surrounding cells and adding anticoagulant preservative
- Can help restore or maintain oxygen-carrying capacity of blood in patients with anemic conditions
- Can correct blood losses during or after surgery
- ABO and Rh matching required before administration

Granulocytes

Granulocyte, or white blood cell, transfusions are rarely indicated; however, they may be used to treat gram-negative sepsis or progressive soft-tissue infection that's unresponsive to an antimicrobial. Human leukocyte antigen compatibility tests are preferable, and Rh matching is required. Daily granulocyte transfusions should be given until the infection resolves or the neutrophil count exceeds 50 mg/ml.

Granulocytes

- Transfusions rarely indicated
- May be used to treat gram-negative sepsis or progressive soft-tissue infection that's unresponsive to antimicrobial therapy
- HLA compatibility preferred; Rh matching required

Fresh frozen plasma

- Prepared by separating plasma from RBCs and freezing it within 6 hours of collection
- Used to treat hemorrhage, expand plasma volume, and correct undetermined coagulation factor deficiencies
- Also used to replace specific clotting factors and correct factor deficiencies resulting from liver disease
- ABO compatibility unnecessary; Rh matching preferred

Cryoprecipitate

- Also called *factor VIII*
- Insoluble portion of plasma recovered from fresh frozen plasma
- Used to treat von Willebrand's disease, hypofibrinogenemia, factor VIII deficiency, hemophilia A, and disseminated intravascular coagulation
- ABO compatibility testing unnecessary

Albumin

- Extracted from plasma
- Contains globulin and other proteins
- Used for acute liver failure, burns, and hypoproteinemia with or without edema
- Also used for surgical patients and neonates with hemolytic disease when crystalloids prove ineffective
- ABO compatibility unnecessary

Fresh frozen plasma

Fresh frozen plasma is prepared by separating the plasma from the RBCs and freezing it within 6 hours of collection. The resulting solution contains plasma proteins, water, fibrinogen, some clotting factors, electrolytes, sugar, vitamins, minerals, hormones, and antibodies.

Fresh frozen plasma is used to treat hemorrhage, expand plasma volume, correct undetermined coagulation factor deficiencies, replace specific clotting factors, and correct factor deficiencies resulting from liver disease. ABO compatibility testing is unnecessary; Rh matching is preferred. Large-volume transfusions of fresh frozen plasma may require correction for hypocalcemia because citric acid in the transfusion binds with and depletes the patient's own serum calcium.

Cryoprecipitate

Cryoprecipitate, also called *factor VIII,* is the insoluble portion of plasma recovered from fresh frozen plasma. It's used to treat von Willebrand's disease, hypofibrinogenemia, factor VIII deficiency (antihemophilic factor), hemophilia A, and disseminated intravascular coagulation. ABO compatibility testing is unnecessary.

Albumin

Albumin, which is available in an isotonic 5% solution or in a hypertonic 25% solution, is extracted from plasma and contains globulin and other proteins. It's used for patients who have acute liver failure, burns, or trauma or those who have had surgery as well as for neonates with hemolytic disease when crystalloids prove ineffective.

As a colloidal solution, albumin's large molecules increase plasma oncotic pressure, coaxing fluid from the interstitial space across normal capillary membranes and into the intravascular space. Albumin may actually do more harm in patients who are suffering from shock by leaking through damaged capillary membranes and dragging intravascular fluid along to worsen interstitial edema. Albumin is also used to treat hypoproteinemia with or without edema. ABO compatibility is unnecessary.

Platelets

Platelets are used for patients who have platelet dysfunctions or thrombocytopenia. They're also used for patients who have had multiple transfusions of stored blood, acute leukemia, or bone marrow abnormalities.

Patients may have febrile or mild allergic reactions to platelet transfusions. Rh matching is preferred.

Autologous blood transfusions

Also called *autotransfusion,* autologous blood transfusion refers to the reinfusion of a patient's own blood or blood components. Indications for autologous blood transfusion include:

✦ elective surgery in which blood has been donated during a period of time leading up to the procedure

✦ elective or nonelective surgery in which anticoagulated blood is withdrawn immediately before the procedure and replaced with colloid or crystalloid volume (In open-heart surgery, the resultant hemodilution helps reduce RBC sludging during periods of induced hypothermia, low flow, and circulatory arrest. Whole blood sequestered outside the cardiopulmonary bypass circuit avoids heart and lung complications. Such blood is simply reinfused into the patient after bypass.)

✦ preoperative hemorrhage or as a continuous intraoperative procedure when considerable blood loss is anticipated. (Heparinized shed blood is aspirated into a filtered reservoir, centrifuged, and saline-washed. RBCs are reinfused.)

Examples of surgeries using autologous blood transfusions include cardiovascular surgery, hip and knee surgeries, liver resection, ruptured ectopic pregnancy, and hemothorax.

Advantages and disadvantages

Autologous blood transfusions are advantageous because they avoid the risk of transfusion reaction, prevent the transmission of disease-causing organisms such as human immunodeficiency virus (HIV), and avoid depleting the local blood supply—but that doesn't mean that they don't have their disadvantages, as well. They require more counseling for donors than other patients who aren't donating their own blood, produce more wasted blood, and have such added expenses as storage, preparation, and testing. Furthermore, some patients—such as those with malignant neoplasms, coagulopathies, excessive hemolysis, or active infections—simply aren't candidates for these transfusions.

Possible complications of autologous blood transfusions include hemolysis, embolus, coagulation disorders, and thrombocytopenia.

Platelets

✦ Used for platelet dysfunctions, thrombocytopenia, multiple transfusions of stored blood, acute leukemia, and bone marrow abnormalities
✦ Rh matching preferred

Autologous blood transfusions

✦ Also called *autotransfusion*
✦ Refers to reinfusion of patient's own blood or blood components

Advantages

✦ Avoid risk of transfusion reaction
✦ Prevent transmission of disease-causing organisms
✦ Avoid depleting local blood supply

Disadvantages

✦ Require more counseling
✦ Produce more wasted blood
✦ Have added expenses (storage, preparation, testing)
✦ Some patients aren't candidates

Administering blood transfusions

- ✦ Safer because of testing for HIV, hepatitis B and C, types I and II T-lymphotropic virus, syphilis, and West Nile virus

Before transfusion

- ✦ Make sure informed consent has been obtained from patient or responsible family member
- ✦ Review facility policy for administering blood
- ✦ Assess patient, documenting vital signs and other pertinent information

ADMINISTERING BLOOD TRANSFUSIONS

Administering a blood transfusion of any type requires cooperation and vigilance on the part of various personnel, from the blood bank technician to the registered nurse at the bedside to the support personnel throughout the health care facility. Concerns have surfaced over the years about the risk of transmitting disease-causing organisms—particularly human immunodeficiency virus (HIV)—through blood transfusions. With HIV-antibody testing being performed on all donated blood and stringent criteria being used to exclude high-risk blood donors, studies now show that HIV transmission through infusion is rare. More specific testing for hepatitis B and hepatitis C viruses, as well as the addition of screening tests for type I and type II T-lymphotropic virus (which can cause infections that may lead to leukemia or neurologic diseases), syphilis, and West Nile virus, have helped to make the blood supply safer.

No matter how safe the blood supply is, however, transfusion reactions can still occur. (See *Guide to blood transfusion reactions,* pages 289 to 291.) Making sure that the administration of a blood transfusion is performed safely requires you to be aware of multiple safeguards before, during, and after the transfusion.

BEFORE THE TRANSFUSION

Before starting a blood transfusion, take these steps:

✦ Make sure the patient or a responsible family member has signed an informed consent form. Explain the procedure to the patient. Many people are still afraid of receiving a blood transfusion because of the fear of contracting HIV. If necessary, educate the patient about the extremely low risk of infection due to highly effective screening procedures.

✦ Make sure that refusal of blood reflects the patient's own decision and not coercion by family members or clergy. If you're caring for a minor or an adult who's incapable of giving their own consent and whose family's religious beliefs preclude the use of blood products (such as Jehovah's Witnesses), consider consulting your facility's legal counsel.

✦ Review your facility's policy for administering blood.

✦ Assess your patient, documenting vital signs and other pertinent information. Notify the physician if the patient has a fever of 100° F (37.8° C) or higher before the transfusion.

Guide to blood transfusion reactions

This chart describes endogenous reactions, those caused by antigen-antibody reactions, and exogenous reactions, those caused by external factors in administered blood.

CAUSES	ASSESSMENT FINDINGS	NURSING INTERVENTIONS
Allergic reaction		
✦ Allergen in donated blood ✦ Donor blood hypersensitive to certain medication	Anaphylaxis (anxiety, chills, facial swelling, laryngeal edema, pruritus, urticaria, wheezing), fever, nausea, vomiting	✦ Stop the infusion. ✦ Give antihistamines as ordered. ✦ Monitor vital signs and continue to assess the patient. ✦ Give epinephrine and corticosteroids as ordered.
Bacterial contamination		
✦ Organisms that survive the cold, such as *Pseudomonas* and *Staphylococcus*	Abdominal cramping, chills, diarrhea, fever, shock, signs of renal failure, vomiting	✦ Stop the infusion. ✦ Give antibiotics, corticosteroids, and epinephrine as prescribed. ✦ Maintain strict blood storage control. ✦ Change the administration set and filter every 4 hours or every 2 units. ✦ Infuse each unit of blood over 2 to 4 hours; stop the infusion if it lasts more than 4 hours. ✦ Maintain sterile technique.
Febrile		
✦ Bacterial lipopolysaccharides ✦ Antileukocyte recipient antibodies directed against donor white blood cells	Chest tightness, chills, cough, facial flushing, fever up to 104° F (40° C) or an increase in temperature of 1° C, flank pain, headache, increased pulse rate, palpitations	✦ Stop the infusion. ✦ Administer antipyretics and antihistamines as ordered. ✦ If the patient needs further transfusions, use frozen red blood cells (RBCs) and a leukocyte filter, and give acetaminophen as ordered.

(continued)

Guide to blood transfusion reactions *(continued)*

CAUSES	ASSESSMENT FINDINGS	NURSING INTERVENTIONS
Hemolytic		
✦ ABO or Rh incompatibility ✦ Intradonor incompatibility ✦ Improper crossmatching ✦ Improperly stored blood	Bloody oozing at infusion site, burning along the vein receiving blood, chest pain, chills, dyspnea, tachycardia, tachypnea, facial flushing, fever, flank pain, nausea, hypotension, hemoglobinuria, oliguria, shock, signs of renal failure	✦ Stop the infusion. ✦ Monitor vital signs, including pulse oximetry, as well as hourly urine output. ✦ Manage shock with I.V. fluids, oxygen, epinephrine, and vasopressors as ordered. ✦ Obtain a posttransfusion reaction blood sample and urine sample for analysis. ✦ Observe for signs of hemorrhage from disseminated intravascular coagulation.
Plasma protein incompatibility		
✦ Immunoglobulin A incompatibility	Abdominal pain, chills, diarrhea, dyspnea, fever, flushing, hypotension	✦ Stop the infusion. ✦ Administer oxygen, fluids, epinephrine, and corticosteroids as ordered.
Bleeding tendencies		
✦ Low platelet count in stored blood, causing thrombocytopenia	Abnormal bleeding and oozing from cuts or breaks in the skin or the gums, abnormal bruising and petechiae	✦ Give platelets, fresh frozen plasma, or cryoprecipitate as ordered. ✦ Monitor platelet count.
Circulatory overload		
✦ Possibly from infusing whole blood too rapidly	Back pain, chest pain or tightness, chills, distended jugular veins, dyspnea, cough, fever, flushed feeling, headache, tachycardia, hypertension, increased central venous pressure, increased plasma volume	✦ Slow or stop the infusion. ✦ Monitor vital signs. ✦ Use packed RBCs instead of whole blood. ✦ Give diuretics as ordered.

Guide to blood transfusion reactions *(continued)*

CAUSES	ASSESSMENT FINDINGS	NURSING INTERVENTIONS
Hypocalcemia		
✦ Citrate toxicity, which occurs when citrate-treated blood is infused too rapidly and binds with calcium, causing a calcium deficiency	Arrhythmias, hypotension, muscle cramps, muscle tremors, nausea, seizures, tingling in fingers, vomiting	✦ Slow or stop the transfusion if ordered. Expect a more severe reaction in hypothermic patients or patients with elevated potassium levels. ✦ Give calcium gluconate I.V. slowly if ordered.
Hypothermia		
✦ Rapid infusion of large amounts of cold blood, which decreases body temperature	Arrhythmias (especially bradycardia), cardiac arrest if core temperature falls below 86° F (30° C), chills, hypotension, shaking	✦ Stop the transfusion. ✦ Warm the patient. ✦ Obtain an electrocardiogram (ECG). ✦ Warm the blood if the transfusion is resumed.
Potassium intoxication		
✦ An abnormally high level of potassium in stored plasma caused by hemolysis of RBCs	Bradycardia, cardiac arrest, diarrhea, ECG changes (such as tall, peaked T waves), flaccidity, nausea, intestinal colic, muscle twitching, oliguria, signs of renal failure	✦ Stop the infusion. ✦ Obtain an ECG and serum electrolyte levels, such as potassium and glucose levels. ✦ Give Kayexalate as ordered. ✦ Give glucose 50% and insulin, bicarbonate, or calcium, as ordered, to force potassium into cells. ✦ Give mannitol, and maintain vigorous hydration to force diuresis and prevent renal damage.

✦ Keep in mind your patient's other treatment needs. If he's receiving an I.V. medication that can't be mixed with blood products, for example, another I.V. line may need to be inserted.

✦ Check the orders for the type of transfusion to be given. (See *Avoiding blood transfusion errors,* page 292.)

✦ Triple-check your patient's identity to ensure that the right patient receives the right transfusion at the right time.

Administering blood transfusions *(continued)*

Before transfusion

- ✦ Check order for type of transfusion to be given
- ✦ Triple-check patient identification to ensure that right patient receives right transfusion at right time

Avoiding blood transfusion errors

To avoid blood transfusion errors, ensure proper identification of the patient and the blood product he's to be given. Also, follow your facility's policy and take these precautions:

- ✦ Match the patient's name, medical record number, ABO and Rh status, and blood bank identification numbers with the label on the blood bag.
- ✦ Check the expiration date.
- ✦ Have another nurse verify the information.
- ✦ Sign the blood slip, filling in the required data. The blood slip will prove useful if the patient develops an adverse reaction.
- ✦ Double-check the physician's order to make sure you're transfusing the correct product.
- ✦ Be sure that the blood was typed and crossmatched within the last 48 hours—a Food and Drug Administration requirement for all blood transfusions.

Administering blood transfusions *(continued)*

Before transfusion

- ✦ Ask patient about prior transfusion reactions
- ✦ Obtain blood from laboratory when ready to hang it
- ✦ Return questionable products to blood bank

During transfusion

- ✦ Maintain sterile technique to protect patient
- ✦ Observe standard precautions to protect yourself

✦ Ask the patient if he has ever had a transfusion reaction and, if so, find out under what conditions the transfusion was given and how the reaction was resolved.

✦ Be sure to cover with the patient the need for the transfusion; the reason for informed consent, if required; risks of transfusion; the amount of time the transfusion should take; related procedures, such as vital sign checks and follow-up blood tests; adverse reactions to watch for and when to report them; and activity restrictions.

✦ Obtain blood from the laboratory when you're ready to hang it. Check the bag for leaks, discoloration, bubbles, and clots. Return questionable products to the blood bank.

✦ Don't store blood in a nursing-unit refrigerator because the temperature may be inaccurate, and the blood could be damaged. Blood that isn't refrigerated for 4 hours or more carries a high risk of bacterial contamination.

✦ If the order calls for blood to be warmed before administration, use a blood-warming device and special tubing. The temperature should be maintained between 89.6° and 98.6° F (32° and 37° C). Blood-warming devices are useful when transfusing large quantities of blood.

During the transfusion

While the transfusion is in progress, take these actions:

✦ Maintain sterile technique to protect the patient.

✦ Observe standard precautions to protect yourself. Wear gloves whenever handling blood products.

✦ Infuse blood products through at least an 18G or 20G I.V. catheter. Never use a smaller-gauge catheter or needle.

✦ Transfuse blood using a Y-type I.V. administration set with filter, and infuse the blood over 2 to 4 hours.

✦ Watch for signs of transfusion complications, including endogenous reactions caused by antigen-antibody reaction in the recipient and exogenous reactions caused by external factors related to blood administration. If a transfusion reaction occurs, the transfusion should be discontinued immediately and appropriate therapy initiated.

✦ When you start the transfusion, remain with the patient and observe him carefully for the first 15 minutes. Most acute adverse reactions occur within that time period, although delayed reactions can occur up to 2 weeks later. Recheck vital signs 15 minutes after hanging the blood, and again every hour.

✦ Use a pressure bag or a specialized infusion pump to administer blood more rapidly, if needed.

✦ Flush with normal saline solution before and after infusing blood products. You may need to flush the I.V. line during the transfusion if the blood is dripping too slowly. Don't use a dextrose solution, which can cause hemolysis, or lactated Ringer's solution, which contains calcium and can clog the tubing.

✦ Filters work best when completely filled with blood. Special filters are available to trap leukocytes, such as leukocyte-depleting filters, or tiny clots and debris that can get through standard filters such as microaggregate filters.

✦ If you're transfusing whole blood, you can reduce the risk of an adverse reaction by adding a microfilter to trap platelets.

Platelet administration

✦ Transfuse platelets over 15 minutes. If the patient's health history includes a platelet transfusion reaction, premedicate with an antipyretic or an antihistamine as ordered.

✦ Avoid giving platelets when the patient is febrile.

✦ Check the platelet count 1 hour after the transfusion ends.

Albumin and other fluid administration

✦ Don't mix albumin with other solutions.

✦ Be aware that albumin may be given as a volume expander until crossmatching for a whole blood transfusion is completed.

✦ Don't use albumin for patients with severe anemia, and give cautiously to patients with a cardiac or pulmonary disorder because heart failure may occur.

Administering blood transfusions *(continued)*

During transfusion

✦ Infuse through at least 18G or 20G I.V. catheter

✦ Transfuse using Y-type I.V. administration set with filter

✦ Infuse over 2 to 4 hours

✦ Watch for signs of complications

✦ When starting to transfuse, remain with patient and observe him carefully for 15 minutes

✦ Flush with normal saline solution before and after infusion; don't use dextrose or lactated Ringer's solution

Platelet administration

✦ Transfuse platelets over 15 minutes

✦ Avoid giving platelets when patient is afebrile

✦ Check platelet count 1 hour after infusion ends

Albumin and other fluid administration

✦ Don't mix albumin with other solutions

✦ Give repeated transfusions of factor VIII every 8 to 10 hours (factor VIII's half life) to maintain normal factor VIII levels

✦ If patient to receive WBCs, agitate blood container to prevent unintentional bolus infusion

✦ *Remember:* WBC transfusions may be given with antibiotic therapy but not with amphotericin B

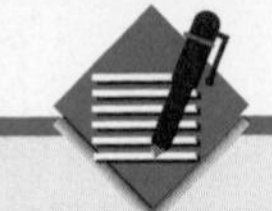

CHARTING CHECKLIST

Documenting blood transfusions

If your patient is receiving a blood transfusion, make sure you document this information:

- ❑ patient identification
- ❑ identification of blood products, including date of expiration
- ❑ vital signs before, during, and after the blood transfusion
- ❑ date, time, type, amount, and duration of the blood transfusion
- ❑ adverse reactions and actions taken
- ❑ patient response, including relevant laboratory test results
- ❑ patient assessment after the blood transfusion
- ❑ patient teaching and patient's response.

✦ Because factor VIII's half-life is 8 to 10 hours, give repeated transfusions (as needed) at those intervals to maintain normal factor VIII levels.
✦ If a patient will receive white blood cells (WBCs), premedicate him with diphenhydramine (Benadryl), if prescribed, and give an antipyretic for fever. Agitate the blood container to prevent cells from settling and unintentional delivery of a bolus infusion. WBC transfusions may be given along with an antibiotic to treat infection, but they shouldn't be given with amphotericin B (Amphocin).

Administering blood transfusions *(continued)*

After transfusion

- ✦ Watch for signs of circulatory overload, especially in elderly patients
- ✦ Obtain laboratory tests as ordered

After the transfusion

After the transfusion, take these actions:
✦ Continue to assess the patient as you remove the blood and tubing, and hang an infusion of normal saline solution to keep the vein open.
✦ Watch for signs of circulatory overload, especially in elderly patients. Carefully monitor the rate of infusion and the I.V. site.
✦ Obtain laboratory tests as ordered to determine the effectiveness of the treatment. The hemoglobin level of an adult patient receiving 1 unit of packed RBCs should increase by 1 g/dl. Hematocrit should increase by 3%. You should see a rise in platelets of 5,000 to 10,000/mm^3 with each unit of platelets infused, and an improvement in prothrombin time and partial thromboplastin time after giving clotting factors.
✦ Document your administration of blood products according to your facility's policy. (See *Documenting blood transfusions.*)

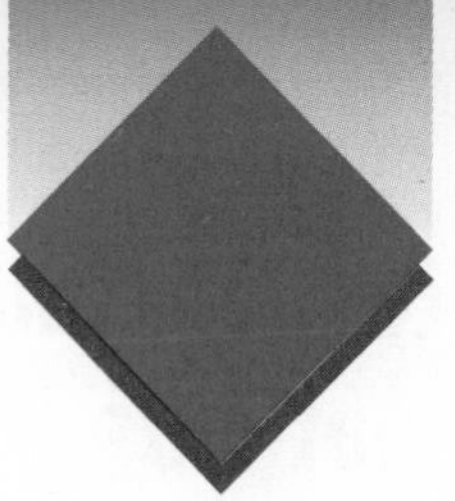

Appendices
Selected references
Index

Common fluid and electrolyte imbalances in pediatric patients

IMBALANCE	CAUSES	SIGNS AND SYMPTOMS	TREATMENT
Hyperkalemia (serum potassium > 5 mEq/L [> 5 mmol/L])	Acute acidosis, hemolysis or rhabdomyolysis, renal failure, excessive administration of I.V. potassium supplement, and Addison's disease	Arrhythmias, weakness, paresthesia, electrocardiogram (ECG) changes (tall, tented T waves; ST segment depression; prolonged PR interval and QRS complex; and absent P waves), nausea, vomiting, hoarseness, flushed skin, intense thirst, and dry, sticky mucous membranes	Dialysis (for renal failure), sodium polystyrene (Kayexalate) (to remove potassium via the GI tract), I.V. calcium gluconate (antagonizes cardiac abnormalities), I.V. insulin or hypertonic dextrose solution (shifts potassium into the cells), bicarbonate (for acidosis), or restricted potassium intake
Hypokalemia (serum potassium < 3.5 mEq/L [< 3.5 mmol/L])	Vomiting, diarrhea, nasogastric suctioning, diuretic use, acute alkalosis, kidney disease, starvation, and malabsorption	Fatigue, muscle weakness, muscle cramping, paralysis, hyporeflexia, hypotension, tachycardia or bradycardia, apathy, drowsiness, irritability, decreased bowel motility, and ECG changes (flattened or inverted T waves, presence of U waves, and ST segment depression)	Oral or I.V. potassium administration (I.V. infusions must be diluted and given slowly)
Hypernatremia (serum sodium > 145 mEq/L [> 145 mmol/L])	Water loss in excess of sodium loss, diabetes insipidus (insufficient antidiuretic hormone [ADH] production or reduced response to ADH), insufficient water intake, diarrhea, vomiting, fever, renal disease, and hyperglycemia	Decreased skin turgor; tachycardia; flushed skin; intense thirst; dry, sticky mucous membranes; hoarseness; nausea; vomiting; decreased blood pressure; confusion; and seizures	Gradual replacement of water (in excess of sodium) or ADH replacement or vasopressin administration (for patients with diabetes insipidus)
Hyponatremia (serum sodium < 138 mEq/L [< 138 mmol/L])	Syndrome of inappropriate antidiuretic hormone, edema (from heart failure), hypotonic fluid replacement (for diarrhea), cystic fibrosis, malnutrition, fever, and excess sweating	Dehydration, dizziness, nausea, abdominal cramps, and apprehension	Sodium replacement, water restriction, diuretic administration, or fluid replacement (with ongoing fluid loss, such as with diarrhea)
Hypovolemia (fluid volume deficit)	Dehydration, vomiting, diarrhea, decreased oral intake, and excessive fluid loss	Thirst, oliguria or anuria, dry mucous membranes, weight loss, sunken eyes, decreased tears, depressed fontanels (in infants), tachycardia, and altered level of consciousness	Oral rehydration (in mild to moderate dehydration), I.V. fluid administration (in severe dehydration), or electrolyte replacement

Common fluid and electrolyte imbalances in elderly patients

IMBALANCE	CAUSES	SIGNS AND SYMPTOMS	TREATMENT
Hyperkalemia (serum potassium > 5 mEq/L [> 5 mmol/L])	Renal failure, impaired tubular function, potassium-conserving diuretic use (in patients with renal insufficiency), rapid I.V. potassium administration, metabolic acidosis, and diabetic ketoacidosis	Arrhythmias, weakness, paresthesia, electrocardiogram (ECG) changes (tall, tented T waves; ST segment depression; prolonged PR interval and QRS complex; shortened QT interval, absent P waves)	Dialysis (for patients with renal failure); sodium polystyrene (Kayexalate) (to remove potassium via the GI tract), I.V. calcium gluconate (antagonizes cardiac abnormalities), I.V. insulin or hypertonic dextrose solution (shifts potassium into the cells), bicarbonate (for patients with acidosis); or potassium intake restriction
Hypokalemia (serum potassium < 3.5 mEq/L [< 3.5 mmol/L])	Vomiting, diarrhea, nasogastric suction, diuretic use, digoxin toxicity, and decreased potassium intake	Fatigue, weakness, confusion, muscle cramps, decreased bowel motility, ECG changes (flattened T waves, presence of U waves, ST segment depression, prolonged PR interval), ventricular tachycardia or fibrillation	Oral or I.V. potassium administration (I.V. infusions must be diluted and given slowly)
Hypernatremia (serum sodium > 145 mEq/L [> 145 mmol/L])	Water deprivation, hypertonic tube feedings without adequate water replacement, diarrhea, and low body weight	Dry mucous membranes, restlessness, irritability, weakness, lethargy, hyperreflexia, seizures, hallucinations, and coma	Gradual infusion of hypotonic electrolyte solution or isotonic saline solution
Hyponatremia (serum sodium < 138 mEq/L [< 138 mmol/L])	Diuretics, loss of GI fluids, kidney disease, excessive water intake, and excessive I.V. fluids or parenteral feedings	Nausea and vomiting, lethargy, confusion, muscle cramps, diarrhea, delirium, weakness, seizures, coma	Gradual sodium replacement, water restriction (1 to 1½ qt [1 to 1.5 L]/day), or discontinuation of diuretic therapy (if ordered)
Hypervolemia (fluid volume excess)	Renal failure, heart failure, cirrhosis, increased oral or I.V. sodium intake, mental confusion, seizures, and coma	Edema, weight gain, jugular vein distention, crackles, shortness of breath, bounding pulse, elevated blood pressure, and increased central venous pressure	Diuretics, fluid restriction (< 1 qt [1 L]/day), sodium restriction, or hemodialysis (for patients with renal failure)
Hypovolemia (fluid volume deficit)	Dehydration, vomiting, diarrhea, fever, polyuria, chronic kidney disease, diabetes mellitus, diuretic use, hot weather, and decreased oral intake secondary to anorexia, nausea, diminished thirst mechanism, or inadequate water intake (common in nursing home patients)	Dry mucous membranes, oliguria or concentrated urine, anuria, postural hypotension, dizziness, weakness, confusion or altered mental status, and possible severe hypotension, increased hemoglobin, hematocrit, blood urea nitrogen, and serum creatinine levels	Fluid administration (may be oral or I.V., depending on degree of deficit and patient's response; a urine output of 30 to 50 ml/hour usually signals adequate renal perfusion)

Selected references

Alexander, M., and Corrigan, A.M. *Core Curriculum for Infusion Nursing,* 3rd ed. Philadelphia: Lippincott Williams & Wilkins, 2004.

Allison, S.P., and Lobo, D.N. "Fluid and Electrolytes in the Elderly," *Current Opinion in Clinical Nutrition and Metabolic Care* 7(1):27-33, January 2004.

Amoore, J., and Adamson, L. "Infusion Devices: Characteristics, Limitations and Risk Management," *Nursing Standard* 17(28):45-52, March-April 2003.

Cartotto, R., et al. "A Prospective Study on the Implications of a Base Deficit During Fluid Resuscitation," *Journal of Burn Care and Rehabilitation* 24(2):75-84, March-April 2003.

Cohen, M.R. "Medication Errors. I.V. Fluid Evaporation: Working Up A Sweat," *Nursing2002* 32(10):14, October 2002.

Cook, L.S. "I.V. Fluid Resuscitation," *Journal of Infusion Nursing* 26(5):296-303, September-October 2003.

Critical Care Challenges: Disorders, Treatments, and Procedures. Philadelphia: Lippincott Williams & Wilkins, 2003.

Critical Care Nursing Made Incredibly Easy, Philadelphia: Lippincott Williams & Wilkins, 2004.

Davidhizar, R., et al. "A Review of the Literature on How Important Water is to the World's Elderly Population," *International Nursing Review* 51(3):159-66, September 2004.

Dudek, S.G. *Nutrition Essentials for Nursing Practice,* 5th ed. Philadelphia: Lippincott Williams & Wilkins, 2005.

Eaton, J. "Detection of Hyponatremia in the PACU," *Journal of Perianesthia Nursing* 18(6):392-97, December 2003.

Fluids & Electrolytes Made Incredibly Easy, 3rd ed. Philadelphia: Lippincott Williams & Wilkins, 2005.

Ford, N.A., et al. "Administration of I.V. Medications Via Soluset," *Pediatric Nursing* 29(4):283-86, 319, July-August 2003.

Hadaway, L.C. "Infusing Without Infecting," *Nursing2003* 33(10):58-63, October 2003.

Hadaway, L.C. "Delivering Multiple Medications via Backpriming," *Nursing2004* 34(3):24, 26, March 2004.

Ignatavicius, D.D., and Workman, M.L. *Medical-Surgical Nursing: Critical Thinking for Collaborative Care,* 4th ed. Philadelphia: W.B. Saunders, 2002.

Heitz, U., and Horne, M.M. *Pocket Guide to Fluid, Electrolyte, and Acid-Base Balance,* 5th ed. St. Louis: Mosby–Year Book, Inc., 2005.

Infusion Nurses Society. *Core Curriculum for Infusion Nursing,* 3rd ed. Philadelphia: Lippincott Williams & Wilkins, 2003.

I.V. Therapy Made Incredibly Easy, 3rd ed. Philadelphia: Lippincott Williams & Wilkins, 2005.

Johnson, R.J., and Feehally, J. *Comprehensive Clinical Nephrology,* 2nd ed. St. Louis: Mosby–Year Book, Inc., 2003.

Just the Facts: Fluids & Electrolytes. Philadelphia: Lippincott Williams & Wilkins, 2005.

Kasper, D.L., et al. *Harrison's Principles of Internal Medicine,* 16th ed. New York: McGraw-Hill Book Co., 2005.

Mims, B.C., et al. *Critical Care Skills: A Clinical Handbook,* 2nd ed. Philadelphia: W. B. Saunders Co., 2004

Morgera, S., et al. "Renal Replacement Therapy with High-Cutoff Hemofilters: Impact of Convection and Diffusion on Cytokine Clearances and Protein Status," *American Journal of Kidney Disease* 43(3):444-53, March 2004.

Nursing2005 Drug Handbook, 25th ed. Philadelphia: Lippincott Williams & Wilkins, 2005.

Potter, P.A., and Perry, A.G. *Fundamentals of Nursing,* 6th ed. St. Louis: Mosby–Year Book, Inc., 2005.

Puglise, K. "Test Your Knowledge: Fluids and Electrolytes," *Journal of Infusion Nursing* 26(3):127-28, May-June 2003.

Schrier, R.W. *Renal and Electrolyte Disorders,* 6th ed. Philadelphia: Lippincott Williams & Wilkins, 2002.

Smeltzer, S.C., and Bare, B.G. *Brunner & Suddarth's Textbook of Medical-Surgical Nursing,* 10th ed. Philadelphia: Lippincott Williams & Wilkins, 2004.

Suhayda, R., and Walton, J.C. "Preventing and Managing Dehydration," *Medsurg Nursing* 11(6):267-78, December 2002.

Swartz, R., et al. "Improving the Delivery of Continuous Renal Replacement Therapy Using Regional Citrate Anticoagulation," *Clinical Nephrology* 61(2):134-43, February 2004.

Teehan, G.S., et al. "Update on Dialytic Management of Acute Renal Failure," *Journal of Intensive Care Medicine* 18(3):130-38, May-June 2003.

Trimble, T. "Peripheral I.V. Starts: Insertion Tips," *Nursing2003* 33(8):17, August 2003.

Trimble, T. "Peripheral I.V. Starts: Securing and Removing the Catheter," *Nursing2003* 33(9):26, September 2003.

Index

---

i refers to an illustration; t refers to a table; **boldface** indicates full-color pages.

i refers to an illustration; t refers to a table; **boldface** indicates full-color pages.

i refers to an illustration; t refers to a table; **boldface** indicates full-color pages.

---

i refers to an illustration; t refers to a table; **boldface** indicates full-color pages.

i refers to an illustration; t refers to a table; **boldface** indicates full-color pages.

i refers to an illustration; t refers to a table; **boldface** indicates full-color pages.

i refers to an illustration; t refers to a table; **boldface** indicates full-color pages.

i refers to an illustration; t refers to a table; **boldface** indicates full-color pages.

i refers to an illustration; t refers to a table; **boldface** indicates full-color pages.

R

S

i refers to an illustration; t refers to a table; **boldface** indicates full-color pages.

---

i refers to an illustration; t refers to a table; **boldface** indicates full-color pages.